Certified Nurse Educator (CNE) Review Manual

Ruth A. Wittmann-Price, PhD, RN, CNS, CNE, CHSE, ANEF, FAAN, is dean of the School of Health Sciences and professor of nursing at Francis Marion University in Florence, South Carolina. She has been an obstetrical/women's health nurse for 38 years. Dr. Wittmann-Price received her AAS and BSN degrees from Felician College, Lodi, New Jersey, and her MS as a perinatal clinical nurse specialist (CNS) from Columbia University, New York, New York. She completed her PhD in nursing at Widener University, Chester, Pennsylvania, and received the Dean's Award for Excellence. She developed a mid-range nursing theory, "Emancipated Decision-Making in Women's Health Care," and has tested her theory in four research studies. International researchers are currently using her theory as the foundation for their studies. Her theory is being used by researchers at the University of Limpopo, South Africa, in their campaign, "Finding Solutions for Africa," which helps women and children. Dr. Wittmann-Price was also the appointed research coordinator for Hahnemann University Hospital in Philadelphia, Pennsylvania, and oversaw the evidence-based practice projects for nursing (2007–2010). Hahnemann University Hospital was granted initial Magnet® designation in December 2009. Dr. Wittmann-Price has taught all levels of nursing students over the past 16 years and has completed an international service-learning trip. Currently, she teaches women's health to baccalaureate students and to students on the MSN nurse educator track. Dr. Wittmann-Price mentors DNP and PhD students and is on several committees at both Drexel University, Philadelphia, Pennsylvania, and Widener University. She has coedited or authored 14 books, contributed chapters to two books, and written over 20 articles. She has presented her research regionally, nationally, and internationally. Dr. Wittmann-Price was inducted into the National League for Nursing Academy of Nurse Educator Fellows in 2013 and became a fellow in the American Academy of Nursing in October 2015.

Maryann Godshall, PhD, CNE, CCRN, CPN, is an assistant clinical professor at Drexel University College of Nursing and Health Professions in Philadelphia, Pennsylvania. She obtained her BSN from Allentown College of St. Francis DeSales, Center Valley, Pennsylvania, and her MSN from DeSales University, Center Valley, Pennsylvania. She has a postmaster's degree in nursing education from Duquesne University, Pittsburgh, Pennsylvania. She completed her PhD at Duquesne University (2014), where her research topic was "Exploring Learning of Pediatric Burn Patients Through Storytelling." Dr. Godshall has been a nurse for more than 20 years and has worked in pediatric critical care, inpatient pediatrics, and pediatric rehabilitation nursing. She holds certifications in both pediatrics and pediatric critical care and has been teaching for over 14 years in both the university and hospital setting. Dr. Godshall is coeditor of *The Certified Nurse Educator (CNE) Review Manual* (2013; Springer Publishing Company), and author of *Fast Facts of Evidence-Based Practice,* Second Edition (2015; Springer Publishing Company). She has published chapters in several books and textbooks, including *Maternal–Child Nursing Care: Optimizing Outcomes for Mothers, Children and Families,* Second Edition (2016), *NCLEX-RN® EXCEL* (2010; Springer Publishing Company), and *Disaster Nursing: A Handbook for Practice* (2009), and has written many journal articles. In 2008, Dr. Godshall won the Nightingale Award of Pennsylvania Nursing Scholarship.

Linda Wilson, PhD, RN, BC, CNE, CHSE-A, ANEF, FAAN, is an assistant dean for special projects, simulation, and certified nurse educator (CNE) accreditation, and an associate clinical professor at Drexel University, College of Nursing and Health Professions, Philadelphia, Pennsylvania. Dr. Wilson completed her BSN at College Misericordia, Dallas, Pennsylvania; her MSN in critical care and trauma at Thomas Jefferson University, Philadelphia, Pennsylvania; and her PhD in nursing research at Rutgers University, Newark, New Jersey. Dr. Wilson has a postgraduate certificate in epidemiology and biostatistical methods from Drexel University and a postgraduate certificate in pain management from the University of California, San Francisco School of Medicine. Dr. Wilson also completed the National Library of Medicine/ Marine Biological Laboratory Biomedical Informatics Fellowship and the Harvard University Institute for Medical Simulation's Comprehensive Workshop and Graduate Course in Medical Simulation. Dr. Wilson has several certifications, including certified post anesthesia nurse (CPAN), certified ambulatory perianesthesia nurse (CAPA), American Nurses Credentialing Center (ANCC) board certification (BC) in nursing professional development, CNE, certified health care simulation educator (CHSE), and certified health care simulation educator–advanced (CHSE-A). Dr. Wilson served as the president of the American Society of Perianesthesia Nurses (2002–2003), and has served as an ANCC Commission on Accreditation Appraiser Site surveyor since 2000. In 2014, Dr. Wilson was inducted into the National League for Nursing (NLN) Academy of Nurse Educator Fellows (ANEF) and was also inducted as a Fellow in the American Academy of Nursing (FAAN).

Certified Nurse Educator (CNE) Review Manual

Third Edition

Ruth A. Wittmann-Price, PhD, RN, CNS, CNE, CHSE, ANEF, FAAN

Maryann Godshall, PhD, CNE, CCRN, CPN

Linda Wilson, PhD, RN, BC, CNE, CHSE-A, ANEF, FAAN

Editors

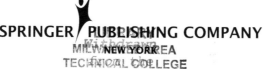

SPRINGER PUBLISHING COMPANY

NEW YORK

Springer Publishing Company, LLC
11 West 42nd Street
New York, NY 10036
www.springerpub.com

Acquisitions Editor: Margaret Zuccarini
Senior Production Editor: Kris Parrish
Composition: diacriTech

ISBN: 978-0-8261-6165-9
e-book ISBN: 978-0-8261-6166-6

16 17 18 19 20 / 5 4 3 2 1

The author and the publisher of this Work have made every effort to use sources believed to be reliable to provide information that is accurate and compatible with the standards generally accepted at the time of publication. The author and publisher shall not be liable for any special, consequential, or exemplary damages resulting, in whole or in part, from the readers' use of, or reliance on, the information contained in this book. The publisher has no responsibility for the persistence or accuracy of URLs for external or third-party Internet websites referred to in this publication and does not guarantee that any content on such websites is, or will remain, accurate or appropriate.

Library of Congress Cataloging-in-Publication Data

Names: Wittmann-Price, Ruth A., editor. | Godshall, Maryann, editor. | Wilson, Linda, 1962- editor.
Title: Certified nurse educator (CNE) review manual / [edited by] Ruth A. Wittmann-Price, Maryann Godshall, Linda Wilson.
Description: 3rd edition. | New York, NY : Springer Publishing Company, LLC, [2017] | Includes bibliographical references and index.
Identifiers: LCCN 2016047389 | ISBN 9780826161659 | ISBN 9780826161666 (e-book)
Subjects: | MESH: Faculty, Nursing | Certification | United States | Problems and Exercises
Classification: LCC RT90 | NLM WY 18.2 | DDC 610.73076—dc23 LC record available at https://lccn.loc.gov/2016047389

Special discounts on bulk quantities of our books are available to corporations, professional associations, pharmaceutical companies, health care organizations, and other qualifying groups. If you are interested in a custom book, including chapters from more than one of our titles, we can provide that service as well.

For details, please contact:
Special Sales Department, Springer Publishing Company, LLC
11 West 42nd Street, 15th Floor, New York, NY 10036-8002
Phone: 877-687-7476 or 212-431-4370; Fax: 212-941-7842
E-mail: sales@springerpub.com

Printed in the United States of America by McNaughton & Gunn.

Contents

Contributors

Diane M. Billings, EdD, RN, FAAN, ANEF   Chancellor's Professor Emeritus, Indiana University School of Nursing, Indianapolis, Indiana

Frances H. Cornelius, PhD, MSN, CNE, RN-BC (Informatics)   Clinical Professor of Nursing, Chair, MSN Advanced Practice Role Department; Chair, Complementary and Integrative Health Programs; Coordinator of Clinical Nursing Informatics Education, Online Learning Council Fellow, College of Nursing and Health Professions, Drexel University, Philadelphia, Pennsylvania

Rosemary Fliszar, PhD, RN, CNE   Director, RN-BSN Program, Assistant Professor, Rider University, Lawrenceville, New Jersey

Tracy P. George, DNP, APRN-BC, CNE   Amy V. Cockcroft Fellow 2016–2017, Assistant Professor of Nursing, School of Health Sciences, Francis Marion University, Florence, South Carolina

Karen K. Gittings, DNP, RN, CNE, Alumnus CCRN   Associate Dean, Associate Professor, School of Health Sciences, Francis Marion University, Florence, South Carolina

Mary Ellen Smith Glasgow, PhD, RN, ANEF, FAAN   Dean and Professor, Duquesne University, School of Nursing, Pittsburgh, Pennsylvania

Maryann Godshall, PhD, CNE, CCRN, CPN   Assistant Clinical Professor of Nursing, College of Nursing and Health Professions, Drexel University, Philadelphia, Pennsylvania

Marylou K. McHugh, EdD, RN, CNE   Associate Clinical Professor, Division of Graduate Nursing, Advanced Role MSN Department, College of Nursing and Health Professions, Drexel University, Philadelphia, Pennsylvania

M. Annie Muller, DNP, RN, APN-BC   Assistant Professor of Nursing, School of Health Sciences, Francis Marion University, Florence, South Carolina

Carol Okupniak, DNP, RN-BC Nursing Informatics   Assistant Clinical Professor of Nursing, College of Nursing and Health Professions, Drexel University, Philadelphia, Pennsylvania

Brenda Reap-Thompson, MSN, RN, CNE   Assistant Clinical Professor of Nursing, College of Nursing and Health Professions, Drexel University, Philadelphia, Pennsylvania

Dorie Weaver, MSN, RN, FSN-BC   Professor of Nursing, Francis Marion University, Florence, South Carolina

Linda Wilson, PhD, RN, BC, CNE, CHSE-A, ANEF, FAAN   Assistant Dean for Special Projects, Simulation and CNE Accreditation, Associate Clinical Professor, College of Nursing and Health Professions, Drexel University, Philadelphia, Pennsylvania

Ruth A. Wittmann-Price, PhD, RN, CNS, CNE, CHSE, ANEF, FAAN   Dean, School of Health Sciences, Professor of Nursing, Francis Marion University, Florence, South Carolina

Foreword

The nursing faculty shortage has been accompanied by a heightened awareness of the important role of educators in schools of nursing and in clinical settings. This awareness has extended beyond nursing education to the general public, with news reports continuing to inform readers about qualified applicants to nursing programs being turned away because of the lack of faculty to teach them. The faculty shortage has occurred for a number of reasons, including fewer graduate students preparing for educator roles to replace the number of faculty who are retiring, difficulties in recruiting clinicians to teach in schools of nursing because of the lower salaries of faculty compared with health care settings, and, until recently, limited numbers of programs to prepare nurse educators. The awareness of the need for nurse educators, combined with the reality of decreasing numbers of faculty, has led to the expansion of master's, doctoral, and certificate programs to prepare nurse educators; development of comprehensive courses on teaching in nursing for graduate students and nurses transitioning to the educator role; and strategies, such as nurse faculty loans, to encourage students to consider a career in nursing education.

Accompanying these trends is the recognition that nursing education has a body of knowledge to be learned, as well as core competencies to be developed for the expert teaching of nursing. Nurse educators need an understanding of learning concepts and theories, strategies for promoting clinical reasoning and higher level thinking skills, deliberate practice and its relationship to developing expertise in psychomotor and clinical skills, and principles for facilitating learner development and socialization. Teachers guide students in achieving the course outcomes, and they need to understand the relationship of those outcomes and the course in which they teach to the overall curriculum. All nursing faculty should know general concepts of curriculum development and their roles and responsibilities in planning the curriculum and courses within it. Across all settings in which students learn, nurse educators must be skilled in planning instruction for students with varying learning needs and abilities, selecting appropriate teaching methods, presenting information effectively to small and large groups of learners, integrating active learning methods within classes and courses, and demonstrating evidence-based clinical teaching skills. Good teaching in the practice setting is essential to promote learning and development of clinical competencies, and for that to take place, the teacher needs to create a supportive learning environment. Nurse educators need a breadth of knowledge and competencies because their roles also may include teaching in simulation and skills laboratories using innovative instructional methods and technologies.

Educators not only teach, but also are responsible for assessing students' learning outcomes and clinical competencies. Assessment is the collection of information about student learning and performance, and provides a basis for identifying learning needs and deciding on instructional activities to promote further learning. Assessment also helps educators confirm that students have met the desired outcomes and developed the necessary clinical competencies. Evaluation is the process of making judgments about those outcomes and competencies, based on the assessment data. Nursing faculty members not only assess student learning and development but also evaluate the program, curriculum, courses, resources, and other aspects to ensure a high-quality education for students. This evaluation is done within a quality improvement framework.

Nurse educators function within institutions and need to understand the environment in which they teach and its effects on their roles and responsibilities. The mission and goals of the setting influence the educator's role. Differences across schools of nursing in tenure and promotion requirements, criteria for appointment and advancement in both tenure and nontenure tracks, and expectations of faculty are striking. To be successful, the teacher needs to understand those requirements and expectations.

Across all settings, the nurse educator is a leader and change agent, participating in efforts to improve nursing education, developing educational innovations, and gaining leadership skills. Once prepared as a nurse educator, one's own learning and professional development continue. Educators need to expand their own knowledge and skills and be committed to participating in career development activities. As faculty members foster the value of lifelong learning among students, so too are faculty lifelong learners.

Decisions made about educational practices should be based on sound evidence, generated through research studies that are of high quality. Much of the current research in nursing education, though, is done with small samples, in one setting, and with questionable tools. We cannot identify best practices in nursing education without high-quality research studies. In some areas of nursing education, however, there is evidence to guide teaching, but how many educators routinely check the literature as a basis for their educational decisions? The role of nurse educator as scholar not only includes conducting research and disseminating findings but also approaching one's teaching by questioning current practices and searching for evidence to answer those questions.

Many health fields offer certifications to acknowledge expertise in a specialty area of practice or role. Similar to certifications in clinical specialties, certification in nursing education is a means for teachers to demonstrate their knowledge about nursing education and expertise in the educator role. The National League for Nursing offers certification in nursing education through its Certified Nurse Educator (CNE) examination. That examination assesses the teacher's knowledge about learning and teaching strategies, learner development and socialization, assessment and evaluation, curriculum development and evaluation, quality improvement as a nurse educator, scholarship in nursing education, and the faculty member's role within an institutional environment and academic community. The CNE examination serves as a means of documenting advanced knowledge, expertise, and competencies in the role of nurse educator.

This book was developed as a resource for nurse educators to prepare themselves to take *and pass* the CNE examination. It includes valuable information for this purpose and also serves as a review of important principles for effective teaching in nursing. The book describes the concepts and principles that define nursing education, describes the core competencies of nurse educators, and provides a perspective of expert teaching in nursing. This book is a valuable resource for nurse educators in preparing for the CNE examination and for aspiring teachers in nursing.

Marilyn H. Oermann, PhD, RN, ANEF, FAAN
Thelma M. Ingles Professor of Nursing
Director of Evaluation and Educational Research
Duke University School of Nursing
Durham, North Carolina
Editor-in-Chief, *Nurse Educator* and *Journal of Nursing Care Quality*

Preface

Through teaching we can touch more patients than ever possible with our own two hands.
—Ruth A. Wittmann-Price

The first two editions of this book assisted many nurse educators in becoming certified. We decided to update and expand the content to keep up with the ever-changing discipline of nursing education. This third edition includes much of the information provided in the first two editions, but we have added a chapter specifically about teaching–learning strategies. This book also incorporates the current National League for Nursing (NLN) Certified Nurse Educator (CNE) test plan and has many new practice questions. Other topics that are prominent in the nursing literature have been added, including flipped classroom, vulnerable populations, global learning activities, and international study. Nurse educators continue to understand that teaching nursing is a rewarding professional career. Witnessing a student or colleague become excited about new information, techniques, or skills is extremely gratifying. The classroom, skills laboratory, simulation laboratory, and clinical realms all fall within the expertise of the nurse educator. These realms are parts of larger systems that nurse educators navigate successfully to accomplish their goal of knowledge development. In any one classroom, laboratory, or clinical setting, facilitating the education of others is not only a rewarding experience but a role that greatly impacts the future of health care.

In the past, nurse educators had no special education about teaching. They were content experts who learned the pedagogy by trial and error. Now, nursing education is recognized as a specialty unto itself that contains a distinct body of knowledge. Like nursing, it is also an applied science. This book highlights areas outlined by the NLN as essential knowledge needed for the nurse educator to excel in the field and pass the CNE examination.

The competencies for nurse educators listed at the beginning of each chapter are taken from the NLN website. *Competency* is defined by *WordNet® 3.0.* (n.d.) as "the quality of being adequately or well qualified physically and intellectually." Competence can be viewed as a minimal skill set or level that must be achieved to pass. *Excellence* means "possessing good qualities in high degree" (*WordNet® 3.0.*, n.d.) and the CNE publicly designates that distinction upon nurse educators.

The CNE was created by our nursing leaders to recognize and capture excellence in nursing education. Since the first examination was offered to 174 candidates as a pencil-and-paper test in Baltimore, Maryland, on September 28, 2005, thousands of nurse educators have passed the examination (NLN, 2016). Those nurse educators proudly display the CNE certification after their names.

To prepare nurse educators for the certification examination, the NLN provides resources that can be accessed from their informative website (http://www.nln.org/facultycertification/index.htm). This book was created because many nurse educators have asked us how we prepared for the first examination in Baltimore in 2005.

This book is a supplement to the materials already available from the NLN and it is developed independently from the NLN in order to further assist nurse educators in gaining confidence about taking the examination. This book is modeled after the NLN's most recently published test plan. Many of the areas in the test plan overlap; therefore, you may find places in this book that have repeated content that is cross-referenced. This replicates the nature of nursing education; it is an interwoven realm of content, context, and process—all of which affects learning. We hope this book captures the essence of information needed for nurse educators to move to a recognized level of excellence. We have put additional references and Teaching Gems in place for those who would like further explanation and exploration of topics and encourage you to investigate these. We have searched for evidence to support our content and, where applicable, have inserted research into each chapter and clearly designated Evidence-Based Teaching Practice boxes to help the reader focus on the evidence discovered by fellow educators. We have also provided case studies at the end of each chapter to promote educational decision making and provided sample test questions that may be similar to those encountered during the CNE examination.

Chapter 1 covers some of the specifics of the CNE examination, describes recertification, and reviews test-taking skills.

Chapter 2 reviews how a nurse educator facilitates learning by assessing the learning needs and skills of the students. It also reviews learner outcomes and teaching strategies and how to adapt them to the student's own experiences. This is important to assess in order to develop an appropriate teaching plan. Another area discussed is how the nurse educator models the role of nurse for the student and helps the student to become motivated and enthusiastic about learning.

Chapter 3 discusses learning strategies. Active and passive learning strategies are reviewed and advantages and disadvantages of each strategy are considered.

Chapter 4 discusses technology in the realm of nursing education. This topic has grown immensely and now needs its own chapter. Technology is used to facilitate learning and this is done by using new innovations that engage the learner along with Web 2.0 tools and Web 3.0 functionality of the World Wide Web.

Chapter 5 is dedicated to online teaching, an ever-growing medium for facilitating learning, especially for the postlicensure nursing learner. Online teaching is just as much an art and science as live classroom teaching is. Often, nurse educators are the leaders in their educational organizations when it comes to online learning.

Chapter 6 demonstrates the competencies needed by nurse educators to facilitate learning in the nursing skills lab. This is an important area of foundational learning for students that is included in most nursing curricula.

Chapter 7 discusses clinical education and the importance of coaching students in facilitating knowledge of professionalism, skill, and interdisciplinary competencies.

Chapter 8 is devoted to simulation and follows the clinical education chapter because the two methods of facilitating learning are very much intertwined. Best practices in human patient simulator (HPS) simulation, standardized patient (SP) simulation, and debriefing are discussed. The new opportunities for certification in simulation are also introduced.

Chapter 9 is devoted to socialization skills of students and speaks to the ever-increasing diversity in culture and styles that affects nursing education. Another important aspect of Chapter 9 is the examination of resources for students who are at risk for any number of individual reasons that affect them perceptually, cognitively, physically, or culturally. Incivility is addressed in relation to today's teaching environment.

Chapter 10 also deals with the second NLN competency for nurse educators, socialization of learners, which is accomplished by describing service learning, international travel, and the global classroom. All socialization methods are described and defined and information is provided that is critical for safe experiences in a nurse's education.

Chapter 11 discusses evaluation strategies used by nurse educators and how they balance the aspects of admission, progression, and retention to ensure good program outcomes. Effective evaluation tools are extremely important in promoting student success and public safety.

Chapter 12 addresses the larger institutional considerations of curriculum design and evaluation. How courses are developed within a curriculum and how the curriculum flows are analyzed. This chapter discusses how the curriculum interfaces with the mission of the institution and the community.

Chapter 13 highlights professional development of nurse educators and how educators navigate their roles and become mentors to the next generation of nurse educators. For educators, learning is lifelong and has increased in intensity exponentially with the accelerating advancements in information and technology. This chapter provides the nurse educator with ideas on how to keep up to date and remain involved in the field of nursing education.

Chapter 14 speaks to the nurse educator's role as a leader who interfaces with the larger community of academics and administrators. This chapter examines nursing's place in the larger systems as well as how nurse educators can effect change in those systems.

Chapter 15 dissects the scholarship needed for nurse educators to stay on top of their game. "Publish or perish" is a phenomenon known to academics that is applicable to nurse educators in an academic setting. This chapter discusses different types of scholarship and professional plans for becoming proficient at publishing and emphasizes the importance of disseminating nursing knowledge.

Chapter 16 discusses interdisciplinary collaboration within the institution for nurse educators. Nursing has a longer history of using standalone schools than it does being part of a larger educational community. Nurse educators have assimilated into the larger community as experts in a field that has the unique components of clinical and didactic education. The professionalism that we bring to the larger academic community has enhanced the standings of many institutions and colleges. Nursing is a visible professional entity that collaborates and contributes to the overall mission of the institution of nursing and to society.

Chapters 17 and **18** include a comprehensive examination and the answers to the chapter questions and the comprehensive examination. These practice questions will assist you to answer correctly on the actual CNE examination.

We have developed this third edition to assist you in your preparation for the CNE examination. Many nurse educators have used previous editions of this book to successfully pass the examination. Our hope is that this is an effective tool to help you reach your goal of recognized excellence. We applaud your efforts as colleagues in the quest to educate the next generation of nurses. We thank you for your efforts to recognize excellence in our field.

Ruth A. Wittmann-Price
Maryann Godshall
Linda Wilson

REFERENCES

Competency. (n.d.). In *WordNet*® *3.0*. Retrieved from http://dictionary.reference.com/browse/competency

Excellence. (n.d.). In *WordNet*® *3.0*. Retrieved from http://dictionary.reference.com/browse/excellence

National League for Nursing. (2016). Certification for nurse educators (CNE). Retrieved from http://www.nln.org/facultycertification/index.htm

Acknowledgments

The three coeditors would like to acknowledge Dr. Frances H. Cornelius for all the excellent information she contributed to this book.

Thank you to all of my students over the years who have taught and continue to teach me a tremendous amount about nursing, life, and humility; and to Angie Pasco, former director of Schuylkill Health School of Nursing, my mentor in nursing education.

—*Ruth A. Wittmann-Price*

To H. Lynn Kane, Helen "Momma" Kane, and Linda Webb, thank you for your amazing friendship and for being my family. To Lou Smith, Evan Babcock, and Steve Johnson, thank you for your wonderful friendship and support. To Elizabeth Diaz, Fabien Pampaloni, and Sam Price, thank you for your endless help, friendship, and support.

—*Linda Wilson*

Introducing the CNE Exam and Its Blueprint

BRENDA REAP-THOMPSON

Nursing is an art: and if it is to be made an art, it requires an exclusive devotion as hard a preparation, as any painter's or sculptor's work; for what is the having to do with dead canvas or dead marble, compared with having to do with the living body, the temple of God's spirit? It is one of the Fine Arts: I had almost said, the finest of Fine Arts.
—Florence Nightingale

LEARNING OUTCOMES

- Identify the processes to best prepare for the Certified Nurse Educator (CNE) examination
- Utilize the tips for success to promote understanding and learning of key concepts
- Demonstrate time-management skills to enhance studying
- Integrate standards from practice into information that is outlined in the CNE test blueprint
- Improve comprehension by eliminating anxiety related to test taking
- Utilize technology to track competencies in preparation for completion of the 5-year recertification activity record

Nurse educator certification comes at a time in history when nursing is actively recruiting advanced practiced nurses into the educational realm. The U.S. Bureau of Labor Statistics (2016) predicts a 26% growth in the employment of RNs from 2014 to 2024. This increase is the direct result of growing chronic conditions, such as diabetes and obesity, the emphasis on preventive care, and the demand for health care services from baby-boom populations. Nursing will continue to expand as health care continues to branch out into community-based primary care and out-patient sites. However, job availability is directly related to the region, number of graduates per year, and the increase in the number of experienced nurses who could have retired but continue to work because of the state of the economy and the diverse employment opportunities in health care. There is an increased demand for nurse practitioners (NPs) in response to the health care movement into the community and the concentration on health promotion and health maintenance as well as on sick-care services. According to the American Nurses Association, NPs play a pivotal role in the future of health care services as primary care providers. The growing emphasis on prevention and public health will continue to create excellent job opportunities for NPs.

The Tri-Council for Nursing, an alliance of the American Association of Colleges of Nursing (AACN), the American Nurses Association, the American Organization of Nurse Executives, and the National League for Nursing (NLN), determined that a more highly educated nursing workforce is critical to delivering safe and effective patient care. This was supported by the Institute of Medicine's (IOM; 2010) *Future of Nursing* report, and is promoted by health care leaders in academia and clinical practice. The evidence-based recommendations in the IOM report call for preparing at least 80% of the RN workforce at the baccalaureate level by 2020. This change in RN preparation has also been encouraged by the nation's Magnet®-designated hospitals (American Nurses Credentialing Center, 2016; Sherman, 2012). According to the AACN data from 2014, this mandate has resulted in a 10.4% increase in RNs enrolling in RN to BSN programs to build on their initial education at the associate degree or diploma level.

WHY BECOME A CNE?

A substantial increase in student nurses is only one factor that summons the urgency for CNE. Another contributing factor, adding to the faculty shortage, is the demographics of the current teaching faculty. The average age of a master's-prepared nurse educator is 57, whereas the average age of those holding doctoral degrees is 61. The percentage of full-time nursing faculty who are age 50 and over is 72%. The national nurse faculty vacancy rate is 8.3% (ANA, 2014).

Becoming a CNE can also enhance the quality of nursing education, which is the foundation needed to promote the culture of safe and effective patient-centered care. At the present time, multiple innovative methods to facilitate learning are being utilized such as enhancing critical thinking and clinical reasoning in the classroom, integrating evidence-based research, utilizing information technology, expanding hands-on service-learning experiences through global initiatives, and providing an interprofessional health care team approach through simulations. The other important aspect of nursing education is incorporating strategies to effectively assess and evaluate the learner within the theoretical and clinical components.

The results of a quantitative study that examined the first-time pass/fail performance of 2,673 academic nurse educators who took the CNE examination determined that a 1-year increase in full-time experience resulted in a 1.05 times greater likelihood of passing the CNE examination. The research also verified that faculty development and mentoring are essential for the development of educators with less than 5 years of full-time experience (Ortelli, 2008).

Many colleges and schools of nursing are recruiting expert nurse clinicians and advanced practice RNs to assist in filling their vacant academic and clinical nurse educator roles. This recruitment process has been fostered by state and foundational funds to supplement nurse educator programs at the master's and doctoral levels. The role development that many nurse educators undergo involves a difficult process of struggling to evolve from being an *expert* clinician to being a *novice* educator. Nursing literature provides ample documentation to demonstrate that being an expert clinician does not provide an educator with the skill set needed to become a successful teacher. Through additional studies that lead to certification in nursing education, expert clinicians can become comfortable in their new role as nurse educators and build their new practice, preparing the next generation of nurses while using proven teaching and learning principles.

> **Teaching Gem:** Nurse educators should consider integrating a learning-styles inventory because this is fundamental in the development of classroom activities and will impact the outcomes of learners (Vinales, 2015).

Indeed, nurse educators with years of experience can validate their expertise and knowledge through certification. These educators are an invaluable resource to the current system, and certified educators are sorely needed as mentors, role models, and visionaries to assist future nurse educators. Educators who complete the core competencies of a CNE are needed to move the profession forward. The following list outlines just a few ways in which that progression will manifest itself:

- Assisting with preparation to create interactive learning environments
- Using versatile education styles to provide quality education for diverse populations of learners
- Developing higher level and alternate format test questions
- Understanding test-item analysis that results in appropriate decision making

The CNE also has an in-depth understanding of the need to balance teaching, research/scholarship, and service, which has become an expectation in nursing academia (Wittmann-Price, 2012).

REACH FOR ACADEMIC EXCELLENCE, BECOME A CNE

Academic excellence often is encouraged through an atmosphere that influences educators to challenge themselves to reach beyond their normal expectations. Nurse educators who support an atmosphere of excellence can thrive, and their success will raise the bar of academic standards within the discipline. Becoming certified as a nurse educator allows faculty to better understand its multifaceted role. This role includes teaching, communicating with learners and colleagues, using information resources, understanding professional practice within the college of nursing and the university, functioning as a change agent, and engaging in scholarly activities. The role is stimulating and encourages educators to be innovative and collaborative in the academic environment.

- Nurse educators who have validated their expertise have the ability to prepare learners who are competent and confident nurses.
- Research and scholarship advanced through publications and presentations will provide a positive impact on pedagogy.
- Involvement in service, such as professional societies or committees at the program, department, college, or university level, will enhance the ability to collaborate and network within the academic community.

Your decision to take the CNE certification examination is a challenging one, which will allow you to test your proficiency as a nurse educator.

> **Teaching Gem:** A great way to display the *scholarship of teaching* for a midlevel career nurse educator is to create a new nursing elective course that will enhance the curriculum.

If peer review is used in the college or university where you teach, consider this as a positive force that will impact your development as a nurse educator.

Table 1.1 presents the content areas contained within the test blueprint and the percentage of each area in the NLN CNE examination (NLN, 2016a).

The following chapters in this CNE preparation guide present a content review for each of the content areas that appear on the CNE examination.

PREPARING FOR THE CNE EXAMINATION

Setting Up a Study Schedule

When you create a study schedule, begin prioritizing the order in which you study the content by using the CNE blueprint, as outlined in Table 1.1. Create a chart and divide your total studying time into eight sections and break up the total studying time into percentages that correlate with the topic's content percentage. The highest percentages of content covered in the examination and the related chapters in this book are as follows:

- Area 1—Facilitate learning (22%; Chapters 2–8)
- Area 6—Engage in scholarship, service, and leadership (21%), which includes
  - Area 6A—Function as a change agent and leader (Chapter 14)
  - Area 6B—Engage in scholarship of teaching (Chapter 15)
  - Area 6C—Function effectively within the institutional environment and the academic community (Chapter 16)

The next-highest percentages of content covered in the examination are:

- Area 4—Participate in curriculum design and evaluation of program outcomes (17%; Chapter 12)
- Area 3—Use assessment strategies (17%; Chapter 11)
- Area 5—Pursue continuous quality improvement in the academic nurse educator role (9%; Chapter 13)
- Area 2—Facilitate learner development and socialization (14%; Chapters 9 and 10)

Employing the aforementioned strategy will help ensure that you will have time to review the areas that represent the highest percentage of questions on the CNE examination. It is also very helpful to attend a CNE review course either in person or via webcast. The course will provide a concentrated review of information such as test development and item analysis, learning needs of special groups, curriculum development, teaching styles, and evaluation of program outcomes. The course presents an opportunity to practice items with educators who are certified and allows time to ask questions. Taking the course will impact your understanding of the key concepts.

Incorporating Key Topics Into Your Review for the CNE Examination

Key topics for inclusion in your review include those in Exhibit 1.1.

TABLE 1.1
Test Plan

CONTENT	PERCENTAGE OF THE EXAMINATION
1. Facilitate learning	22
2. Facilitate learner development and socialization	14
3. Use assessment and evaluation strategies	17
4. Participate in curriculum design and evaluation of program outcomes	17
5. Pursue continuous quality improvement in the academic nurse educator role	9
6. Engage in scholarship, service, and leadership A. Function as a change agent and leader B. Engage in scholarship of teaching C. Function effectively within the institutional environment and the academic community	21

Source: NLN (2016a).

EXHIBIT 1.1

Key Topics to Include in Your Review

Teaching styles—authoritarian, Socratic, heuristic, and behavioral	Teaching–learning process
Active learning	Cooperative learning and testing
Self-directed learning	Planning clinical learning experiences
Critical thinking activities—classroom and clinical	Characteristics of learners (cultural, traditional, nontraditional, and educationally disadvantaged)

(continued)

EXHIBIT 1.1

Key Topics to Include in Your Review *(continued)*

Domains—cognitive, psychomotor, and affective	Promotion of professional responsibility by self-assessment and peer review
Graduation and retention rates	Academic appeals process
Bloom's taxonomy	Test blueprint
Norm- and criterion-referenced tests	Formative and summative evaluation
Test validity	Test reliability
Item discrimination ratio	Point-biserial correlation
Item difficulty	Program standards—federal laws, state regulations, professional accreditation—the Commission on Collegiate Nursing Education (CCNE) and the Accreditation Commission for Education in Nursing (ACEN)
Credentialing—American Association of Colleges of Nursing (AACN)	Curriculum—mission statement, conceptual framework, level objectives, behavioral objectives, and evaluation of learning outcomes (theoretical and clinical)
Curriculum evaluation—internal and external	Family Educational Rights and Privacy Act (FERPA)/Buckley Amendment
Audio conferencing	Video streaming
Synchronous and asynchronous methods of instruction	Types of leadership
Scholarship of discovery	Scholarship of teaching
Scholarship of practice (application)	Scholarship of integration

EVIDENCE-BASED TEACHING PRACTICE

Incorporating a culture of safety and interprofessional communication into the nursing curriculum may save lives (Davis, Harris, Mahishi, Bartholomew, & Kenward, 2016).

> **EVIDENCE-BASED TEACHING PRACTICE**
>
> Prepare for emerging technology such as genetics, less invasive and more accurate diagnostic and treatment tools, three-dimensional printing, and robotics. Technology will make an impact on human life and change the practice of nursing within the next decade (Huston, 2013).

Planning and Registering for the CNE Examination Using the NLN Website to Establish Your Eligibility

Verify that you meet the eligibility requirements to take the examination. These requirements are listed on the NLN website.

- Access the NLN website: www.nln.org.

  Click on "Certification for Nurse Educators."

  - Print the *Certified Nurse Educator CNE 2016 Candidate Handbook* (NLN, 2016a), which includes the detailed test blueprint (outlines specific information under each of the six content areas) and list of recommended texts and journals.

- Order the Self-Assessment Examination (SAE).

  - This 65-item practice examination has multiple-choice questions with available rationales. Although it is half the length of the certification examination, it correlates with the content categories and cognitive complexity item distribution in the certification examination. The score report, calculated in each of the six areas, can be used to focus your review. Candidates have access to the examination for 60 days from the date of purchase. (Note: There is a fee for this optional practice test.)

- Register to take the CNE examination.

  - Registration deadlines can be found on the website so make sure you register in advance because you will need this confirmation prior to scheduling the test location, date, and time. The notice of eligibility may take up to 3 weeks to arrive after completing the registration.

  - Current fees are available on the NLN website.

  - Your faculty administrator can provide you with information about reimbursement for the examination fee.

NUTS AND BOLTS OF THE CNE EXAMINATION

Become Familiar With the CNE Examination

- The examination has 150 items; 130 are operational, and 20 are pretest items that do not count toward the score.
- Items contain four options of multiple-choice questions that are within the cognitive levels of recall, application, and analysis.

- Three hours are allotted to complete the examination, which includes a short tutorial.
- This allows approximately 72 seconds for each question.
- Avoid rapid guessing on the examination.
- Read questions carefully and answer items at a consistent pace.
- Focus on important words in the question to improve your focus.
- Answer all questions to increase your chance of being successful.

Examination Items Requiring Additional Time
- Information about learner grades that require math calculations
- Information about test item analysis that require a comparison of data

Become Familiar With Electronic Testing Advantages

- If you are unsure of an answer, you can bookmark the question and return to it when you have completed the remainder of the examination.
- Arrows, to page forward or backward during the examination, provide the ability to return to a question and change the answer. However, as educators, we are aware that the first choice is usually correct.

TIPS FOR SUCCESS

Incorporate Strategies to Ease the Fear of Test Anxiety

It is normal for a nurse educator to feel anxious about taking the CNE examination.

- Anxiety is a natural response to the new challenges in our lives.
- Some anxiety will produce a heightened awareness and may improve test taking, whereas anxiety that is uncontrolled will impede the ability to think critically.
- Everyone who takes tests experiences anxiety; however, recognizing and controlling anxiety is an important key.

Some strategies that can be used to ease test anxiety include the following:

1. Reducing anxiety related to time constraints
   * Schedule the examination when you have a semester that is less stressful.
   * Start a study group with other educators and plan to meet once a week for 2 hours.
   * Use the detailed test plan to divide assignments.

     – Each faculty member can complete an assignment and share notes with the group.
     – Faculty members can also share the sources of information recommended by the NLN.

2. Reducing anxiety related to not having recent experience in test taking
   * After reviewing the content for the examination, complete as many test questions as possible, including the practice examination from the NLN.
   * Self-evaluation will assist you in refocusing on specific content.
   * Practice will increase your confidence.

3. Reducing anxiety related to previous experience with testing difficulty
   * Stop negative thoughts that begin with "what if."
   * Strategies, such as positive self-talk, daily exercise, yoga, and meditation, have all been proven to decrease anxiety.
   * Practice these strategies on a regular basis so that decreasing anxiety becomes easy to achieve.
   * Engage in activities that you find relaxing on the evening prior to the examination, such as watching a movie or going to dinner with friends.

EVIDENCE-BASED TEACHING PRACTICE

Testing anxiety can be reduced by guided imagery, guided reflection, music, aromatherapy, and relaxation breathing. Also study and focus groups can be of assistance before a tesing situation (Gibson, 2014).

UTILIZE LEARNING STRATEGIES

Remember by Comparison

An example of remembering by comparison is determining what information is the same and what is different among a variety of areas of information. This learning strategy focuses on the differences. An example of this learning strategy using Boyer's model of scholarship is remembering that all four types of scholarship include peer-reviewed articles, research, and grant awards. However, there are distinct differences among the four areas as described here.

Scholarship of Discovery

The scholarship of discovery is the discovery of new knowledge (Boyer, 1990). A scientific finding is integrated into the application and integration process of health care. Examples are peer-reviewed publications of research, theory, or philosophical essays and grant awards in support of research or scholarship. Discovery includes primary empirical research, historical research, theory development, and testing. It includes work that receives state, regional, national, and international recognition.

Scholarship of Teaching

The scholarship of teaching has transpired into an active learning environment in which the nurse educator uses a variety of teaching methods to provide learners with the ability to discuss, collaborate, and explore. The curriculum has been developed to reflect a global, diverse population. Examples are peer-reviewed publications of research related to *teaching methodology* or *learning outcomes* and grant awards in support of teaching and learning. It includes state, regional, national, and international recognition.

Scholarship of Practice (Application)

The scholarship of application is the ability to apply theory to practice. This process of clinical reasoning and intervention results in positive patient outcomes. It can also be related to defining and resolving health problems of a community. Examples are peer-reviewed publications of research, case studies, technical applications or other practice issues, and grant awards in support of practice. It includes state, regional, national, and international recognition.

Scholarship of Integration

The scholarship of integration is becoming common practice as it involves providing an interprofessional health care team approach for critical analysis and integration of ideas to research complex health problems. Because of the dynamics and experience of various disciplines, the result is a comprehensive holistic solution. Examples are peer-reviewed publications of research, policy analysis, case studies, integrative reviews of literature, interdisciplinary grant awards, copyrights, licenses, patents, and products for sale.

> **Teaching Gem:** Nick (2016) discusses the need for nurse educators to "go global." There is a great need for international professional development about many nurse educators topics such as clinical trends, evidence-based practice, online searching of databases, and learning active teaching–learning strategies.

Publication of nursing knowledge is an expectation of a nurse educator's role and can be accomplished through persistence in writing and the mind-set that dissemination is a responsibility. Just like all other skills, practice with the assistance of mentors is invaluable for the writing process (Oermann & Hays, 2011).

Develop Mnemonic Devices

Develop mnemonics if a memory aid is needed; however, using mnemonics may be less useful in some situations in which may be easier to just remember the facts. For example, when the nurse educator is developing a test, the BOBCAT mnemonic can provide guidance to develop the test appropriately. This mnemonic stands for

- **B**lueprint
- **O**bjectives of the course content
- **B**loom's taxonomy
- **C**lient needs categories (National Council of State Boards of Nursing [NCSBN], 2016)
- **A**nalysis of data
- **T**est results and changes for the future

In summary: A **b**lueprint is developed from the **o**bjectives of the course. **B**loom's taxonomy is used to develop questions at higher cognitive levels such as application and analysis. Client needs areas of NCLEX-RN® (National Council Licensure Examination for Registered Nurses; NCSBN, 2016) are necessary to guide educators teaching in an undergraduate prelicensure program to construct questions in the eight areas, such as management of care, safety and infection control, health promotion and maintenance, and reduction of risk potential, to name a few. Analysis of data is performed, and test results are determined. After the results of the test are reviewed, revisions to items should be completed so they can be used in the future.

Relate New Information to Be Learned to Information Already Mastered

Learning new information is easier if it can be related to information or facts that are already understood. An example of this learning strategy is illustrated next. Many times test validity and test reliability become confused. If you understand what test validity means, *you only need to add to your memory the information about reliability.*

- *Validity* means the test is measuring the information it is supposed to measure. It is "valid." The test blueprint is used to developed questions related to the objectives of the course; this ensures validity.
- *Reliability* refers to the consistency of the test scores. The test's reliability can be improved by making changes to the items so that they are more discriminating.

Correlate Testing With Practice

Examine your own activities as an educator and relate them to the content in the questions. This will be helpful in developing a complete understanding of the information. You will find that your experience will be very helpful in answering questions. Many examples of how to correlate your own experience with the content to be learned are presented in Exhibit 1.2.

EXHIBIT 1.2	
Correlating Experience	
QUESTION CONTENT	**EDUCATOR EXPERIENCE**
Create opportunities for the learners to develop their own critical thinking skills.	Learners can develop critical thinking skills by participating in the following assignments: writing a teaching plan, developing a concept map, discussing a case study, completing an exercise in delegation or prioritization in the clinical area, or making decisions in the simulation laboratory.
Use information technologies to support the teaching–learning process.	Specific materials may be taught more effectively by using technology. It may be advantageous for learners to create a video in response to a clinical situation, participate in synchronous *or asynchronous* discussions, work in a group to develop a Wikipedia article.

(continued)

EXHIBIT 1.2

Correlating Experience (*continued*)

QUESTION CONTENT	EDUCATOR EXPERIENCE
Respond effectively to unexpected events that affect the clinical and/or classroom instruction.	Collect all the information, including anecdotal records if the event occurred at the clinical site. Clarify professional behavior as outlined in the Code of Ethics for Nurses with Interpretive Statement and Nursing: Scope and Standards of Practice. Utilize conflict resolution, if indicated. Refer the student to the Student Conduct Committee, if indicated.
Identify learning styles and unique learning needs of students from culturally diverse backgrounds.	Many students speak English as a second language (ESL). The development of communication and active learning in the classroom may assist these students with understanding information such as: 1. Discussing cultural beliefs related to a specific disease, as this can impact client care in the clinical setting 2. Using a team approach by having students in small groups answer questions in class 3. Gaming, such as playing Jeopardy in the classroom, to review content
Provide input for the development of nursing program standards and policies regarding: 1. Admission 2. Progression 3. Graduation	If you have not had the opportunity to work with the admissions, academic progression, or graduation committees in your college of nursing, then request permission to review the minutes or attend meetings. Involvement in these committees promotes a clear understanding of the process. Admission criteria are usually posted on the school's website and include Scholastic Aptitude Test scores, entrance examination scores, grade point average (GPA), and Test of English as a Foreign Language (TOEFL) requirements for students born in non-English-speaking countries. The progression committee determines whether a student should be permitted to continue in the program after failure of a course or courses. The committee may overturn a decision if the student had extenuating circumstances, such as a serious illness or death in the family. The students may also go through the academic appeals process to overturn a grade they believe to be inaccurate. The committee also takes into account the student's grades in prerequisite and corequisite courses when making a decision. Graduation occurs when the learner completes the minimum number of credits specified for the degree and his or her GPA is within the program standards. A student must also complete the clinical requirements for courses with a satisfactory rating in the clinical component.

(*continued*)

EXHIBIT 1.2

Correlating Experience (*continued*)

QUESTION CONTENT	EDUCATOR EXPERIENCE
Participate in curriculum development or revision.	Read and compare the mission statements and philosophy statements of the university and the college of nursing. Review the level objectives and the behavioral objectives in the nursing program curriculum. Level objectives are reflective of the progressive competence of the students within the goals and philosophy of the program. Behavioral objectives drive the design for the courses with a focus on learning outcomes. The curriculum is updated as needed *and should be reviewed annually* to incorporate changes in the student body and the community, the use of technology, and current health care trends. The goal is to improve program outcomes.
Use feedback gained from self, peer, and learner evaluations to improve role effectiveness.	Self-evaluation can assist faculty members in determining their own needs, such as preparation for class, organization, teaching strategy development, and test development. Learners may have a need for the enhancement of information or clinical opportunities that are not recognized by the educator. Student evaluations can be used to improve the course. Peer evaluations can be helpful; however, they can also cause conflict among faculty members. The educator should have specific guidelines designated for the evaluation, and the date of the didactic evaluation should be decided by both faculty members.
Use legal and ethical principles to influence, design, and implement policies and procedures related to learners, educators, and the educational environment.	Legal issues can include: 1. Cosigning documentation in the clinical area 2. Providing care that results in an injury to the client or the learner 3. Completion of an incident report 4. Cheating during an examination 5. Plagiarism on a class assignment 6. Dismissal of a student from the program The college should have policies addressing these issues. In addition, students are protected by the U.S. Constitution's Bill of Rights. The First Amendment protects freedom of religion, press, speech, and the right to assemble. The Fourth Amendment provides protection against unreasonable search and seizure.

(continued)

EXHIBIT 1.2	
Correlating Experience (*continued*)	
QUESTION CONTENT	EDUCATOR EXPERIENCE
Use evidence-based resources to improve and support teaching.	Evidence-based resources can be used in the classroom or clinical setting by 1. Scheduling an assignment in which one group of learners takes a turn discussing a research article related to the content presented in the classroom that week 2. Providing evidence-based articles to learners in the clinical area who have down time; the learner(s) will take time to review the article and present the information during the postconference period
Participate in departmental and institutional committees.	Examples of committees within the nursing department include faculty affairs, student affairs, scholarship and innovation, educator resources, and technology. Some examples of committees within an institution include faculty and governance, faculty finance, green initiative, and sustainability.

CRITICAL THINKING QUESTION

What should a novice nurse educator look for when searching and interviewing for an academic position?

EVIDENCE-BASED TEACHING PRACTICE

Byrne and Welch (2016) studied the motivation of nurse educators to take the CNE examination and variables that predicated success. Statistical analysis did not demonstrate any significant difference in test scores when comparing roles (faculty vs. new graduate) and years of teaching indicating the need for future research related to significant variables that predict test success.

HOW TO RENEW YOUR CERTIFICATION AFTER 5 YEARS

After you pass the CNE examination, you will feel elated and glad you will not need to think about it for another 5 years. However, you will have to think about it if you are going to record renewal credits (RCs).

There are two options for renewal:

1. Document 50 RCs that must be related to at least five of the NLN nurse educator core competencies. The credits earned must be distributed over the 5-year renewal period.
2. Register and pass the CNE exam prior to the expiration date located on your certificate.

Simplify the recertification process with three steps:

1. Download the activity record form from the NLN (2016b) website after you pass the examination. Complete the form when you meet any of the competencies. Each competency includes the specific activity, date, RC, and the outcome. It is much easier to complete the form immediately instead of trying to locate the information years later. *RC is awarded when organized professional activities are employed to enhance professional development as a nurse educator.* The educator must have submissions in at least five competencies in order to reflect the full academic role.

RC conversion examples:

One university college course (three semester hours) = 15 RC

One continuing education unit (CEU) = 1 RC

One hour of faculty development or scholarship = 1 RC

Access the NLN website for a full list of activities, the credit conversion table and sample completion form.

2. Keep the hard copies of certificates of attendance in a folder. Scan these documents into a folder in your electronic PDF documents so you have an additional copy in case the original copies become lost or damaged within the 5 years. These supporting documents only need to be sent if requested by the Academic Nurse Educator Certification Program (ANECP). The NLN Certification Program randomly selects a percentage for audit.
3. Submit the information approximately 8 to 10 weeks before the due date. The certification period begins on the date you passed the examination. The certification period ends on the expiration date located on the current CNE certificate.

If you fail to satisfy the recertification requirements prior to the conclusion of the cycle, you will be placed on an inactive list and you will receive a suspension notice. Failure to satisfy the requirements within 1 year results in termination of the certification. During the suspension period, faculty who are suspended may not represent themselves as certified by the NLN.

Table 1.2 can assist you with determining the activities that meet each competency. Please note that activities for recertification may overlap into more than one competency.

TABLE 1.2
Examples of Activities for Each Competency

COMPETENCY	ACTIVITIES MAY INCLUDE BUT ARE NOT LIMITED TO
Facilitate learning	• Creating innovative teaching–learning activities—Collaborative ventures with community partners • Using evidence-based practice or information technology
Facilitate learner development and socialization	• Assist students to develop as nurses and integrate expected values and behaviors; an example would be development of a simulation experience • Identify individual learning styles and needs for culturally diverse, at risk, or physically challenged learners • Assist learners to engage in thoughtful constructive self- or peer evaluation
Use assessment and evaluation strategies	• Create appropriate assessment instruments to evaluate learner outcomes • Design tools for assessing clinical practice • Provide input for the development of program policies regarding admission, progression, or graduation
Participate in curriculum design and evaluation of program outcomes	• Design curricula that reflect trends while preparing graduates to function in the health care environment • Develop or update courses to reflect the theoretical framework of curricula • Support educational goals through community partnership
Pursue continuous quality improvement in the nurse educator role	• Develop and maintain competence in the multidimensional role; examples would be attending conferences, seminars, workshops • Mentor and support faculty colleagues in the role of academic nurse educators • Engage in activities that promote role socialization; an example would be participation in a nursing organization • Use feedback from self, peers, learners, and/or administration for improvement
Function as a change agent and leader	• Provide an active service within a nursing service organization, association, or committee • Work within a special panel or think tank for an educational issue • Represent nursing education within an intradisciplinary work group
Engage in scholarship	• Develop an area of expertise within the academic educator role • Share expertise with colleagues; examples would be publications or presentations
Function within the educational environment	• Collaborate with other disciplines to enhance the academic environment • Participate in committee work on the departmental or institutional level

Source: NLN (2016a).

CASE STUDIES

CASE STUDY 1.1

Olivia is an NP with 4 years of experience as a clinical educator in women's health. She recently took a full-time position in a small private college and is responsible for the didactic portion of the women's health course. She is feeling overwhelmed with preparing information for class and developing questions for examinations. Olivia is concerned because the learners do not agree with the correct answers on exams. Olivia fears that discussing this information with her mentor will indicate that she is unsuccessful in her new role.

Should Olivia discuss this issue with her mentor?

How should Olivia approach this issue with the learners?

What data should Olivia be viewing to determine whether the questions are discriminating?

CASE STUDY 1.2

Mark has 10 years of experience in critical care nursing and also worked for 3 years in quality improvement. He accepted a position in a midsized university and developed some learner-centered activities for class. The program director believes that Mark should lecture to be sure the learners are provided with the information and then use the learner-centered activities if time allows.

How should Mark respond to the program director?

How can Mark evaluate whether the learner-centered activities have positive outcomes?

REFERENCES

American Nurses Association. (2014). The nursing workforce 2014: Growth, salaries, education demographics & trends. Retrieved from http://www.nursingworld .org/mainmenucategories/thepracticeofprofessionalnursing/workforce/fast-facts -2014-nursing-workforce.pdf

American Nurses Credentialing Center. (2012). Magnet recognition overview. Retrieved from http://www.nursecredentialing.org/Magnet/ProgramOverview

Boyer, E. (1990). *Scholarship reconsidered: Priorities of the professoriate*. Princeton, NJ: Carnegie Foundation for the Advancement of Teaching.

Byrne, M., & Welch, S. (2016). CNE certification drive and exam results. *Nursing Education Perspectives, 37*(4), 221–223. doi:10.5480/14-1408

Davis, K. K., Harris, K. G., Mahishi, V., Bartholomew, E. G., & Kenward, K. (2016). Perceptions of culture of safety in hemodialysis centers. *Nephrology Nursing Journal, 43*(2), 119–182.

Gibson, H. A. (2014). A conceptual view of test anxiety. *Nursing Forum, 49*(4), 267–277.

Huston, C. (2013). The impact of emerging technology on nursing care: Warp speed ahead. *Online Journal of Issues in Nursing, 18*(2), 1. doi:10.3912/OJIN.Vol18No02Man01

Institute of Medicine. (2010). *The future of nursing: Leading change, advancing health*. Washington, DC: National Academies Press. Retrieved from http://www.nationalacademies.org/ HMD/Reports/2010/The-Future-of-Nursing-Leading-Change-Advancing-Health.aspx

National Council of State Boards of Nursing. (2016). Test plans. Retrieved from https://www.ncsbn.org/test-plans.htm

National League for Nursing. (2016a). Certified nurse educator (CNE) 2016 candidate handbook. Retrieved from http://www.nln.org/docs/default-source/professional-development-programs/certified-nurse-educator-%28cne%29-examination-candidate-handbook.pdf?sfvrsn=2. Republished with permission of National League for Nursing, from Nurse Educator Core Competency 2013 year: permission conveyed through Copyright Clearance Center, Inc.

National League for Nursing. (2016b). Renewal. Retrieved from http://www.nln.org/certification/recertification/index.htm

Nick, J. M. (2016). Tips for nurse educators who want to go global. *Reflections on Nursing Leadership, 42*(1), 1–4.

Oermann, M. H., & Hays, J. (2011). *Writing for publication in nursing* (2nd ed.). New York, NY: Springer Publishing.

Ortelli, T. (2008). Headlines from the NLN. Characteristics of candidates who have taken the certified nurse educator (CNE) examination: A two-year review. *Nursing Education Perspectives, 29*(2), 120–121.

Sherman, R. (2012). An 80% BSN prepared nursing workforce by 2020? [Blog.] Retrieved from http://www.emergingrnleader.com/80bsnworkforce2020

U.S. Bureau of Labor Statistics, U.S. Department of Labor. (2016). Occupational outlook handbook: Registered nurses. Retrieved from http://www.bls.gov/ooh/healthcare/registered-nurses.htm

Vinales, J. J. (2015). The learning environment and learning styles: A guide for mentors. *British Journal of Nursing, 24*(8), 454–457. doi:10.12968/bjon.2015.24.8.454

Wittmann-Price, R. A. (2012). *Fast facts for developing a nursing academic portfolio.* New York, NY: Springer Publishing.

Facilitating Learning in the Classroom Setting

RUTH A. WITTMANN-PRICE

Strive for excellence, not perfection.
—H. Jackson Brown, Jr.

This chapter addresses the Certified Nurse Educator Exam Content Area 1: Facilitate Learning (National League for Nursing [NLN], 2016, p. 5).

- Content Area 1 is 22% of the examination
- It is estimated that there will be approximately 33 questions from Content Area 1

LEARNING OUTCOMES

- Discuss the theoretical and philosophical underpinnings of nursing education
- Compare behaviorism and constructivism
- Describe learning and motivation
- Contrast andragogy with pedagogy
- Evaluate the evidence on critical thinking and metacognition
- Demonstrate classroom organization and management

Nursing education today is more exciting and challenging than ever before. Gone are the days of a homogeneous classroom of learners who respond unquestioningly to lockstep teaching and learning methods. Now nurse educators facilitate learning for students of all ages; from many different lifestyles, ethnic, and cultural backgrounds; with different generational characteristics; and, most important, with different learning styles. The overarching goal is that every learner deserves nurse educators who can best facilitate the learner's journey toward becoming a successful, professional nurse. Educational expertise is needed to assist students to become competent and caring professional nurses. To accomplish the goal of successful career transitions from learner to nurse or from nurse to advanced practice nurse, faculty must facilitate the development of clinical decision-making skills and inspire lifelong learning. Only well-educated nurse educators can prepare nursing professionals who provide quality and value-based patient care to meet the needs of the current health care environment.

EDUCATIONAL PHILOSOPHIES

A positive learning environment must be established to facilitate students' knowledge acquisition. This is accomplished when the learning environment is built on sound philosophical foundations. These foundations:

- Are never stagnant and change as the larger social system matures
- Provide the foundations on which learning theories and educational pedagogies can be built
- Consider the branch of philosophy that addresses why we teach, how we teach, and what the goals of education are for learners and society (Wortham, 2011)

CRITICAL THINKING

If *ontology* is concerned with becoming and what is actual and real and *epistemology* is concerned about theories of knowledge, how do these two concepts interact in your teaching philosophy (Hurlock, 2002)?

Teaching philosophies of academic nurse educators (ANE) are developed over time and each is personal to each educator. Personal philosophies are developed from educational philosophies and are used in the development of professional portfolios (Felicilda-Reynaldo & Utley, 2015).

LEARNING THEORIES

"*Teaching* is what the educator provides the learner in terms of goals, methods, objectives, and outcomes. *Learning* refers to the processes by which the learner changes skills, knowledge, and dispositions through a planned experience" (Kaakinen & Arwood, 2009, p. 1). How people learn and how they store, connect, discover, and retrieve information and skills have been well studied and formalized into many theoretical frameworks. These frameworks try to explain the connection between knowledge and the human brain, a truly interesting subject that affects learners every day.

Educational philosophy guides learning theories, and there is some overlap in terms and ideas from among them. Philosophies are driven by *metaphysics*, the study of what is real; *epistemology*, the study of what is knowledge and truth; and *axiology*, the study of what is good (Valiga, 2012). Theories have more defined concepts and are more applicable to the teaching situation than philosophies are. The learning theories discussed today in nursing are mainly *constructivism* and *behaviorism*. In Table 2.1, philosophical foundations are broken down into brief descriptions of general philosophies, sometimes referred to as "worldviews," educational philosophies, and the corresponding teaching–learning theories.

TABLE 2.1

Worldview Philosophies, Educational Philosophies, and Teaching–Learning Theories

WORLDVIEW PHILOSOPHIES	EDUCATIONAL PHILOSOPHIES	TEACHING–LEARNING THEORIES
TRADITIONAL PHILOSOPHIES AND THEORIES		
Idealism (Plato, Socrates) • Ideas are important • People would like to live in a perfect world	**Perennialism** (Thomas Aquinas) • Traditional educational style that is teacher centered • Liberal education is valued • Studies should include great thinkers of the past • Prepare learners for adult life • Reading, writing, and arithmetic are important	**Information Processing** (Gagne, 1970) • Describes how information is received, stored, and processed in the mind • Learning is a function of the brain (sometimes called brain-based learning) • Humans process information and store it in memory • Memory is achieved by sensory input, which goes to short-term memory (working memory), which is then stored, if significant, in long-term memory, in which information may be forgotten but is never lost completely
Realism (Positivism) (Aristotle) • The world is orderly • Science can be viewed objectively and analyzed • Develop knowledge that is value and context-free (K. V. Mann, 2011)	**Essentialism** (Bagley, Hirsh) • Traditional educational approach that develops learners' minds through knowledge passed to the learner from the educator • A core curriculum is valued, as are democracy and cultural heritage • Physical world is the true reality • Learners should appreciate the masterworks of art and literature • Learners need critical thinking skills to help society • Teacher-directed learning	**Behaviorism** (Pavlov, Watson, Skinner) • Stimulus and response are the basis for learning • The environment develops the person • Requires behavior modification and classroom management • Positive reinforcement is used to encourage acceptable behavior • Generated the idea of "programmed learning" • Tyler (1949) introduced behavioral objectives in education • Faculty decides on the educational experience • Nursing education is still steeped in behaviorism today (lockstep curriculum) **Social Learning Theory or Social Cognitive Theory** (Bandura, 1997) • Perception of confidence in oneself in the situation (self-efficacy) • Positive expectations are the incentives • Bandura's term *reciprocal determinism* means that the world and the person's behavior cause each other • Feedback to the learner is important • Self-efficacy is based on four principles: 　◦ Enactive mastery experiences or the learner's own history of successes 　◦ Vicarious experiences or the observed behaviors of a role model being successful at a task 　◦ Verbal persuasion or telling someone that he or she will be successful 　◦ Physiological states or the person's "gut feeling" that he or she can succeed (K. V. Mann, 2011)

(continued)

TABLE 2.1
Worldview Philosophies, Educational Philosophies, and Teaching–Learning Theories (*continued*)

WORLDVIEW PHILOSOPHIES	EDUCATIONAL PHILOSOPHIES	TEACHING–LEARNING THEORIES
POSTSTRUCTURALISM OR MODERN PHILOSOPHIES AND THEORIES		

Pragmatism (Dewey, Pierce)
• Ideas can be tested scientifically
• The human experience is important
• Influenced by social reform and the growth of citizenship in early 19th century
	Progressivism (Dewey)
	• School mimics society
	• Real-life curriculum and problem-solving exercises are the most important
	• Attend to and optimize inquisitive, active learning
	• Experiential learning takes place in the classroom
	• Learners have choices about what to learn
	• Learners are engaged in group and peer learning
	• Education experiences are learner centered
		Constructivism (Piaget, Vygotsky)
		• "Active" learning theory
		• Learning is built by the learner and is built on previous knowledge and in the reality of the learner
		• Attributes of constructivism include:
		  ◦ Learning is actively constructed through interaction with the environment, and it is marked by reflection and actions
		  ◦ The learner tries to make sense out of his or her perceptions and experiences (K. V. Mann, 2011)
		  ◦ Doing is learning
		  ◦ Social negotiation is a part of learning
		  ◦ Supports multiple perspectives on subjects
		  ◦ Taking ownership of learning is important
		  ◦ Be self-aware and reflective in the knowledge-acquisition process
		  ◦ The goals are problem solving, reasoning, critical thinking, and the active and reflective use of knowledge
		  ◦ Most important, it is learner-focused (Brandon & All, 2010)
		Piaget (1972) described cognitive learning as a process of:
		• Accommodation
		• Assimilation
		• Equilibration
		Knowles's (1980) adult learning theory (andragogy)
		• Supports constructivism because it also builds on the learner's previous experiences (more information about andragogy can be found later in this chapter)
		Situated Learning Theory
		• Closely linked with constructivism
		• Reality based
		• Learner is an active participant in learning
		• Especially helpful when applied to clinical practice (K. V. Mann, 2011)
		Experiential Learning Theory
		Experimental learning theory (ELT) is a framework for learning whereby students reflect on what they are doing. It is usually hands-on and the outcome is minimized and the process is what is reflected upon. It is defined as "the process whereby knowledge is created through the transformation of experience. Knowledge results from the combination of grasping and transforming experience" (Kolb, 1984, p. 41)

TABLE 2.1
Worldview Philosophies, Educational Philosophies, and Teaching–Learning Theories (*continued*)

WORLDVIEW PHILOSOPHIES	EDUCATIONAL PHILOSOPHIES	TEACHING–LEARNING THEORIES
		There are four major concepts within the theory: • Concrete experience (CE) or those experiences built from reality • Abstract conceptualization (AC) or thinking about an experience • Reflective observation (RO) or taking in the experience • Active experimentation (AE) using hands-on experiences to learn (Kolb, Boyatzis, & Mainemelis, 1999)
Existentialism (Kierkegaard, Satre) • Seeks individual meaning in life • Schools hold social ideals • Perception of the individual is reality • No one can know us as we know ourselves • Education of the whole person is the goal • Subject matter takes second place to the development of a positive self-concept, self-knowledge, and self-responsibility • Learners have great latitude in choosing subject matter	**Reconstructionism/Critical Theory** (Habermas, Freire) • School is important for social change • School alone can prepare a learner for life • Includes the way educators construct or influence learning • Contains not only knowledge but also considers power • It includes constructing privilege, social identity, and cultural practices (Schultz, 2010) **Emancipatory Education** (Freire, 1970) • Education is a microsystem of society • Educators are cultural workers who profess freedom through an equalized classroom • Both educators and students are learners through true dialogue **Feminism** • Personal knowledge is a true knowledge • Power in the classroom must be analyzed • No human being should be marginalized • Places a great emphasis on empowerment and the learners' voices • Empirical knowledge is only one type of knowledge • Also uses narrative pedagogy (Welch, 2011)	**Humanism** (Rogers, Maslow) • Human beings are autonomous, and the dignity of human beings is most important • Self-actualization and education lead to individual happiness • A nursing approach can be found in Bevis and Watson's (1989) *Toward a Caring Curriculum* **Narrative Pedagogy** (Diekelmann, 2005) A phenomenological pedagogy • Focus is on the meaning and significance of teaching through phenomenology pedagogies such as narratives and storytelling • Builds experiences that stray from a formal, competency-based, outcome education format • Develops deeper thinking and finds meaning in lived experiences • Bases understanding on interpreting not memorizing • Students and faculty learn from each other (Ironside, 2014)

Adapted from Chinn (2007).

CRITICAL THINKING QUESTION

What belief(s) or philosophies speak to you as a nursing educator?

EVIDENCE-BASED TEACHING PRACTICE

Medina and Draugalis (2013) describe nine evidence-based steps to developing a teaching philosophy. The steps include:
1. Prepare an introduction
2. Describe teaching beliefs
3. Explain the importance of beliefs
4. Provide evidence based on educational theory
5. Describe teaching methods
6. Describe methods of learning assessment
7. Provide feedback summary
8. Prepare strong conclusion
9. Include references

THEORY OF MEANINGFUL LEARNING

Sousa, Formiga, Oliveira, Costa, and Soares (2015) describe "meaningful learning" as a learning theory that was developed by Ausubel (1962), which describes how learning must make sense personally to the learner. The *Theory of Meaningful Learning* proposes that knowledge must be interesting to the learner and be grounded in past experiences. The learner uses knowledge to develop new and unique meaning. The theory discusses receptiveness of the learner and discovery. Active teaching strategies increase individualized knowledge discovery. The Theory of Meaningful Learning is akin to the constructivist theoretical assumptions.

MODELS SPECIFIC TO NURSING

Teaching Gem: When a class begins with learning objectives (behaviorism) and reviews the anatomy and physiology before the patient condition (constructivism) is discussed, two learning theories are integrated.

There are two classic nursing models that have been significant in nursing education for the past several decades and are widely used as the theoretical foundations for many nursing studies and curricula, and learning activity development. They are Barbara Carper's (1978) "ways of knowing" and Patricia Benner's (1982) "novice to expert theory." Both will be reviewed in brief.

Carper (1978) described four ways that nurses understand practice situations, and they are:

1. Empirical or scientific knowledge (includes evidence-based practice [EBP])
2. Personal knowledge or understanding how you would feel in the patient's position

3. Ethical knowledge or attitudes and understanding of moral decisions
4. Aesthetic knowledge or understanding the situation of the patient at the moment

Munhall (1993) added the fifth way of knowing: *unknowing* or understanding that the nurse cannot know everything about the patient and must place himself or herself in a position willing to learn from the patient's perspective.

EVIDENCE-BASED TEACHING PRACTICE

Newham, Curzio, Carr, and Terry (2014) used Carper's ways of knowing to discuss junior nurses' activities and to recognize that today knowledge is primarily based on Carper's (1978) empirical knowing with a focus on quantitative data that have measurable outcomes. Empirical knowledge is goal directed and time limited and therefore easy to evaluate but it may also "devalue" the other important modes of nursing knowledge.

Benner (1982) described five levels of nursing expertise patterned on studies of how nurses grow in their role, and they include:
Novice—a beginner with no experience

- Relies on general rules to help perform tasks
- Rules are context free, independent of specific cases, and applied universally
- Behavior is limited and inflexible

Advanced beginner—a person who is at the point of demonstrating acceptable performance and

- Has gained prior experience in actual situations to recognize some patterns
- Uses principles based on experiences that begin to be formulated to guide actions

Competent—typically a nurse with 2 to 3 years' experience in the same role and

- Is aware of long-term goals
- Has a perspective about planning care with conscious, abstract, and analytical thinking
- Has greater efficiency and organization

Proficient—a nurse who perceives and understands situations as a whole and

- Understands patients holistically and has improved decision making
- Learns from experiences what to expect in certain situations
- Can be flexible and modify plans

Expert—a nurse who no longer relies on principles, rules, or guidelines to understand patient needs and determine actions and

- Has an intuitive grasp of practice situations
- Is flexible and highly proficient

EVIDENCE-BASED TEACHING PRACTICE

Thomas and colleagues (2015) reported that a study in the NLN simulation leadership group identified a lack of theory foundation for simulation expertise in faculty. They subsequently developed a "tool kit" based on Benner's theory to assist faculty in reaching an expert level as a simulation educator.

Dr. Patricia Benner has also been the primary author of a literature review and analysis contained in the book *Educating Nurses: A Call for Radical Transformation* (2009), which was funded by the Carnegie and Atlantic philanthropies. After a thorough historical and current review of nursing education, the following significant recommendations were made:

- Use teaching to integrate knowledge into the practice setting
- Decrease the division between classroom and clinical knowledge
- Emphasize clinical reasoning and multiple ways of thinking along with critical thinking
- Focus on the formation of professional identity along with socialization

DEEP, SURFACE, AND STRATEGIC LEARNING

Deep learning is a term first described by Marton and Saljo (1976) to refer to a learning approach and type of knowledge acquisition. The approach a learner takes to information presented in the classroom can be classified into three types of learning styles: deep, surface, and strategic.

1. A deep learning approach is accomplished when a learner addresses material with the intent to understand both the concepts and meaning of the information.
   * The learner relates new ideas to existing experiences and formulates links in long-term memory.
   * The motivation for a deep learning approach is primarily intrinsic, created from the learner's interest and desire to understand the relevance of the information to applied practice.
   * A type of deep learning is utilizing tangible everyday household objects to link new concepts to promote deep learning in an effort to link the concept to long-term memory (Wittmann-Price & Godshall, 2009).
2. A surface learning, or atomistic, approach facilitates learning by:
   * Memorization of facts and details. Surface learning is similar to rote learning in that the learner assimilates information presented at face value.
   * Motivation for surface learning, which is primarily extrinsic, is driven by either the learner's fear of failing or the desire to complete the course successfully.
3. A strategic learning approach; using this learning approach, the learner does what is needed to complete a course. Strategic learning is a mixture of both deep and surface learning techniques (Wittmann-Price & Godshall, 2009).
   * All three approaches to learning can be measured by the Approaches and Study Skills Inventory for Students (ASSIST; Ramsden & Entwistle, 1981).

EVIDENCE-BASED TEACHING PRACTICE

Heid (2015) developed an online clinical postconference pilot study to evaluate the development of deep learning through the use of clinical scenarios and guided discussion. Senior nursing students were provided with online clinical postconference activities for 30 minutes each week. Evaluations of students' satisfaction, integration of nursing concepts, and application from practice to theory were positive.

Mirghani, Ezimokhai, Shaban, and van Berkel (2014) used the 20-question Biggs two-factor Study Process Questionnaire (SPQ) with medical students ($N = 214$). Students in their first and second years of school demonstrated a significantly higher surface learning score and students in their final 2 years had a significantly higher deep learning score. This study has implications for nursing and how information is provided and retained. Building a knowledge base may be necessary as a foundation for connecting information.

MOTIVATIONAL THEORIES

Not only do nurse educators need to know how learners acquire information, they also need to know why they learn. What are their motivating factors? Motivation has been linked to learner retention and success. Many variables affect motivation; motivation can be influenced by the need for achievement or curiosity, or it can be a function of the situation at hand or a person's ability. A learner's *locus of control* can be *extrinsically* or *intrinsically motivated*. Motivation includes a student's goals, beliefs, perceptions, and expectations (Hanifi, Parvizy, & Joolaee, 2013).

EVIDENCE-BASED TEACHING PRACTICE

Hanifi and colleagues (2013) completed a grounded study about nursing students' motivation in clinical learning experiences ($N = 16$) and found that three themes emerged as demotivating factors: (a) social conditions, (b) encountering clinical education challenges, and (c) looking for an escape from nursing or merely tolerating nursing.

Nesje (2015) studied nursing graduate retention in relation to prosocial motivational factors, which is described as becoming a nurse because it is a calling. The researcher surveyed 160 nursing students in their final year of education and then again 3 years later and prosocial motivators were significantly associated with career commitment.

- Extrinsic motivations are those based on external variables, such as grades or earning money, and in today's environment there are many social pressures for students to become nurses.
- Intrinsic motivation has to do with the feeling of accomplishment, of learning for the sake of learning, or the feeling that being a nurse is something the learner always wanted to do. Hanifi and colleagues (2013) identified internal motivators as spiritual, selflessness, and serving people and they assist students to stay in nursing (Nesje, 2015). Intrinsic motivation is correlated with *self-determination*

theory, developed by Deci and Ryan (Deci, Eghrari, Patrick, & Leone, 1994). According to the theory, humans have three types of needs:

* To feel competent
* To feel related
* To feel autonomous

ARCS Model

Keller (1987) talks about the factors that educators can implement to motivate learners in the *ARCS model*:

A—Attention (keeping the learner's attention through stimulus changes in the classroom or clinical setting)

R—Relevance (make the information relevant to the learner's goals)

C—Confidence (make expectations clear so the learner will engage in learning)

S—Satisfaction (have appropriate consequences for the learner's new skills)

EVIDENCE-BASED TEACHING PRACTICE

Stockdale, Sinclair, and Kernohan (2014) applied the ARCS motivational theory to the process of patient education and found that it significantly increased patients' motivation to follow their planned goal.

Brophy Model

Brophy (1986) listed the following methods by which motivation is formed:

* Modeling
* Communication of expectations
* Direct instruction
* Socialization by parents and educators

Vroom's Expectancy Model

Vroom's expectancy model (VEM) describes what people want and whether they are positioned to obtain it. The Vroom model describes three concepts:

1. Force (F)—The amount of effort a person will put into reaching a goal
2. Valence (V)—How attractive the goal is to the person
3. Expectancy (E)—The possibility of the goal being achieved

The VEM model is $F = V \times E$ (Vroom, 1964).

Belongingness

Belongingness is conceptually related to motivation. Students, like all people, have a need to belong or be part of the group. Belongingness is instrumental in students' achievement, retention, self-esteem, self-directed learning (SDL), and self-efficacy. Without belongingness, students are at risk for attrition (Ashktorab et al., 2015). Vinales (2015) describes nursing students' belongingness in relation to building empowerment through increasing competency and confidence using a nurse role model. Hasanvand, Ashktorab, and Seyedfatemi (2014) report that students will conform to the norm in clinical learning experiences in order to gain a feeling of belongingness. Levett-Jones and Lathlean (2008) have completed landmark studies on belongingness and have identified themes about learning, which assist learners to either succeed or disengage; these are listed in Exhibit 2.1.

Lottes (2008) uses a formula that she calls *FIRE UP* to enhance learners' classroom motivation. This motivational strategy is shown in Exhibit 2.2.

Change

Change and motivation are interwoven concepts—one is dependent on the other. Change (learning new information, skills, or values) does not happen unless a

---

EXHIBIT 2.1

Themes About Learning

Theme A = Motivation to learn—being accepted and valued as a learner
Theme B = SDL assists in building confidence
Theme C = Anxiety is a barrier to learning
Theme D = Confidence to ask questions

EXHIBIT 2.2

Lottes' FIRE UP Motivational Strategy

F: be Funny—Use light entertainment to increase attention
I: be Interesting—Use graphics to help learners focus
R: be Real—Remember that you were a nursing student once
E: Engage them—Use active learning techniques
U: be Unique—Use an individual style in the classroom
P: be Passionate—Of course, love what you do

Source: Lottes (2008). Reprinted with permission of SLACK Inc.

CRITICAL THINKING QUESTION

What was your motivation for going back to school to become a nurse educator or for studying for the Certified Nurse Educator examination? Was it intrinsically or extrinsically motivated?

TABLE 2.2
Andragogy and Pedagogy

EDUCATIONAL ELEMENT	ANDRAGOGY	PEDAGOGY
Demands of learning	Learners have life demands besides school	Learners can devote more time to the demands of learning because responsibilities are minimal
Role of instructor	Learners are autonomous and self-directed Educators facilitate the learning but do not supply all the facts	Teacher-centered because the educator directs the learning Often uses surface learning
Life experiences	Learners have a tremendous amount of life experience Learners connect the learning to their knowledge base Learners must recognize the value of the learning	Learners do not have the knowledge base to make the connections between new knowledge and life experiences without facilitation
Purpose for learning	Learners have a goal in sight for their learning	Learners cannot always see the long-term necessity of information
Permanence of learning	Learning is self-initiated and tends to last a long time	Learning is compulsory and tends to disappear shortly after instruction

learner is motivated; therefore, an unmotivated learner most likely will not change. Change theories are well-described in Chapter 14.

Pedagogy and Andragogy

Pedagogy is generally defined as the art and science of teaching. It refers to the manner in which educators instruct, and its development was intended for children. *Andragogy* refers to the art and science of teaching adults (Knowles, 1980). Differences in the learning styles of students are discussed in detail in Chapter 9. Table 2.2 discusses the differences between andragogy and pedagogy.

TEACHING STYLES AND EFFECTIVENESS

Every ANE has his or her own style of teaching; teaching styles have been classified by many different methods. Nurse educators rarely subscribe to just one teaching style. Most educators use a variety of styles, even within a single learning session. This mixed approach can appeal to the variety of learning styles and can improve learning outcomes. Reflecting on the type of style that you use most encourages self-understanding and may serve to improve your effectiveness.

Several attributes contribute to teaching effectiveness. One attribute is immediate feedback and another is encouraging active learning (Aljezawi & Albashtawy, 2015). Also identified as an effective teaching style is the use of methods that enhance critical thinking such as concept mapping, questioning, and case studies (Lin, Han, Pan, & Chen, 2015).

EVIDENCE-BASED TEACHING PRACTICE

Gardner (2014) completed a phenomenological study with nurse educators ($N = 8$) who were in their role at least 5 years. The nurse educators chosen for the study had the reputation of being an effective teacher. The researchers identified themes: (a) becoming a nurse educator, (b) finding support, (c) developing a teaching style, (d) gaining confidence and competence, (e) teaching and learning as partnership, (f) being part of a bigger picture, (g) the best and the worst experiences, and (h) looking toward the future. The participants were found to engage learners, be flexible in changing their teaching methods to meet the needs of the students, and they shared their teaching experiences with other nurse educators.

Following are some of the ways teaching styles are categorized. Also included are good teaching behaviors and personality traits for educators that experts consider most effective.

Grasha's Classification of Teaching Styles

Grasha's (1996) classification defines teaching styles as expert, formal authority, demonstrator, facilitator, and delegator. The characteristics of each teaching style are unique and are listed in Table 2.3.

TABLE 2.3
Grasha's Teaching Styles

STYLE	CHARACTERISTICS
Expert	Educator uses his or her vast knowledge base to inform learners and challenges them to be well prepared. This can be intimidating to the learner.
Formal authority	This style puts the educator in control of the learners' knowledge acquisition. The educator is not concerned with student–teacher relationships, but rather focuses on the content to be delivered.
Demonstrator or personal model	The educator coaches, demonstrates, and encourages a more active learning approach.
Facilitator	Learner centered; active learning strategies are encouraged. The accountability for learning is placed on the learner.
Delegator	The educator role is that of a consultant, and the learners are encouraged to direct the entire learning process.

Source: Grasha (1996). Reprinted with permission of Carol Grasha.

Quirk's Classification of Teaching Styles

Quirk (1994) categorizes teaching styles into four distinct types:

1. Assertive—An assertive style is usually content specific and drives home information.
2. Suggestive—Educator uses experiences to describe a concept and then requests the learners research more information on the subject.
3. Collaborative—Educator uses skills to promote problem solving and a higher level of thinking in the learners.
4. Facilitative—Educators using this style often challenge the learners to reflect and use affective learning. Educators challenge learners to ask ethical questions and to demonstrate skill with interpersonal relationships and professional behavior.

Kelly's Teaching Effectiveness

Kelly (2008) also studied learners' perceptions of teaching effectiveness and found that the three most important attributes were:

1. Teacher knowledge
2. Feedback
3. Communication skills

House, Chassie, and Spohn's Teaching Behaviors

House, Chassie, and Spohn (1999) provide examples of the following behaviors and their effect on learners:

- Making eye contact can encourage learner participation in class.
- Positive facial expressions that elicit a positive learner response, such as head nodding, can assist learners in feeling comfortable speaking in class, whereas negative gestures, such as frowning, can discourage learner class participation.
- Vocal tone is very important and can easily portray underlying feelings and encourage or discourage learner participation.

Choo's Characteristics of Educators

Choo (1996) lists some of the characteristics of educators that are positive and promote learning:

- Values learning
- Exhibits a caring relationship
- Provides learner independence
- Facilitates questioning
- Tries different approaches
- Accepts the differences among learners

Koshenin's Positive Teacher–Learner Relationship Attributes

Koshenin (2004) identified five themes in the mentoring teacher–learner relationship that are worthy of note, because they can be conceptually transferred into the classroom. They are as follows:

- Worry about the learner's adjustment
- The pervasive experience of the relationship
- The feeling of mutual learning
- Worry about the learning results
- Disappointment in the lack of cooperation between the school and field (or the classroom and the larger organization of academia)

Hicks and Burkus's Master Teachers

Hicks and Burkus (2011) describe attributes of "master teachers," which include:

- Clear communication—oral and written
- Positive role modeling
- Professionalism demonstrated in lifelong learning and scholarship
- Reflective practice and making adjustments for improvement
- Use of philosophical, epistemological, and ontological influences in their practice of education

Story and Butts's Four "Cs"

Story and Butts (2010) discuss teaching delivery in the framework of the important four "Cs":

1. Caring—Learners need to know that educators truly care about them
2. Comedy—Humor is used to "demystify" the heavy content proposed to learners in the classroom
3. Creativity—Creative learning activities, such as food examples and role-play, are integrated into the lessons
4. Challenge—Maintain high expectations and the learners will reach them

Mann's 11 Practical Tips

A. S. Mann (2004) provides 11 practical tips for new college educators, which are designed to assist with their transition into academia. They are:

1. Do not use a red pen to correct work.
2. Provide breaks for long classes.
3. Review test answers in writing, if requested.
4. Take roll call to emphasize the importance of being present.

5. Set boundaries.

6. Evaluate the advice of others and be yourself.

7. Write down your expectations.

8. Do not change textbooks during a course.

9. Attend any and all in-services you can about teaching.

10. Teach to the learners' level.

11. Prepare for the next year every year.

The Myers–Briggs Type Indicator

The educator's personality also affects instruction. The Myers–Briggs Type Indicator (MBTI) measures Jung's (1921) 16 personality types by classifying them into four bipolar dimensions.

1. Extroversion/introversion

2. Sensing/intuition

3. Thinking/feeling

4. Judgment/perception (Plonien, 2015)

Besides cognitive evaluations of grades and standardized test scores, students' personality types may indicate success in higher education. Noncognitive indicators can be another variable to predict educational success (Stacey & Kurunathan, 2015). Using the MBTI as a self-knowledge tool is a mechanism to enhance communication, leadership, and conflict-resolution skills in nursing (Plonien, 2015).

EVIDENCE-BASED TEACHING PRACTICE

Herinckx, Munkvold, Winter, and Tanner (2014) developed a Classroom Effectiveness Teaching Scale, which has 27 items divided into four dimensions. Two of the dimensions assess the learning environment and the effectiveness of using evidence-based teaching practices (EBTPs) to promote deep learning in the classroom. The scale was developed as part of the Oregon Consortium for Nursing Education (OCNE).

Silver, Hanson, and Strong (1996) developed a Teaching Style Inventory (TSI) based on Jung's theory of psychological types, or personality types. It tests the educator's propensity for one of four types:

1. Sensing thinking

2. Sensing feeling

3. Intuitive thinking

4. Intuitive feeling

FACULTY INCIVILITY

Incivility penetrates all aspects of nursing and most educational and health care organizations have adopted a zero-tolerance policy. *Incivility* has been defined as behaviors that include disrespect and promote conflict. Uncivil behavior increases stress among the members of a group. Incivility and workload stress often go hand-in-hand (Clark, Olender, Kenski, & Cardoni, 2013).

Clark, Barbosa-Leiker, Gill, and Nguyen (2015) identified the following incivil behaviors:

- Complaining
- Lying
- Gossiping
- Using abusive language
- Insubordination
- Scapegoating

EVIDENCE-BASED TEACHING PRACTICE

Clark and colleagues (2013) studied faculty incivility in a national study that included 40 states. Faculty surveyed ($N = 588$) perceived incivility as a moderate to severe problem. The participants described incivility as setting a coworker up to fail, making rude remarks, putting others down, personally attacking others, making threatening comments, resisting change, failing to perform one's share of the workload, distracting others by using media devices during meetings, and refusing to communicate on work-related issues.

Incivility in the educational workplace often goes unreported because of fear of retaliation, lack of support from administrators, and lack of clear policies (Clark et al., 2013). learner incivility toward nurse educators is addressed in Chapter 9.

Zsohar and Smith (2006) have composed a list of the "top-10 don'ts" for class-room teaching, as these very well may be perceived as being incivil to learners.

1. Don't be late for class.
2. Don't pretend knowledge.
3. Don't read or repeat information that is easily accessible to the learner.
4. Don't bring personal baggage into class.
5. Don't come unprepared with excuses for a lack of preparation.
6. Don't be confrontational.
7. Don't interrupt.
8. Don't devalue the content taught by colleagues.
9. Don't be inconsistent with expectations.
10. Don't forget to be passionate about teaching.

LEARNING OUTCOMES VERSUS LEARNING OBJECTIVES

Historically, nursing education has used objectives for learning since Tyler's landmark book, *Basic Principles of Curriculum and Instruction* (1949), encouraged educators to develop behavioral objectives to organize their teaching. Therefore, objectives are part of the behavioral paradigm. To standardize the format of objectives, educators have incorporated the action verbs outlined in Bloom's taxonomy, which has since been revised.

Most teaching sessions begin with objectives or learning outcomes to frame the content or experience. *Objectives* and *learning outcomes* are two terms used often in nursing education; the differences between the terms may, on the surface, be slight, but they depict two approaches to evaluating learning that have emerged in recent years.

1. An objective speaks to the process; therefore, it is teacher centric.
2. An outcome, on the other hand, speaks to the product, thus, it is learner centric (Wittmann-Price & Fasolka, 2010).

Changing from objectives to outcomes is truly more of a conceptual change than an operational change. Some nurse educators have simply switched words but not their thought processes. Others believe that neither objectives nor outcomes give us the freedom needed to encourage learners to think critically (Bevis & Watson, 1989; Diekelmann, 1997). Nursing education leaders have rightfully questioned the use of objectives within today's postmodern educational philosophy environment because:

- All learning is not displayed in behavior
- By predetermining objectives or outcomes, the depth and breadth of the learners' experiences may be squelched

It is difficult at best to package the human intellect into a modifiable mold for convenience in grouping, evaluating, and justifying what is being taught or presented and what a learner carries forth from the experience.

Developing learning outcomes is done on many levels in academia. Outcomes are more general at the institutional level, and more specific at the course level. Learning outcomes will vary depending on the level for which they are being developed: the entire school, a program, levels within a program, and the course-specific level. Clinical courses can have two sets of outcomes: one set for the theory portion of the course and the second set for the clinical portion. Because most educational institutions still describe learning in terms of outcomes, sample formulas used to write the objectives are is depicted in Table 2.4.

Bloom's Taxonomy

Bloom's *Taxonomy of Educational Objectives* (Bloom, Englehart, Furst, Hill, & Drathwohl, 1956) describes an end behavior (see Table 2.5). The taxonomy uses "behavioral terms" to divide learning into leveled achievement, from knowledge acquisition to the synthesis of new ideas (Novotny & Griffin, 2006).

TABLE 2.4
Learning Outcomes

ANTECEDENT	LEARNER	VERB DESCRIBING BEHAVIOR	CONTENT	CONTEXT	CRITERIA
By the end of this session	The learner will	Demonstrate	Sterile gloving	In clinical settings	100% of the time
By the end of this session	The learner will	Compare	Different cultures	Related to childbearing experiences	By Interviewing two culturally different patients

TABLE 2.5
Bloom's Taxonomy

LEVEL	CONCEPT	VERBS USED WHEN WRITING LEARNING OUTCOMES
Creating (formerly called *synthesis*)	Judgment, selection	Arrange, assemble, collect, compose, construct, create, design, develop, formulate, manage, organize, plan, prepare, propose, set up
Evaluating (formerly called *evaluation*)	Productive thinking, novelty	Argue, assess, attach, choose, compare, defend, estimate, judge, predict, rate, core, select, support, value, evaluate
Analyzing (formerly called *analysis*)	Induction deduction, logical order	Analyze, appraise, calculate, categorize, compare, contrast, criticize, differentiate, discriminate, distinguish, examine, experiment, question, test
Applying (formerly called *application*)	Solution, application	Apply, choose, demonstrate, dramatize, employ, illustrate, interpret, operate, practice, schedule, sketch, solve, use, write
Understanding (formerly called *comprehension*)	Memory, repetition, description	Classify, describe, discuss, explain, express, identify, indicate, locate, recognize, report, restate, review, select, translate
Remembering (formerly called *knowledge*)	Explanation, comparison, illustration	Arrange, define, duplicate, label, list, memorize, name, order, recognize, relate, recall, repeat, reproduce, state

Learning Domains

Learning is discussed as a process that takes place in three domains: cognitive, affective, and psychomotor. Learners in nursing programs are evaluated for growth in all three domains. Bloom's taxonomy (see Table 2.5) identifies learning mainly in the cognitive domain. Psychomotor domains are not difficult to evaluate because they produce an observable behavior change. Many times this change is related to procedures and skills. The affective domain of learning is more difficult to assess because it is related to judgment and values (Partusch, 2007). Wong and Driscoll (2008) describe the learning development of the affective domain in stages, which are:

1. Receiving—when learners attend, listen, watch, and recognize
2. Responding—when learners answer, discuss, respond, reply, and participate
3. Valuing—when learners accept, adopt, initiate, or have a preference
4. Organizing—This is conceptualized as formulating, integrating, modifying, and systematizing
5. Internalizing—This occurs when learners commit, exemplify, and incorporate into practice

Gagne's Conditions of Learning

Gagne (1970) reinforced the need for objectives by stating that objectives are the second event in the nine conditions of learning (Table 2.6). He characterized objectives as a useful step to inform a learner of what is to be achieved. Using objectives served to organize the teaching- and-learning process while the discipline of nursing was in its growing stage of intense curriculum development (Miner, Mallow, Theeke, & Barnes, 2015). Gagne's steps for instruction are a classic list of tasks that is still referenced today.

TABLE 2.6
Gagne's Conditions of Learning

INSTRUCTIONAL EVENT	OPERATIONALIZATION OF EVENT
1. Gain attention of the learner	Stimuli activate receptors
2. Inform learners of objectives	Sets expectations for the learner
3. Stimulate recall of prior learning	Activates short-term memory and the retrieval of information by asking questions
4. Present the content	Presents content with features that can be remembered

(continued)

TABLE 2.6
Gagne's Conditions of Learning (*continued*)

INSTRUCTIONAL EVENT	OPERATIONALIZATION OF EVENT
5. Provide "learning guidance"	Assists the learner to organize the information for long-term memory
6. Elicit performance (practice)	Asks learners to perform to enhance encoding and verification
7. Provide appropriate feedback	Encourages performance
8. Assess performance	Evaluates learning
9. Enhance retention and transfer	Review periodically to decrease memory loss of information

DEVELOPING A LESSON PLAN

Lesson plans are not often spoken about in higher education to the same extent they are in primary education. In higher education, lesson plans often simply consist of a chart showing what learning the educator expects to facilitate during a specific time period and how that learning facilitation is going to be accomplished. Saad, Chung, and Dawson (2014) state:

> Lesson plans are written notes stating the specific objectives, the method of delivery and timelines associated with the delivery of lesson content. Another purpose of a lesson plan is to assist teachers in structuring the teaching and learning for teachers and students alike. Planning is essential to make sure the objectives of lessons are achieved. (p. 408)

An example of a lesson plan is shown in Exhibit 2.3

EVIDENCE-BASED TEACHING PRACTICE

Saad and colleagues (2014) used lesson-planning software and compared its use to manual or traditional lesson planning and found that the software saved a significant amount of time for the faculty in developing, retrieving, and editing lesson plans.

EXHIBIT 2.3

Lesson Plan

LEARNING OUTCOMES	RELATED COURSE OBJECTIVES	CONTENT OUTLINE	TIME	ASSIGNMENT	TEACHING STRATEGY	EQUIPMENT NEEDED	EVALUATION
Discuss hyperbilirubinemia in the preterm infant	Understand the physiological needs of the high-risk infant	1. Physiological jaundice 2. Pathological jaundice 3. Diagnostic tools 4. Nursing interventions	45 minutes	Case study using bilirubin graph	Lecture with case study and clicker questions	Audience response system (project Bilirubin graphs) for each learner	Five multiple-choice or alternative type questions on test 3
Compare Rh and ABO blood group incompatibilities	Understand the physiological needs of the high-risk infant	1. Rh sensitivity 2. ABO matching	30 minutes	None	PowerPoint presentation then use quick Jeopardy game	Easel and flip chart for game	Three multiple-choice or alternative type questions on test 3

Simulation learning experiences also use lesson plans to determine the objectives, time, methods, equipment, and roles needed during a simulation scenario (Venkatasalu, Kelleher, & Shao, 2015).

CRITICAL THINKING AND METACOGNITION

Critical thinking, as an educational concept, can be traced back to 1941 when Glaser defined composites of knowledge. Other historical developments about the concept of critical thinking include:

- In 1989, NLN recognized the inclusion of critical thinking as a specific criterion for the accreditation of nursing programs.
- Miller and Malcolm (1990) adapted Glaser's definition into a model for critical thinking and advised educators to pay closer attention to learners' mental processes.
- In the early days of concept development, educators were concerned with finding an appropriate definition for *critical thinking* in order to evaluate its development within learners.
- A multitude of definitions arose, and some of the more prominent ones are listed in Table 2.7.

Nurse educators can *role-model critical thinking* and *create opportunities for learners to develop their own critical thinking skills* by asking higher level questions and "thinking out loud," or dialoguing about an issue from different perspectives in order to synthesize a solution. The authors of *The ISNA Bulletin* (Indiana State Nurses Foundation & Indiana State Nurses Association, 2014) define attributes or characteristics that enhance and deter critical thinking; these are listed in Table 2.8.

TABLE 2.7
Descriptions of Critical Thinking

AUTHOR	DESCRIPTION OF CRITICAL THINKING
Facione, Facione, and Sanchez (1994)	Critical thinking is the process of purposeful, self-regulating judgment.
Paul and Elder (2007)	Attitudes are central, rather than peripheral, to critical thinking, as are independence, confidence, and responsibility, which are needed to arrive at one's own judgment.
Bandman and Bandman (1995)	Critical thinking is the rational examination of ideas, inferences, assumptions, principles, arguments, conclusions, issues, statements, beliefs, and actions. It covers scientific reasoning and includes the nursing process, decision making, and reasoning in controversial issues. It also includes deductive, inductive, informal, and practical reasoning.

TABLE 2.8
Attributes or Characteristics That Enhance and Deter Critical Thinking

CHARACTERISTICS OF CRITICAL THINKING	CHARACTERISTICS THAT DETER CRITICAL THINKING

• Universal intellectual standards are upheld and include:
  ◦ Clarity
  ◦ Accuracy
  ◦ Precision
  ◦ Relevance
  ◦ Depth
  ◦ Breath
  ◦ Logic
• Intellectual humility as opposed to intellectual arrogance
• Intellectual courage as opposed to intellectual cowardice
• Intellectual empathy as opposed to intellectual narrow-mindedness
• Intellectual autonomy as opposed to intellectual conformity
• Intellectual integrity as opposed to intellectual hypocrisy
• Intellectual perseverance as opposed to intellectual laziness
• Confidence in reason as opposed to distrust of reason and evidence
• Fair-mindedness as opposed to intellectual unfairness
• Reasoning
• Divergent thinking
• Creativity
• Clarification
	• Egocentrism fallacy
	  ◦ It's true because I believe it.
	  ◦ It's true because we believe it.
	  ◦ It's true because I want to believe it.
	  ◦ It's true because I have always believed it.
	  ◦ It's true because it is in my selfish interest to believe it.
	• Omniscience fallacy
	• Omnipotence fallacy
	• Invulnerability fallacy
	• The halo effect

Source: Indiana State Nurses Foundation & Indiana State Nurses Association (2014).

Ritchie and Smith (2015) propose that critical thinking is the seventh "C" needed in community health nursing along with:

1. Care
2. Compassion
3. Competence
4. Communication
5. Courage
6. Commitment
7. Critical thinking

Walker (2003) reviewed some of the teaching strategies that enhance critical thinking and suggests that they include:

- Questioning that promotes the evaluation and synthesis of facts
- Classroom discussions and debates with open negotiation
- Short, focused writing assignments such as
  * Summarize five major points in a chapter
  * Discuss the essence of the chapter using a metaphor
  * Explain the chapter to your neighbor, who has a high school education
  * How does the chapter affect your life, personally or professionally?
- Using case studies—use of case studies has been reported as a learning strategy to increase critical thinking skills (Falco, 2009; Popil, 2012)
- Reflective journaling (Raterink, 2016)
- Analytical writing (Price, 2015)
- Concept mapping (Yeo, 2014)

EVIDENCE-BASED TEACHING PRACTICE

Ahn and Yeom (2014) studied the relationship of moral sensitivity and **critical thinking** disposition among baccalaureate **nursing** students ($N = 142$) in Korea. Mean scores on the Moral Sensitivity Questionnaire (K-MSQ) were 2.83 out of 7 and mean scores on the **Critical Thinking** Disposition Questionnaire (CTDQ) were and 3.70 out of 5, which suggests a need to increase content in moral development. In addition, **stronger CTDQ scores were found in students who viewed nursing as a lifelong career as opposed to those who considered being a bedside nurse as a short-term goal.**

EVIDENCE-BASED TEACHING PRACTICE

Shin, Ma, Park, Ji, and Kim (2015) studied the relationship of pediatric simulation learning experiences with the development of critical thinking skills in undergraduate nursing students ($N = 237$). The results of using the simulation software on three university sites were measured with Yoon's **Critical Thinking** Disposition tool (2004) used to measure students' critical thinking abilities. Results demonstrated that it took three exposures to the simulation software to show a critical thinking gain in the prudence, systematicity, healthy skepticism, and intellectual eagerness subcategories.

Assessment of learners' critical thinking skills has been completed by use of several different tools. Two of the most widely used tools are:

- The California Critical Thinking Disposition Inventory; this tool evaluates seven "habits of the mind":

  1. Truth seeking
  2. Open-mindedness
  3. Analyticity
  4. Systematicity
  5. Self-confidence
  6. Inquisitiveness
  7. Cognitive maturity

- The Watson-Glaser Critical Thinking Appraisal (1964); this tool offers three different forms of the instrument, and the newest version has 16 scenarios and 40 items. There are five subcategories:

  1. Inference
  2. Recognition of assumptions
  3. Deduction
  4. Interpretation
  5. Evaluation (Romeo, 2010)

EVIDENCE-BASED TEACHING PRACTICE

Kowalczyk, Hackworth, and Case-Smith (2012) surveyed program directors (*N* = 317) about the use of critical thinking strategies in education, and all identified it as an important component in education. The study also identified the following barriers to using critical thinking strategies:
- The need to deliver a large amount of information to cover content
- Learner concerns of getting a good grade versus actually learning the content
- Insufficient time for instructors to learn new teaching methods
- Lack of learner motivation to become critical thinkers

Mindfulness

Mindfulness is a term related to critical thinking. *The ISNA Bulletin* (Indiana State Nurses Foundation & Indiana State Nurses Association, 2014) defines *mindfulness* as: "You are engaged with a certain activity, focused and actively thinking about whatever it is you are undertaking at the moment" (p. 6).

Metacognition

Metacognition is a concept that is from critical thinking. "Metacognition is an active process of knowing, or being acutely aware of one's cognitive state with the ability to complete a given task" (Hsu & Hsieh, 2014, p. 234). *Metacognition* refers to evaluating your own learning and ideas and being able to change them to understand and promote your own learning success.

EVIDENCE-BASED TEACHING PRACTICE

Hsu and Hsieh (2014) completed a study to examine the influence of demographic, learning involvement, and learning performance variables on metacognition of RN to BSN nursing students ($N = 99$). The correlational study using analysis of online dialogues, the Case Analysis Self Evaluation Scale, and the Blended Learning Satisfaction Scale found that all the performance variables were significant independent predictors of metacognition and accounted for over 50% of the variance in metacognition.

EVIDENCE-BASED TEACHING PRACTICE

The foundations of evidence-based teaching practice (EBTP) are analogous to EBP. Nurse educators use the same method of synthesizing and appraising evidence in order to draw a conclusion or develop an opinion that is grounded and derived from logical, common ideas in the literature (Hicks & Butkus, 2011).

Kalb, O'Conner-Von, Brockway, Rierson, and Sendelbach (2015) surveyed nursing education program administrators and faculty ($N = 551$) in a national study on the use of EBTP in their programs. EBTP was considered in the areas of teaching, learning, and program development. Participants all perceived EBTP as an important element in their teaching and EBTP needs to be continuously emphasized and resourced. This supports the finding of Patterson and Klein (2012) that identifies institutional barriers to using EBTP.

Ferguson and Day (2005) state that nursing education still needs much more quantitative and qualitative research to improve the science of nursing education. EBTP is based on four elements:

1. Evidence—both quantitative and qualitative
2. Professional judgment—nurse educators' decision-making ability
3. Values of learners as clients—using judgment appropriately by getting to understand learners
4. Resource issues—money, time, and space

EVIDENCE-BASED TEACHING PRACTICE

Felicilda-Reynaldo and Utley (2015) studied the teaching philosophies of 375 ANE using a mixed-method survey. The researchers found that although EBP was mentioned numerous times, only 44 ANE incorporated EBP into their teaching philosophies.

Faculty development about identifying and using EBTP is a need in many nursing programs. Understanding the significance and the need to use best practices in teaching is a nursing educational priority (Long et al., 2014).

CLASSROOM MANAGEMENT

The underpinning of positive classroom management is respect for the learners. Once an atmosphere of trust and respect is established, there should be very few classroom-management issues. Classroom management is also very different today when compared to the past, because of large class sizes and the advent of new technologies. Both of these issues have implications for classroom management. Chickering and Gamson's (1987) seven principles of good teaching practice are as follows:

1. Encourage contact between learners and educators
2. Develop reciprocity and cooperation among learners
3. Encourage active learning
4. Give prompt feedback
5. Emphasize time on task
6. Communicate high expectations
7. Respect diverse talents and ways of learning

Classroom management also includes deterring cheating. A literature review of 43 articles done by Stonecypher and Willson (2014) regarding academic misconduct recommends faculty consider the following methods to maintain integrity in the classroom:

- Publish detailed integrity policies
- Ensure students and faculty know the policies
- Provide test security
- Use proctors
- Use high-level test questions
- Ensure personal property is not out in the open

According to Mulligan (2007), there are four pillars of classroom management:

Pillar 1: Educators should use instructional strategies (active learning strategies) that motivate and keep learners interested and engaged.

Pillar 2: Educators need to use instructional time wisely and take a proactive approach to teaching by making the learners accountable for their learning.

Pillar 3: Social behaviors that need attention and correction should be done immediately, face to face, and privately.

Pillar 4: Educators need to create a flexible environment that adjusts to the learners' needs. For example, a learner with attention deficits may be less disruptive if placed up front and center.

Learners' use of technology in the classroom has also become a concern for nurse educators. Establishing "ground rules" early in the course and communicating them clearly may assist in maintaining classroom management. Educational technology is addressed in Chapter 3.

CLOSING AND NOT JUST "ENDING" A COURSE

"So the course is over. I enter my office, turn on the light, and begin to consider how I will facilitate closure for the next group of students. Just like caring for a patient, the process starts well before I ever meet them" (Yonge, Lee, & Luhanga, 2006, p. 151).

CASE STUDIES

CASE STUDY 2.1

Marcia is a new faculty member at a small baccalaureate school of nursing. She is full time, tenure track, and working on her doctoral degree. Marcia is assigned a mentor and a 12-credit semester teaching load, which is normal for many institutions. She meets with her mentor, who goes over her syllabus with her. The mentor asks Marcia why she has so many assignments in a clinical course. Marcia states that she believes that the learners' writing skills are lacking and they need writing assignments. If you were the mentor and saw a novice place 50% of the clinical course grade on writing assignments, how would you handle it?

CASE STUDY 2.2

A seasoned faculty member has been placed in the accelerated prelicensure learner curriculum. There are a large number of learners, and she has 10 clinical groups with seven different adjunct instructors. She uses the same syllabus that she used for the traditional prelicensure undergraduates, whom she taught successfully last semester. An assignment on the syllabus of the accelerated prelicensure learners is to pick a patient and create a complete care plan for him or her, including assessment, diagnoses, planning implementation, and evaluation format. The writing criteria state that the plan should be in American Psychological Association (APA) format and approximately 10 to 12 pages long. The instructor gives the learners a rubric, and the majority of learners complete the assignment on time. At the end of the semester, the educator is taken aback that the learners had so many negative comments about the care plan assignment. If you were the educator, how would you alter the assignment yet still ensure that you meet the course learning outcomes of developing a plan of care for a complex patient?

PRACTICE QUESTIONS

1. The nurse administrator observes a new faculty member in the classroom. The faculty member uses active learning strategies and provides the students with time to ask questions, but two students in the back of the class continue to look at the mobile phone devices in their laps and exchange comments to each other. Constructive advice about the classroom observation that the nurse administrator can provide would be:

   A. Address the behavior during the next class session

   B. Ask all students to put their phones at the front of the classroom on the table

   C. Provide additional active learning activities to keep all students engaged

   D. Request the students sit up front with a seat in between them

2. The nurse educator is developing a test and would like to increase the number of evaluation questions. The best format to promote evaluative thinking in students would be to add:

A. Fill-in multiple blanks

B. Hot spot

C. Display question

D. Select all that apply

3. A nurse educator has submitted a syllabus with the following student learning outcomes. Which learning outcome is written at the lowest level of Bloom's taxonomy?

A. Demonstrate caring to geriatric patients

B. Discuss common health care concerns of geriatric patients

C. Evaluate geriatric patients' understanding of home safety

D. Formulate a plan of care for a geriatric patient

4. During a curriculum meeting, the certified health care simulation educator states, "This semester we will do objective structured clinical examinations (OSCEs)." The philosophical foundations for this analysis would best fit:

A. Narrative pedagogy

B. Behaviorism

C. Constructivism

D. Feminism

5. During a faculty interview, the nurse educator candidate states that a preferred learning activity to facilitate learner understanding is looking at the historical roots of oppression. What nursing educational philosophy or theory is indicated by this learning activity?

A. Narrative pedagogy

B. Behaviorism

C. Constructivism

D. Feminism

6. A nursing faculty group is revising the core values of the undergraduate nursing program. The group wants to add the values of individualism and self-reflection. These values best reflect which of the following educational theories?

A. Narrative pedagogy

B. Behaviorism

C. Constructivism

D. Feminism

7. A faculty group is concerned about students' clinical decision-making ability and is revising its clinical learning evaluation tool using a graded scale from one (1) to four (4) with one (1) being dependent on the instructor for assistance, two (2) needing frequent cues, three (3) needing occasional cues and preforming

safely, and four (4) performing safely and independently. The best policy to support the tool would be:

A. Have the students reach a three (3) on each criterion by the end of each semester

B. Have the students reach level one (1) in the first trimester and work up to level four (4) in the last trimester

C. Alter the passing score depending on the specific clinical skill

D. Have students predetermine the level they want to achieve and then compare the outcomes at the end of the semester

8. When interviewing for a job, a nurse educator candidate verbalizes her concerns about students having a good science and math foundation. This nurse educator most likely subscribes to the philosophy of:

A. Phenomenology

B. Emancipatory education

C. Narrative pedagogy

D. Constructivism

9. A new faculty member who has come directly from a practice setting is chronically late for meetings and often does not answer e-mails in a timely manner. The faculty member does a good job with her class and contributes to committee work. The nurse administrator should address this behavior because it may be interpreted as:

A. A knowledge deficit

B. Poor role transition

C. Poor work ethic

D. Incivility

10. The educational nurse administrator tracks the attrition rates of the nursing educational program and finds that minority students are dismissed during their junior year at twice the number of nonminority students. The faculty discusses strategies for decreasing minority student attrition and decides the best method would be:

A. Reexamine the admission criteria

B. Start a one-to-one faculty–student tutoring program

C. Identify high-risk students in their sophomore year and have them go part-time their junior year

D. Establish a minority student nursing club that meets monthly and provides social events

REFERENCES

Ahn, S., & Yeom, H. (2014). Moral sensitivity and critical thinking disposition of nursing students in Korea. *International Journal of Nursing Practice, 20*(5), 482–489. doi:10.1111/ijn.12185

Aljezawi, M., & Albashtawy, M. (2015). Quiz game teaching format versus didactic lectures. *British Journal of Nursing, 24*(2), 86–92. doi:10.12968/bjon.2015.24.2.86

Ashktorab, T., Hasanvand, S., Seyedfatemi, N., Zayeri, F., Levett-Jones, T., & Pournia, Y. (2015). Psychometric testing of the Persian version of the Belongingness Scale—Clinical placement experience. *Nurse Education Today, 35*(3), 439–443. doi:10.1016/j.nedt.2014.11.006

Ausubel, D. P. (1962). A subsumption theory of meaningful verbal learning and retention. *Journal of General Psychology, 66*, 213–244.

Bandman, E. L., & Bandman, B. (1995). *Critical thinking in nursing* (2nd ed.). Norwalk, CT: Appleton & Lange.

Bandura, A. (1997). *Self-efficacy: The exercise of control.* New York, NY: W. H. Freeman.

Benner, P. (1982). From novice to expert. *American Journal of Nursing, 82*(3), 402–407.

Bevis, E., & Watson, J. (1989). *Toward a caring curriculum: A new pedagogy for nursing.* New York, NY: National Nursing League Publications.

Bloom, B., Englehart, M., Furst, E., Hill, W., & Drathwohl, D. (Eds.). (1956). *Taxonomy of educational objectives.* New York, NY: Longmans, Green.

Brandon, A. F., & All, A. C. (2010). Constructivism theory analysis and application to curricula. *Nursing Education Perspectives, 31*(2), 89–92.

Brophy, J. (1986). *On motivating students. Occasional paper no. 101.* East Lansing: Institute for Research on Teaching, Michigan State University.

Carper, B. A. (1978). Fundamental patterns of knowing in nursing. *Advances in Nursing Science, 1*(1), 13–24.

Chickering, A. W., & Gamson, Z. F. (1987). Seven principles for good practice in undergraduate education. *Wingspread Journal, 9*(2), 1–7.

Chinn, P. (2007). Philosophical foundations for excellence in nursing. In B. Moyer & R. A. Wittmann-Price (Eds.), *Nursing education: Foundations of practice excellence* (pp. 15–28). Philadelphia, PA: F. A. Davis.

Choo, L. A. (1996). Reflections: Learning at work. *Professional Nurse, Singapore, 23*(3), 8–11.

Clark, C. M., Olender, L., Kenski, D., & Cardoni, C. (2013). Exploring and addressing faculty-to-faculty incivility: A national perspective and literature review. *Journal of Nursing Education, 52*(4), 211–218. doi:10.3928/01484834-20130319-01

Clark, C. M., Barbosa-Leiker, C., Gill, L. M., & Nguyen, D. (2015). Revision and psychometric testing of the incivility in nursing education (INE) survey: Introducing the INE-R. *Journal of Nursing Education, 54*(6), 306–315. doi:10.3928/01484834-20150515-01

Deci, E., Eghrari, H., Patrick, B. C., & Leone, D. R. (1994). Facilitating internalization: The self-determination theory perspective. *Journal of Personality, 62*(1), 119–142. doi:10.1111/j.1467-6494.1994.tb00797.x

Diekelmann, N. L. (1997). Creating a new pedagogy for nursing. *Journal of Nursing Education, 36*(4), 147–148.

Diekelmann, N. L. (2005). Engaging the students and the teacher: Co-creating substantive form with narrative pedagogy. *Journal of Nursing Education, 44*(6), 249–252.

Facione, N. C., Facione, P. A., & Sanchez, C. A. (1994). Critical thinking disposition as a measure of competent judgment: The development of the California Critical Disposition Inventory. *Journal of Nursing Education, 33*, 345–350.

Falco, P. A. (2009). Teaching nursing critical thinking strategies to nursing students. *Metas de Enfermería, 12*(9), 68–72.

Felicilda-Reynaldo, R. F. D., & Utley, R. (2015). Reflections of evidence-based practice in nurse educators' teaching philosophy statements. *Nursing Education Perspectives, 36*(2), 89–95. doi:10.5480/13-1176

Freire, P. (1970). *Pedagogy of the oppressed.* New York, NY: Continuum.

Ferguson, L., & Day, R. A. (2005). Evidence-based nursing education: Myth or reality? *Journal of Nursing Education, 44*(3), 107–115.

Gagne, R. (1970). *The conditions of learning* (2nd ed.). New York, NY: Holt, Rinehart and Winston.

Gardner, S. S. (2014). From learning to teach to teaching effectiveness: Nurse educators describe their experiences. *Nursing Education Perspectives, 35*(2), 106–111. doi:10.5480/12-821.1

Grasha, A. F. (1996). *Teaching with styles.* Pittsburgh, PA: Alliance Publishers.

Hanifi, N., Parvizy, S., & Joolaee, S. (2013). Motivational journey of Iranian bachelor of nursing students during clinical education: A grounded theory study. *Nursing & Health Sciences, 15*(3), 340–345. doi:10.1111/nhs.12041

Hasanvand, S., Ashktorab, T., & Seyedfatemi, N. (2014). Conformity with clinical setting among nursing students as a way to achieve belongingness: A qualitative study. *Iranian Journal of Medical Education, 14*(3), 216–231.

Heid, C. L. (2015). Fostering deep learning: An on-line clinical postconference pilot study. *Teaching & Learning in Nursing, 10*(3), 124–127.

Herinckx, H., Munkvold, J. P., Winter, E., & Tanner, C. A. (2014). A measure to evaluate classroom teaching practices in nursing. *Nursing Education Perspectives, 35*(1), 30–36. doi:10.5480/11-535.1

Hicks, N. A., & Burkus, E. (2011). Knowledge development for master teachers. *Journal of Theory Construction and Testing, 15*(2), 32–35.

House, B. M., Chassie, M. B., & Spohn, B. B. (1999). Questioning: An essential ingredient in effective teaching. *Journal of Continuing Education in Nursing, 21*(5), 196–201.

Hsu, L., & Hsieh, S. (2014). Factors affecting metacognition of undergraduate nursing students in a blended learning environment. *International Journal of Nursing Practice, 20*(3), 233–241. doi:10.1111/ijn.12131

Hurlock, D. (2002). The possibility of an interdisciplinary poetic pedagogy: Re-conceiving knowing and being. *History of Intellectual Culture, 2*(1). Retrieved from http://www.ucalgary.ca/hic/files/hic/hurlock_article.pdf

Ironside, P. (2014). Enabling narrative pedagogy: Inviting, waiting, and letting be. *Nursing Education Perspectives, 35*(4), 212–218. doi:10.5480/13-1125.1

Indiana State Nurses Foundation & Indiana State Nurses Association. (2014). Developing a nursing IQ—Part 1. Characteristics of critical thinking: What critical thinkers do, what critical thinkers do not do. *ISNA Bulletin, 41*(1), 6–14.

Jung, C. G. (1921). Psychological types. In R. F. C. Hull (Ed.), *The collected works of C. G. Jung* (Vol. 6, Bollingen Series XX, H. G. Baynes, Trans.). Princeton, NJ: Princeton University Press.

Kaakinen, J., & Arwood, E. (2009). Systematic review of nursing simulation literature for use of learning theory. *International Journal of Nursing Education Scholarship, 6*(1), 1–20. doi:10.2202/1548-923X.1688

Kalb, K. A., O'Conner-Von, S. K., Brockway, C., Rierson, C., & Sendelbach, S. (2015). Evidence-based teaching practice in nursing education: Faculty perspectives and practices. *Nursing Education Perspectives, 36*(4), 212–219. doi:10.5480/14-1472

Keller, J. M. (1987). Development and use of the ARCS model of motivational design. *Journal of Instructional Development, 10*(3), 2–10.

Kelly, C. (2008). Students' perceptions of effective clinical teaching revisited. *Nurse Education Today, 27*(8), 885–892.

Knowles, M. (1980). *The modern practice of adult education.* Chicago, IL: Follett.

Kolb, D. A. (1984). *Experiential learning: Experience as the source of learning and development.* Upper Saddle River, NJ: Prentice-Hall.

Kolb, D. A., Boyatzis, R. E., & Mainemelis, C. (1999). *Experiential learning theory: Previous research and new directions.* Cleveland, OH: Department of Organizational Behavior, Weatherhead School of Management, Case Western Reserve University. Retrieved from http://www.d.umn.edu/~kgilbert/educ5165-731/Readings/experiential-learning-theory.pdf

Koshenin, L. (2004). A nurse's role in mentoring a foreign student. *Sairaanhoitaja, 77*(11), 18–21.

Kowalczyk, N., Hackworth, R., & Case-Smith, J. (2012). Perceptions of the use of critical thinking teaching methods. *Radiologic Technology, 83*(3), 226–236.

Levett-Jones, T., & Lathlean, J. (2008). Belongingness: A prerequisite for nursing students' clinical learning. *Nurse Education in Practice, 8*(2), 103–111.

Lin, C., Han, C., Pan, I., & Chen, L. (2015). The teaching–learning approach and critical thinking development: A qualitative exploration of Taiwanese nursing students. *Journal of Professional Nursing, 31*(2), 149–157. doi:10.1016/j.profnurs.2014.07.001

Long, C. R., Ackerman, D. L., Hammerschlag, R., Delagran, L., Peterson, D. H., Berlin, M., & Evans, R. L. (2014). Faculty development initiatives to advance research literacy and evidence-based practice at CAM academic institutions. *Journal of Alternative & Complementary Medicine, 20*(7), 563–570. doi:10.1089/acm.2013.0385

Lottes, N. C. (2008). FIRE UP: Tips for engaging student learning. *Journal of Nursing Education, 47*(7), 331–332.

Mann, A. S. (2004). Eleven tips for the new college teacher. *Journal of Nursing Education, 43*(9), 389–390.

Mann, K. V. (2011). Theoretical perspectives in medical education: Past experience and future possibilities. *Medical Education, 45*, 60–68. doi:10.1111/j.1365-2923.2010.03757.x

Marton, F., & Saljo, R. (1976). On qualitative differences in learning: I—Outcome and process. *British Journal of Educational Psychology, 46*(1), 4–11.

Medina, M. S., & Draugalis, J. R. (2013). Writing a teaching philosophy: An evidence-based approach. *American Journal of Health-System Pharmacy, 70*, 191–193. doi:10.2146/ajhp120418

Miller, M. A., & Malcolm, N. S. (1990). Critical thinking in the nursing curriculum. *Nursing & Health Care, 11*(2), 67–73

Miner, A., Mallow, J., Theeke, L., & Barnes, E. (2015). Using Gagne's 9 events of instruction to enhance student performance and course evaluations in undergraduate nursing course. *Nurse Educator, 40*(3), 152–154. doi:10.1097/NNE.0000000000000138

Mirghani, H. M., Ezimokhai, M., Shaban, S., & van Berkel, H. J. M. (2014). Superficial and deep learning approaches among medical students in an interdisciplinary integrated curriculum. *Education for Health: Change in Learning and Practice, 27*(1), 10–14. doi:10.4103/1357-6283.134293

Mulligan, R. (2007). Management strategies in the educational setting. In B. Moyer & R. A. Wittmann-Price (Eds.), *Teaching nursing: Foundations of practice excellence* (pp. 109–125). Philadelphia, PA: F. A. Davis.

Munhall, P. L. (1993). Unknowing: Toward another pattern of knowing in nursing. *Nursing Outlook, 41*(3), 125–128.

National League for Nursing. (2016). Certified nurse educator (CNE) candidate handbook 2016. Retrieved from http://www.nln.org/docs/default-source/professionaldevelopment-programs/certified-nurse-educator-%28cne%29-examination-candidate-handbook.pdf?sfvrsn=2

Nesje, K. (2015). Nursing students' prosocial motivation: Does it predict professional commitment and involvement in the job? *Journal of Advanced Nursing, 71*(1), 115–125. doi:10.1111/jan.12456

Newham, R., Curzio, J., Carr, G., & Terry, L. (2014). Contemporary nursing wisdom in the UK and ethical knowing: Difficulties in conceptualising the ethics of nursing. *Nursing Philosophy, 15*, 50–56. doi:10.1111/nup.12028

Novotny, J., & Griffin, M. T. (2006). *A nuts-and-bolts approach to teaching nursing.* New York, NY: Springer Publishing.

Partusch, M. (2007). Assessment and evaluation strategies. In B. A. Moyer & R. A. Wittmann-Price (Eds.), *Nursing education: Foundations of practice excellence* (pp. 213–227). Philadelphia, PA: F. A. Davis.

Patterson, B. J., & Klein, J. M. (2012). Evidence for teaching: What are faculty using? *Nursing Education Perspectives, 33*(4), 240–245.

Paul, R., & Elder, L. (2007). Critical thinking: The nature of critical and creative thought. *Journal of Developmental Education, 32*(2), 34–35.

Piaget, J. (1972). *The psychology of the child.* New York, NY: Basic Books.

Plonien, C. (2015). Preoperative leadership: Using personality indicators to enhance nurse leader communication. *AORN Journal, 102*(1), 74–80. doi:10.1016/j.aorn.2015.05.001

Popil, I. (2012). Promotion of critical thinking by using case studies as teaching method. *Nurse Education Today, 31*(2), 204–207. doi:10.1016/j.nedt.2010.06.002

Price, B. (2015). Applying critical thinking to nursing. *Nursing Standard, 29*(51), 49–58. doi:10.7748/ns.29.51.49.e10005

Quirk, M. E. (1994). *How to learn and teach in medical school: A learner-centered approach.* New York, NY: Charles C. Thomas.

Ramsden, P., & Entwistle, N. J. (1981). Effects of academic departments on students' approaches to studying. *British Journal of Educational Psychology, 51*, 368–383.

Raterink, G. (2016). Reflective journaling for critical thinking development in advanced practice registered nurse students. *Journal of Nursing Education, 55*(2), 101–104. doi:10.3928/01484834-20160114-08

Ritchie, G., & Smith, C. (2015). Critical thinking in community nursing: Is this the 7th C? *British Journal of Community Health, 20*(12), 578–579. doi:10.12968/bjcn.2015.20.12.578

Romeo, E. M. (2010). Quantitative research on critical thinking and predicting nursing students' NCLEX-RN performance. *Journal of Nursing Education, 49*(7), 378–386. doi:10.3928/01484834-20100331-05

Saad, A., Chung, P. W. H., & Dwson, C. W. (2014). Effectiveness of a case-based system in lesson planning. *Journal of Computer Assisted Learning, 30*(5), 408–424.

Schultz, J. R. (2010). The scholar-practitioner: A philosophy of leadership. *Scholar-Practitioner Quarterly, 4*(1), 52–64.

Shin, H., Ma, H., Park, J., Ji, E. S., & Kim, B. H. (2015). The effect of simulation courseware on critical thinking in undergraduate nursing students: Multi-site pre-post study. *Nurse Education Today, 35*(4), 537–542. doi:10.1016/j.nedt.2014.12.004

Silver, H., Hanson, J. R., & Strong, R. W. (1996). *Teaching styles & strategies (Unity in diversity series, Manual no. 2).* Alexandria, VA: Silver and Strong.

Sousa A. T. O., Formiga, N. S., Oliveira, S. H. S., Costa, M. M. L., & Soares, M. J. G. O. (2015). Using the theory of meaningful learning in nursing education. *Revista Brasilieira de Enfermagem, 68*(4), 626–635. doi:10.1590/0034-7167.2015680420i

Stacey, D. G., & Kurunathan, T. M. (2015). Noncognitive indicators as critical predictors of students' performance in dental school. *Journal of Dental Education, 79*(12), 1402–1410.

Stockdale, J., Sinclair, M., & Kernohan, W. G. (2014). Applying the ARCS design model to breastfeeding advice by midwives in order to motivate mothers to personalise their experience. *Evidence Based Midwifery, 12*(1), 4–10.

Stonecypher, K., & Willson, P. (2014). Academic policies and practices to deter cheating in nursing education. *Nursing Education Perspectives, 35*(3), 167–179. doi:10.5480/12-1028.1

Story, L., & Butts, J. B. (2010). Compelling teaching with the four Cs: Caring, comedy, creativity, and challenging. *Journal of Nursing Education, 49*(5), 291–294. doi:10.3928/01484834-20100115-08

Thomas, C. M., Sievers, L. D., Kellgren, M., Manning, S. J., Rojas, D. E., & Gamblian, V. C. (2015). Developing a theory-based simulation educator resource. *Nursing Education Perspectives, 36*(5), 340–342. doi:10.5480/15-1673

Tyler, R. W. (1949). *Basic principles of curriculum and instruction.* Chicago, IL: University of Chicago Press.

Valiga, T. M. (2012). Philosophical foundations of the curriculum. In D. Billings & J. A. Halstead (Eds.), *Teaching in nursing: A guild for faculty* (4th ed., pp. 107–118). St. Louis, MO: Elsevier Saunders.

Venkatasalu, M. R., Kelleher, M., & Shao, C. H. (2015). Reported clinical outcomes of high-fidelity simulation versus classroom-based end-of-life care education. *International Journal of Palliative Nursing, 21*(4), 179–186. doi:10.12968/ijpn.2015.21.4.179

Vinales, J. J. (2015). The mentor as a role model and the importance of belongingness. *British Journal of Nursing, 24*(10), 532–535. doi:10.12968/bjon.2015.24.10.532

Vroom, V. (1964). *Work and motivation.* New York, NY: Wiley.

Walker, S. (2003). Active learning strategies to promote critical thinking. *Journal of Athletic Training, 38*(3), 263–267.

Watson, G., & Glaser, E. M. (1964). *Watson–Glaser critical thinking appraisal manual*. New York, NY: Harcourt, Brace & World.

Welch, S. (2011). Nursing caps to feminist pedagogy: Transformation of nursing education. *Teaching and Learning in Nursing, 6*(3), 102–106. doi:10.1016/j.teln.2010.12.002

Wittmann-Price, R. A., & Fasolka, B. (2010). Objectives and outcomes: The fundamental difference. *Nursing Education Perspective, 31*(4), 233–236. doi:10.1043/1536-5026-31.4.233

Wittmann-Price, R. A., & Godshall, M. (2009). Strategies to promote deep learning in clinical nursing courses. *Nurse Educator, 34*(5), 214–216.

Wong, C. K., & Driscoll, M. (2008). A modified jigsaw method: An active learning strategy to develop the cognitive and affective domains through curricular review. *Journal of Physical Therapy Education, 21*(3), 15–23.

Wortham, S. (2011). What does philosophy have to offer education, and who should be offering it? *Educational Theory, 61*(6), 727–741.

Yeo, C. M. (2014). Concept mapping: A strategy to improve critical thinking. *Singapore Nursing Journal, 41*(3), 2–7.

Yonge, O., Lee, H., & Luhanga, F. (2006). Closing and not just ending a course. *Nurse Educator, 31*(4), 151–153.

Yoon, J. (2004). *Development of an instrument for the measurement of critical thinking disposition in nursing* (master's thesis). The Catholic University of Education, Seoul, Korea.

Zsohar, H., & Smith, J. A. (2006). Faculty issues. Top ten list of don'ts in classroom teaching. *Nurse Educator, 31*(4), 144–146.

Teaching and Learning Strategies

KAREN K. GITTINGS AND RUTH A. WITTMANN-PRICE

Those who know, do. Those that understand, teach.

—Aristotle

This chapter addresses the Certified Nurse Educator Exam Content Area 1: Facilitate Learning (National League for Nursing [NLN], 2016, p. 5).

- Content Area 1 is 22% of the examination
- It is estimated that there will be approximately 33 questions from Content Area 1

LEARNING OUTCOMES

- Differentiate between teaching strategies and learning activities
- Contrast passive and active learning
- Identify key points for effective PowerPoint presentations
- Identify advantages and disadvantages of various passive learning strategies
- Describe advantages and disadvantages of various active learning strategies
- Discuss flipping the classroom and associated challenges

TEACHING STRATEGIES AND LEARNING ACTIVITIES

The teaching–learning process involves the planning and implementation of experiences that are designed to lead to the achievement of student learning outcomes. These learning experiences can be thought of in terms of teaching strategies and learning activities. Although these terms are sometimes used interchangeably, the difference is in their focus.

- Teaching strategies, also referred to as *methods* or *techniques*, are teacher-centered activities. These strategies are used by faculty when teaching.
- Learning activities focus more on the learner. Faculty design strategies that enhance learner involvement and participation.

With the emphasis increasingly on learner-centered instruction, learning activities are being used to encourage student involvement. This places more of a responsibility on the learner for the acquisition of knowledge (Scheckel, 2012).

PASSIVE AND ACTIVE LEARNING

Learning activities can be further categorized as passive or active. With passive learning, learners take in information through their senses to be recalled at a later date. This mode of learning is still used commonly in today's classrooms. With active learning, learners are more engaged and are encouraged to participate in the acquisition of knowledge. Active learning can lead to improved retention and better understanding (Scheckel, 2012).

Passive Learning Advantages

- Faculty are able to present large amounts of information.
- Faculty have greater control over the learning environment.
- Learners often prefer this method because of previous experience.
- Important concepts are identified for learners.
- Learners may feel less anxious with a method familiar to them (Scheckel, 2012).

Passive Learning Disadvantages

- Leaves little time for questions or discussion.
- Faculty may not know whether learners understand the information presented.
- Requires little effort from learners.
- Does not facilitate application of concepts or use of higher level thinking (Scheckel, 2012).

CRITICAL THINKING QUESTION

Role modeling is a passive-teaching strategy that can be used to influence the attitude of learners. What other active-learning strategy is effective for learning in the affective domain?

Active Learning Advantages

- Increased attentiveness in the learning environment
- Improved retention of content
- Deeper understanding of the information
- Improved critical-thinking and problem-solving skills (Scheckel, 2012)

Active Learning Disadvantages

- Learners may be resistant to change.
- Learners may view these strategies as requiring extra work.
- Faculty may be resistant to change from their patterns of teaching and learning.
- Faculty may be concerned about student evaluations, especially if they are non-tenured (Scheckel, 2012).

LECTURE

Lecture, which is a type of passive learning, is still most commonly used in today's classroom. Nurse educators have to cover large amounts of content within their courses. Lecturing allows the educator to control the pace and flow of the class so that instructional goals for each specific class time can be achieved. Despite using lecture as a primary teaching strategy, most educators supplement with visual slides or audio files. Microsoft's PowerPoint is a very popular tool that has replaced the transparencies of the past. Instead of learners hurriedly trying to write notes and keep up, the challenge today is to not provide every note, which would lessen learner engagement. There are many other learning strategies that can be employed in the classroom to increase learner participation in their own knowledge acquisition.

EVIDENCE-BASED TEACHING PRACTICE

In a study conducted by Innes and Main (2013), the researchers set out to determine whether the use of personal response systems (PRS) enhanced education in nursing and midwifery lectures. "Of the 91 respondents, 95% found the PRS added interest to lectures, 78% found that it generated group discussion, 90% said it improved their understanding, 93% enjoyed using the system, and 93% would like to use it again in their learning" (Innes & Main, 2013, p. 20). Although the use of PRS requires additional preparation by the educator and extra delivery time in the classroom, evidence suggests that its use provides increased understanding.

POWERPOINT

Many educators use PowerPoint presentations to supplement lectures in the classroom, but few have received any guidance on how to use PowerPoint effectively. Learners can become quickly bored, particularly when slides are busy and the educator proceeds to read directly from the slides. Because PowerPoint is likely here to stay, it is important that educators learn how to develop presentations that are effective for student learning (Lim, 2012).

Keys to Effective Presentations

- Choose simple slide designs.
- Titles should be short and succinct.
- Font should contrast with the background and be easily readable (larger than 32).
- Follow the 6-by-6 rule—no more than six bullets per slide and six words per bullet.
- Begin with objectives.
- Limit one idea per slide if possible.
- Include graphics to facilitate understanding (no more than one per slide).
- Use multiple strategies to engage the learners (websites, videos, discussions, and polls).
- Slides should serve as an outline only.
- Limit talking to 1 to 2 minutes per slide.
- Never read directly from slides.
- Printouts should contain less information than the presentation to keep learners engaged (Dusaj, 2013).

> **Teaching Gem:**
> First impressions are made within the first 10 minutes of any presentation. One should always dress one level higher the audience. A professional appearance conveys credibility, authority, and expertise (Hayne & McDaniel, 2013).

PowerPoint is only as effective as the educator presenting; the presenter must stay cognizant of how the audience (learners) is responding and adapt accordingly. Other active learning strategies should be incorporated to keep the learners engaged. Prezi is an alternative to PowerPoint that uses a large canvas rather than individual slides; the presenter can zoom in to specific parts to emphasize points (Tables 3.1 and 3.2).

TABLE 3.1
Passive Learning Strategies

STRATEGY	DESCRIPTION	ADVANTAGES	DISADVANTAGES
Lecture	Educator presents the content. May include audio or visual aids and/or handouts.	• Clarifies complex information for the learner • Efficient for covering large amounts of information (Rowles, 2012) • An inspiring teacher can engage learners and keep their attention • Can be made more engaging by breaking up the lecture with other activities (Hagler & Morris, 2015) • Highlights main ideas and summarizes data • Effective for cognitive learning (K. Fitzgerald & Keyes, 2014) • Educator serves as role model for critical thinking and problem solving • Opportunity for learners to develop listening skills (DeYoung, 2015)	• Minimal learner engagement • Initial lengthy faculty preparation (Rowles, 2012) • Learners are unlikely to retain information when they are not actively engaged (Hagler & Morris, 2015) • Mostly ineffective with affective and psychomotor learning • All learners are taught the same despite differing abilities and limitations (K. Fitzgerald & Keyes, 2014) • Focuses more on the teaching of facts and less on analytical thinking • Effective for primarily auditory, linguistic learners • Loss of attention occurs over time (DeYoung, 2015)
Demonstration	Educator shows the learner how to perform a specific skill.	• Facilitates understanding (Rowles, 2012) • Effective for visual learners (Hagler & Morris, 2015)	• Learners may get bored (Rowles, 2012) • Limited to small groups so that all can observe (K. Fitzgerald & Keyes, 2014)
Reading	It is the learner's responsibility to read assigned chapters that relate to course content.	• Provides an opportunity to understand, interpret, and apply information • Strategies exist to improve reading comprehension (Hagler & Morris, 2015)	• May be difficult to learn through this method • Often difficult for learners to complete all of the assigned readings (Hagler & Morris, 2015)
Role modeling	Educators model behaviors.	• Effective for affective learning • Influences attitudes of learners • Potential to instill socially desired behaviors (K. Fitzgerald & Keyes, 2014)	• Requires a positive relationship between the educator and learner • May result in unacceptable behaviors if the role model has a negative influence (K. Fitzgerald & Keyes, 2014)

TABLE 3.2
Active Learning Strategies

STRATEGY	DESCRIPTION	ADVANTAGES	DISADVANTAGES
Algorithms	Step-by-step process for problem solving	• Assists learners in identifying the most relevant information • Develops problem-solving abilities • Effective in teaching complex procedures (Rowles, 2012)	• Time-consuming for faculty to develop • Steps must be easy to understand • Learners need instruction in use (Rowles, 2012)
Audience response systems (ARS)/ clickers	Electronic polling system that provides instant results	• Instant feedback available • May be used for attendance or to gauge learner understanding of the material • Similar systems available using Internet sites or smartphones (Zwirn & Muehlenkord, 2012) • Learners are more motivated to prepare for class • Allows learners to practice NCLEX®(National Council Licensure Examination) style questions with the instructor • Increases two-way communication in the classroom (Mareno, Bremner, & Emerson, 2010)	• Some cost involved for clickers • Instructors need to learn the technology • May be distracting (Mareno et al., 2010)
Case study/Case report	Application of nursing content and theory to analyze real-life situations	• Promotes critical thinking • Helps learners make the connection between didactic and practice events • Learners can practice problem solving (Rowles, 2012)	• Time-consuming for faculty to develop • Complex cases may be difficult to write • May be less effective when learners are not prepared for class (Rowles, 2012)
Clinical conferences/ online conferences	Small-group discussions that occur pre-, mid-, or postclinical experiences.	• Assists learners to connect theory to practice • Promotes clinical decision making and critical thinking • Increases learner confidence (Stokes & Kost, 2012)	• More effective if planned in advance (Stokes & Kost, 2012)

(continued)

TABLE 3.2
Active Learning Strategies *(continued)*

STRATEGY	DESCRIPTION	ADVANTAGES	DISADVANTAGES
Collaborative/ cooperative learning	Learners work on assignments in teams.	• Encourages teamwork • Learners are held accountable for their work, plus that of the group • Useful with large projects (Rowles, 2012) • Increases retention and promotes deeper learning • Learners also learn group skills (Hagler & Morris, 2015) • Strengthens communication skills (DeYoung, 2015)	• Learners are often resistant to group work • Some learners may not participate to group standards • Potential scheduling conflicts (Rowles, 2012) • Educators must plan and create a highly structured group environment (Hagler & Morris, 2015)
Debate	A logical argument and defense of a position aimed at demonstrating the truth or falsity of the matter.	• Learners are exposed to the intricacy and complexity of health care decision making • Broadens views • Improves communication • Team building (Rowles, 2012) • May be used to promote thinking about ethical or controversial issues (Hagler & Morris, 2015)	• Requires extensive knowledge of the subject matter • Lengthy learner preparation time • May increase learner anxiety • Increases time committed to group work (Rowles, 2012)
Debriefing	Faculty assist learners to reflect on clinical experiences; often used with simulation.	• Learners are guided to reflect on the experience and their feelings (Jefferies & Clochesy, 2012) • Opportunity to review actions and clinical decisions and discuss ways to improve (Jefferies, Dreifuerst, Aschenbrenner, Adamson, & Schram, 2015)	• Faculty need training to provide effective debriefing • Should not be used to provide additional information or to lecture on mistakes (Jefferies & Clochesy, 2012)

Flipped classroom	Learners complete learning activities prior to coming to class so that active learning can occur in the classroom; swaps lecture for active learning time.	• More focused learning can occur in the classroom • Facilitates collaboration and team work • Higher learning occurs (Connors & Tally, 2015)	• Learners are accountable for prework, which may lead to discontent • Requires a change in mind-set of the learners and faculty (Connors & Tally, 2015)
Games	Learners compete against self, a game, peers, or a computer.	• Effective for cognitive and affective learning • Fun for learners • Assists the learner to connect theory to practice • Provides immediate feedback (Rowles, 2012) • Improves retention • Engages learners even when the content is repetitive or dry (K. Fitzgerald & Keyes, 2014) • Increases interaction among learners (DeYoung, 2015)	• May take a significant amount of time from class • Faculty may lose control of the classroom • Difficult to evaluate individual learning (Rowles, 2012) • If subject is not reinforced, the message may be lost • Competition may deter some learners (Carifa & Goodin, 2011) • May require additional, adaptable space • Potentially creates a noisy environment (K. Fitzgerald & Keyes, 2014)
Grand rounds	Educator discusses patient problems and nursing care.	• Facilitates exchange of ideas among faculty, learners, and nursing staff (Stokes & Kost, 2012) • Encourages critical thinking and problem solving • Collaboration with the health care team is enhanced • Improves communication (Woodley, 2015)	• Requires planning • Patient permission should be obtained (Stokes & Kost, 2012)

(continued)

TABLE 3.2
Active Learning Strategies (*continued*)

STRATEGY	DESCRIPTION	ADVANTAGES	DISADVANTAGES
Group discussions/ seminar	Students and educator meet to discuss specific topics and share ideas.	• Peer sharing occurs • Problems can be discussed and solved as a group • Faculty serve as role models (Rowles, 2012) • Group participants are better able to clarify their own thoughts and beliefs when faced with the ideas of others (Hagler & Morris, 2015) • Promotes deeper understanding and longer retention of information • Promotes positive interpersonal relationships • Effective for learning in the affective and cognitive domains (K. Fitzgerald & Keyes, 2014) • Attitudes can be changed (DeYoung, 2015)	• Learners must be prepared with knowledge of the topic • Some learners may be reluctant to speak and participate • Difficult to evaluate student learning in those not participating • Discussions may be dominated by one or two people (Rowles, 2012) • Learners may not be able to decipher the important points to remember (Hagler & Morris, 2015) • More time-consuming to transmit information • Most effective with small-size groups (K. Fitzgerald & Keyes, 2014)
Group projects	Cooperative project in which learners work together to achieve a common goal.	• Increases long-term retention • Encourages critical thinking and problem solving • Requires negotiation and collaboration • Decreases the amount of work required of any individual learner • Learners experience conflict resolution, compromise, and trust building (Ward-Smith, Peterson, & Schmer, 2010)	• The work may be divided unevenly resulting in a few people doing all the work • Learners may only learn the portion that they worked on • Conflict may occur • Scheduling time to work together may be a challenge (Ward-Smith et al., 2010)
Humor	The use of comical situations or comments to highlight important points and enhance learning.	• Increases learner interest in the topic • May improve retention • Enhances learner–teacher rapport • Reduces boredom and tension (Rowles, 2012)	• May be inappropriate • May be demeaning if used inappropriately • May interfere with the learner–teacher relationship • Learners may find it distracting (Rowles, 2012)

Strategy	Description	Benefits	Challenges/Considerations
Imagery	Forming a mental picture or rehearsing in one's mind before taking action.	• Enhances learning of psychomotor skills (Rowles, 2012)	• Requires more time than just practice of skills • Faculty need to fully understand the strategy before educating learners in its use • Stress may interfere with effective use (Rowles, 2012)
Jigsaw	Group learning in which each member of the group is given a packet of information to learn and share with the rest of the group so that all benefit.	• Learners work together for success • Each group member is accountable for his or her portion (Moyer & Wittmann-Price, 2008)	• Time-consuming for faculty to develop • The packets/work must be evenly divided • Learners may complain that they are teaching themselves (Moyer & Wittmann-Price, 2008)
Learning circles	Learners get together to discuss a focused topic in order to learn from each other; usually peer based with a facilitator.	• Promotes equality • Promotes open discussions (Walker, Henderson, Cooke, & Creedy, 2010)	• Takes time to plan and arrange • Learners must be self-directed (Walker et al., 2010)
Learning contracts	Written contract between an individual learner and teacher specifying what needs to be accomplished to meet course outcomes.	• Effective for adult learners • Builds on prior knowledge and experiences • Learners can work at their own pace (Rowles, 2012) • May be used to clarify expectations for learners not meeting course requirements • Often used for practicum courses or precepted clinical experiences (Hagler & Morris, 2015)	• Learners must be independent, self-motivated, and self-disciplined • Time-consuming if faculty have a large number of learners with individualized contracts • Learners may need instruction on developing contracts (Rowles, 2012)

(continued)

TABLE 3.2
Active Learning Strategies (*continued*)

STRATEGY	DESCRIPTION	ADVANTAGES	DISADVANTAGES
Literature analogies/ newspaper analysis	Literature is used to clarify nursing concepts and to identify similarities and differences.	• Learners can relate unfamiliar concepts with those that are more familiar (Rowles, 2012)	• Difficult and time-consuming for faculty to locate relevant literature • Learners may be unable to see the relationships (Rowles, 2012)
Mind mapping/ concept maps	Concepts and subconcepts are diagrammed to visually demonstrate relationships.	• Effective for visual learners • Improves understanding of complex information • Encourages analytical thinking (Rowles, 2012) • Learners make connections between concepts and describe relationships (Hagler & Morris, 2015)	• May initially be time-consuming until learners are practiced in organizing the concepts • Faculty may be unfamiliar with this strategy and also require instruction in its use (Rowles, 2012)
One-to-one instruction/ tutoring	Face-to-face interaction designed to meet the needs of the learner; may be formal or informal.	• Experience is unique to the learner • Retention is improved when information is given in small amounts • Content and pace of instruction is adapted to the learner's needs • Effective for learning in the cognitive, affective, and psychomotor domains • Provides immediate feedback for the learner (K. Fitzgerald & Keyes, 2014)	• Labor intensive • Time-consuming for the educator • Isolates the learner (K. Fitzgerald & Keyes, 2014)
Podcasts/ vodcasts/ enhanced podcasts	Audio or video that is available over the Internet; may be played with iPods, e.g., includes PowerPoints with voice-over narration.	• May be used to record lectures • Provides an opportunity for learners to relisten to course information outside the classroom • May be used for inclement weather or faculty illness • May be utilized to explain assignments in online courses (Friesth, 2012)	• Requires some faculty training • Requires iPod or other mobile device if used in mobile format • Access to high-speed Internet required • Learners may be more inclined to miss class (Friesth, 2012)

Portfolio/ electronic portfolios	Electronic or printed documents that are evidence of learning; may be used to demonstrate best work or growth.	• Encourages learners to self-reflect • Documents progress of learner's work • Effective with independent, self-directed learners (Rowles, 2012) • Electronic portfolios are easy to store and update (Oermann & Gaberson, 2014)	• May become overly large if guidelines for inclusion are not provided • Learners need guidance on what to include • Time-consuming for faculty to review • May be costly (Rowles, 2012)
Poster	Electronic or printed document that may include text, graphs, or pictures to represent a concept.	• Permits learners to be creative • Complex ideas can be conveyed in a concise format • Learners can learn from each other • Can be graded by faculty easily and quickly (Rowles, 2012)	• Supplies may be costly • May be frustrating for some learners who lack creativity (Rowles, 2012)
Problem-based learning	A curriculum approach in which clinical problems and professional issues are used to organize the content.	• Develops critical thinking and clinical decision-making • Effective with teams and group work • Can be used with interdisciplinary groups • Increases learner responsibility for learning (Rowles, 2012)	• Extensive time commitment for faculty to learn to develop problems • Unfamiliar to most learners; requires extended orientation to learner expectations • Difficult to use in larger classes (Rowles, 2012)
Questioning/ Socratic questioning	Queries about content designed to elicit a response; questioning to explore complex ideas or analyze concepts.	• Can be planned or used spontaneously • Promotes clinical decision making with high-level questions • Encourages discussion and multiple points of view • Strengthens test-taking abilities (Rowles, 2012) • Can be used to review content (DeYoung, 2015)	• Learners must understand the content • Faculty must be prepared to deliver questions that require more than a statement of the facts • Learners may feel threatened • May take a significant amount of class time in order to give learners sufficient time to formulate an answer (Rowles, 2012)

(continued)

TABLE 3.2
Active Learning Strategies (continued)

STRATEGY	DESCRIPTION	ADVANTAGES	DISADVANTAGES
Reflection/ journaling/ blogs	Electronic or written record of personal experiences related to specific content.	• Learners are better able to connect classroom learning with clinical experiences • Encourages critical thinking • Faculty have better insight into student learning (Rowles, 2012) • Means of reflecting and expressing feelings (Oermann & Gaberson, 2014) • Effective for learning in the cognitive and affective domains (Moyer & Wittmann-Price, 2008)	• Learners may view this as busywork if the objectives are not clear • Learner issues may manifest that require faculty intervention • Learners may minimize the assignment and invest little time • Time-consuming for faculty to read and provide feedback (Rowles, 2012)
Return demonstration	This requires the learner to repeat a skill that was previously demonstrated.	• Increases retention • Facilitates understanding • Novices are able to model expert technique (Rowles, 2012) • Effective for the kinesthetic learner (Hagler & Morris, 2015) • Confidence and competence are increased through repetition and frequent feedback (K. Fitzgerald & Keyes, 2014)	• Learners master skills at different speeds • Learners may get bored with waiting • Requires supervision, supplies, and space • Costs (Rowles, 2012) • Takes a considerable amount of time for learners to practice and educators to monitor • Groups must be kept small to allow for practice and close supervision (K. Fitzgerald & Keyes, 2014)
Role play	Enactment of a specific role, usually unscripted, whereby others are observing and analyzing the demonstration.	• Learning occurs through observation and discussion • Promotes understanding of human behaviors • Peer review • Improves decision making (Rowles, 2012) • Effective for learning in the affective domain (Moyer & Wittmann-Price, 2008) • Provides opportunity to explore attitudes and beliefs (K. Fitzgerald & Keyes, 2014) • Improves interpersonal and communication skills (DeYoung, 2015)	• Learners may not want to participate • Time investment needed for faculty to develop scenarios • May take a significant amount of class time (Rowles, 2012) • May reinforce stereotypical behavior (Moyer & Wittmann-Price, 2008) • May appear unrealistic if overly dramatic (K. Fitzgerald & Keyes, 2014)

Self-learning packet/ module/ reusable learning objects (RLO)	Content is presented in sections that permit the learner to progress forward if he or she has demonstrated mastery, often through pretests/ posttests.	• Students have more control over their learning • Self-directed and paced • Flexible (Rowles, 2012) • May be used to introduce new content or reinforce/clarify existing content • May be used for learner prework when flipping the classroom (Hagler & Morris, 2015)	• Learners may procrastinate • Time-consuming to prepare • Learners may not be sufficiently motivated (Rowles, 2012)
Service learning	A form of experiential learning that occurs outside the traditional classroom.	• Facilitates application of knowledge to the real world • Encourages civic involvement • Promotes problem solving (Hagler & Morris, 2015) • Incorporates reflective practice (Preheim & Foss, 2015)	• Requires extensive planning to ensure that learning outcomes can be met • Time-consuming for the faculty to plan and develop experiences and monitor for effectiveness (Hagler & Morris, 2015)
Simulation	A situation that is designed to mimic real-life clinical experiences.	• Learners can practice in a safe environment • No harm occurs to the patient • Learners can experience situations seldom seen • Immediate feedback is provided • Increases critical thinking • Encourages teamwork (Scheckel, 2012) • Effective for cognitive, psychomotor, and affective learning • Promotes increased autonomy and independence (Yuan, Williams, & Fang, 2011)	• Faculty must develop or search for scenarios • Learning outcomes need to be clear for each simulation • Only a small number of learners can actively participate in each session • Equipment is expensive to purchase and maintain • Requires physical space and technical support (Scheckel, 2012) • Mixed results on whether confidence and competence are increased • Validated measurement tools for simulation are in demand (Yuan et al., 2011)

(continued)

TABLE 3.2
Active Learning Strategies (continued)

STRATEGY	DESCRIPTION	ADVANTAGES	DISADVANTAGES
Social writing tools/wikis	A single document developed by a group that can be edited by each member.	• Promotes collaboration among group members • Thinking and writing skills are further developed (Halstead & Billings, 2012) • Facilitates group work without needing face-to-face meetings • Individual learner contributions can be seen using the history function (DeYoung, 2015)	• An open wiki would be accessible by the public (Sopczyk, 2014) • Learners may be reluctant to critique or edit the work of others • Learners who procrastinate impact the work of the group (DeYoung, 2015)
Standardized patient (SP)	Live actors portray patients in a realistic clinical simulation.	• Effective for improving communication and/or physical-assessment skills • Learners can experience a situation not often seen in the clinical environment • Increases confidence • Increases long-term retention of material (Rowles, 2012) • Learners receive written and oral feedback (Oermann & Gaberson, 2014)	• Need to be cautious to involve all learners • Must be realistic for knowledge to transfer to real life • Actors must be trained • May be costly (Rowles, 2012)
Storytelling/dialogue/narrative pedagogy	This is a conversation between at least two people in which relevant stories are shared.	• Encourages reflection and analysis • Reinforces affective learning • Heightens caring behaviors (Rowles, 2012)	• Faculty must keep stories relevant and realistic • Stories may lead to peer sharing, which can become lengthy and cause learners to lose focus (Rowles, 2012)
Team-based learning	Learners work on assignments in groups, taking accountability for the quality of their own work and that of the group.	• Can be used in larger classes • Enhances team building (Rowles, 2012) • Introduces peer assessment and accountability • Improves knowledge scores and learning outcomes (Fatmi, Hartling, Hillier, Campbell, & Oswald, 2013)	• Learners and faculty need time to learn this strategy • May be challenging for groups to schedule time to work on assignments outside of class time • Conflict may interfere with effective group functioning (Rowles, 2012) • Learner reactions may be mixed • Learners may see this strategy as adding to their workload (Fatmi et al., 2013)

Think–pair–share	A type of cooperative learning whereby the educator asks a question, allows time for the learners to think, pairs up learners for discussion, and then requests that the collaborative response be shared with the class.	• Increases learner engagement • Improves understanding of difficult content • Encourages collaboration • Enhances interpersonal and small-group skills (D. Fitzgerald, 2013)	• Requires learners to come to class prepared • Learners may initially be resistant to the additional work required (D. Fitzgerald, 2013)
Top 10 list	Learners prioritize topics from their reading in a list format.	• Helps learner to organize, prioritize, and compare their results with others (Beitz & Snarponis, 2006)	• Learners will probably prioritize differently (Beitz & Snarponis, 2006)
Unfolding case studies	Learners follow a patient through a series of events and, using the data provided, make decisions related to the patient's care; usually integrated into individual lessons.	• Develops critical thinking and clinical decision making • Assists in making connections between theory and practice (Oermann & Gaberson, 2014) • Effective with teams and group work • Can be used with interdisciplinary groups • Increases learner responsibility for learning (Rowles, 2012)	• Extensive time commitment needed for faculty to develop realistic, challenging cases • Difficult to use in larger classes (Rowles, 2012)

(continued)

TABLE 3.2
Active Learning Strategies (continued)

STRATEGY	DESCRIPTION	ADVANTAGES	DISADVANTAGES
Vignettes	Hypothetical situation that simulates real-life experiences.	• Used to explore attitudes, beliefs, and perceptions • Facilitates discussion (Wright, Heathcote, & Wibberley, 2014)	• Learners may be reluctant to share personal feelings • Cannot entirely replicate real-life (Wright et al., 2014)
Virtual reality/worlds/clinical experiences	Computer-based, three-dimensional technology that creates virtual clinical environments or practicums; e.g., Second Life.	• Provides distance clinical experiences • Can also be used as classrooms and meeting spaces • Learners gain practice skills, demonstrate professional behaviors, and learn teamwork and collaboration • Useful when clinical sites are limited as in rural areas (Stokes & Kost, 2012; Zwirn & Muehlenkord, 2012) • Learners can gain experience with culturally diverse patients (DeYoung, 2015)	• Expensive • Faculty and learners need to be oriented to use (Zwirn & Muehlenkord, 2012)
Warm-up/start-up exercises	Activities used to check reading assignments at the beginning of class; may count toward grade.	• Encourages learners to read before class	• Takes class time
Webinars	Internet-based web conference that attendees join via telephone or computer.	• Effective for distance teaching or meetings • Allows discussion and interaction (Sopczyk, 2014)	• Requires technological expertise • Background noise can become a problem (Sopczyk, 2014)

Writing/research paper	The act of conveying ideas or knowledge through the written word in the form of scholarly papers, journals, etc.	• Promotes critical thinking • Students learn to organize their ideas • Enhances communication skills (Rowles, 2012)	• Grading can be subjective • Time-consuming for both learners and faculty • Does not lend itself well to use in large classes
YouTube/DVDs	Films or video clips used to enhance content.	• Appeals to younger learners • Discussions can enhance learning and encourage critical thinking (Rowles, 2012) • Effective for demonstration of psychomotor skills • Usually inexpensive (Hainsworth & Keyes, 2014)	• May be time-consuming for faculty to locate relevant videos • Faculty must review videos for accuracy and appropriateness for all learners • Longer films or clips may take up a significant amount of class time (Rowles, 2012) • Passive unless the educator is involved (DeYoung, 2015)

FLIPPED CLASSROOMS

The flipped or inverted classroom has generated much interest in recent years because it is a learner-centered approach with the potential to keep learners actively engaged in the learning process. In flipping the classroom, learners are required to review content and complete prework before coming to class. In the classroom, active learning strategies are used to assist learners in developing higher order thinking and problem-solving skills (Betihavas, Bridgman, Kornhaber, & Cross, 2016).

Although many nurse educators continue to use the traditional lecture as the primary mode of transmission of information, it is well recognized that for learners to retain and apply the information, they must be actively engaged in their learning. Nursing students, in particular, must learn how to think critically, solve problems, and apply theory to practice. The recognition of the importance of student-centered learning has led to the increased use of active learning strategies, including flipped classrooms (Betihavas et al., 2016).

> **Teaching Gem:** Team-based learning and unfolding case studies are two strategies that lend themselves well to use in the flipped classroom. Learners are divided into small groups (4–6) to work through unfolding case studies. After the group has had time to work together, the full class can come back together to further discuss the case. This enhances team building and clinical decision-making.

Most research into the effectiveness of flipped classrooms has been done in the disciplines of pharmacology and medicine. In a systematic review by Betihavas and colleagues (2016), five studies of flipped classrooms used in nursing education showed evidence of mixed results on academic performance and student satisfaction. Several challenges in implementing flipped classrooms were identified.

Student Challenges

- Difficulty in adjusting
- Unable to see the value
- Increased preparation time
- Dissatisfaction with group work (Betihavas et al., 2016)

Faculty Challenges

- Inexperience
- Increased preparation time (Betihavas et al., 2016)

Despite a limited number of studies in using flipped classrooms in nursing education, most studies in the health disciplines support the use of this learner-centered approach to prepare learners for practice. Although learners may be less satisfied with this approach, likely related to increased workload, several studies have reported improved academic performance. Flipped classrooms increase the opportunity for students to learn higher level thinking, which can facilitate their transition to practice (Betihavas et al., 2016).

EVIDENCE-BASED TEACHING PRACTICE

Della Ratta (2015) flipped the classroom in two fundamental nursing courses at a public university. Learners prepared for class by completing assigned readings and reviewing narrated PowerPoint lectures. In the classroom, using the principles of team-based learning, learners worked through case studies and clinical scenarios. Learners were found to have developed teamwork and collaborative skills. Quantitatively, learner scores on a standardized fundamentals test given at the end of the semester were significantly higher than previous semesters in which the classroom was not flipped.

CASE STUDIES

CASE STUDY 3.1

Amanda was recently hired to teach Adult Health III to 50 senior level baccalaureate students. She is a recent graduate of a nurse educator program. Amanda has taught as a clinical instructor for two semesters, but she has no other academic teaching experience. In planning for her course, Amanda has decided to include journaling as a method of evaluation worth 20% of the student's grade. As her mentor, do you have any concerns with this? How would you advise Amanda?

CASE STUDY 3.2

Marcey is a recent MSN graduate hired to run the simulation laboratory. She is very excited to expand the use of simulation in the prelicensure BSN program. She would like to collaborate with the theater department to use students as SPs. As her mentor, Marcey has asked you to assist with the planning. What important issues need to be considered and addressed in moving forward with this project?

PRACTICE QUESTIONS

1. A nurse educator is interested in using a learning strategy that will allow learners to self-reflect and examine their feelings about the clinical experience. A colleague suggests that she consider incorporating:

   A. Journaling

   B. Concept maps

   C. Group discussions

   D. Socratic questioning

2. A novice adjunct clinical instructor is observed questioning learners in the clinical setting. What would cause the course coordinator to intervene?

   A. The instructor questions the learners privately, away from other staff

   B. Questions are asked that only require a statement of the facts

   C. Learners are questioned about medications before administering them

   D. The instructor asks questions of the clinical group in postconference

3. A nurse educator teaching the professional course for the first time has decided to have learners begin a portfolio they will build on throughout the nursing program. What should the educator consider in adopting this learning strategy?

   A. Portfolios should not be graded

   B. Learners should include a sample of work from each course

   C. Guidelines for inclusion should be provided to the learners

   D. There is no time commitment for the faculty

4. A clinical practicum-based nurse educator needs to teach all the intensive care unit (ICU) nurses about a change in the process for obtaining blood cultures. What strategy would be most effective for allowing a large number of nurses to learn the information while on duty?

   A. Return demonstration

   B. Self-learning packet

   C. Group discussion

   D. YouTube video

5. A novice nurse educator who has returned from a faculty development conference is sharing what she has learned about active learning strategies with other faculty. What statement by the novice would require you to intervene?

   A. "Learners will have a deeper understanding of the information"

   B. "Active learning improves problem-solving skills"

   C. "Lecture using PowerPoint slides is one type of active learning strategy"

   D. "Learners will be more engaged in the classroom"

6. A nurse educator is interested in assessing her students' understanding of course content as she is teaching. One method that is not time intensive and provides immediate feedback is:

   A. Audience response systems

   B. Debate

   C. Think–pair–share

   D. Group discussion

7. A mental health educator is planning to use theater students as standardized patients (SPs) to teach nursing students effective communication skills. It is most important to:

   A. Use only senior-level theater students

   B. Allow the nursing students to choose who will be a part of the simulation

   C. Train the theater students so they are familiar with their roles and expectations

   D. Encourage over-dramatization by the theater students

8. After returning from a conference and learning about various teaching and learning strategies, a nurse educator is interested in flipping the classroom in one of her courses. When explaining this to her colleagues, what statement would require her mentor to intervene?

    A. "Using this method, I will be able to focus on key concepts in the classroom"

    B. "I can place the learners in groups so they benefit from peer learning"

    C. "Learners will love this method because there is no increase in work for them"

    D. "This is an opportunity for learners to use and develop higher level thinking skills"

9. A nurse educator is designing a learning activity for students to examine their attitudes and beliefs about caring for transgender patients. This would be best facilitated through:

    A. Reading

    B. Case studies

    C. YouTube video

    D. Role playing

10. A novice educator expresses concern to her mentor that her students are not reading their textbooks. One method that could be used for testing each student's preparation for class would be:

    A. Warm-up exercises

    B. Think–pair–share

    C. Self-learning module

    D. Questioning

REFERENCES

Beitz, J., & Snarponis, J. (2006). Strategies for online teaching and learning. *Nurse Educator, 31*(1), 20–24.

Betihavas, V., Bridgman, H., Kornhaber, R., & Cross, M. (2016). The evidence for flipping out: A systematic review of the flipped classroom in nursing education. *Nurse Education Today, 38,* 15–21.

Carifa, L., & Goodin, H. J. (2011). Using games to provide interactive perioperative education. *AORN Journal, 94*(4), 370–376. doi:10.1016/j.aorn.2011.01.018

Connors, H. B., & Tally, K. (2015). Integrating technology in education. In M. H. Oermann (Ed.), *Teaching in nursing and role of the educator* (pp. 61–81). New York, NY: Springer Publishing.

Della Ratta, C. B. (2015). Flipping the classroom with team-based learning in undergraduate nursing education. *Nurse Educator, 40*(2), 71–74.

DeYoung, S. (2015). *Teaching strategies for nurse educators* (3rd ed.). New York, NY: Pearson.

Dusaj, T. K. (2013). Pump up your PowerPoint® presentations. *American Nurse Today, 8*(7), 43–46.

Fatmi, M., Hartling, L., Hillier, T., Campbell, S., & Oswald, A. E. (2013). The effectiveness of team-based learning on learning outcomes in health professions education: BEME guide no. 30. *Medical Teacher, 35,* e1608–e1624. doi:10.3109/0142159X.2013.849802

Fitzgerald, D. (2013). Employing think-pair-share in associate degree nursing. *Teaching and Learning in Nursing, 8*(3), 88–90.

Fitzgerald, K., & Keyes, K. (2014). Instructional methods and settings. In S. B. Bastable (Ed.), *Nurse as educator: Principles of teaching and learning for nursing practice* (4th ed., pp. 469–515). Burlington, MA: Jones & Bartlett.

Friesth, B. M. (2012). Teaching and learning at a distance. In D. M. Billings & J. A. Halstead (Eds.), *Teaching in nursing: A guide for faculty* (pp. 386–400). St. Louis, MO: Elsevier Saunders.

Hagler, D., & Morris, B. (2015). Teaching methods. In M. H. Oermann (Ed.), *Teaching in nursing and role of the educator* (pp. 35–59). New York, NY: Springer Publishing.

Hainsworth, D., & Keyes, K. (2014). Instructional materials. In S. B. Bastable (Ed.), *Nurse as educator: Principles of teaching and learning for nursing practice* (4th ed., pp. 518–558). Burlington, MA: Jones & Bartlett.

Halstead, J. A., & Billings, D. M. (2012). Teaching and learning in online learning communities. In D. M. Billings & J. A. Halstead (Eds.), *Teaching in nursing: A guide for faculty* (pp. 401–421). St. Louis, MO: Elsevier Saunders.

Hayne, A. N., & McDaniel, G. S. (2013). Presentation rubric: Improving faculty professional presentations. *Nursing Forum, 48*(4), 289–294.

Innes, G., & Main, M. (2013). Improving learning with personal response systems. *Nursing Times, 109*(13), 20–22.

Jefferies, P. R., & Clochesy, J. M. (2012). Clinical simulations: An experiential, student-centered pedagogical approach. In D. M. Billings & J. A. Halstead (Eds.), *Teaching in nursing: A guide for faculty* (pp. 352–368). St. Louis, MO: Elsevier Saunders.

Jefferies, P. R., Dreifuerst, K. T., Aschenbrenner, D. S., Adamson, K. A., & Schram, A. P. (2015). Clinical simulations in nursing education: Overview, essentials, and the evidence. In M. H. Oermann (Ed.), *Teaching in nursing and role of the educator* (pp. 83–101). New York, NY: Springer Publishing.

Lim, F. A. (2012). Wake up to better PowerPoint presentations. *Nursing, 42*(2), 46–48.

Mareno, N., Bremner, M., & Emerson, C. (2010). The use of audience response systems in nursing education: Best practices guidelines. *International Journal of Nursing Education Scholarship, 7*(1), 1–17. doi:10.2202/1548-923X.2049

Moyer, B. A., & Wittmann-Price, R. A. (2008). *Nursing education: Foundations for practice excellence.* Philadelphia, PA: F. A. Davis.

Oermann, M. H., & Gaberson, K. B. (2014). *Evaluation and testing in nursing education.* New York, NY: Springer Publishing.

Preheim, G., & Foss, K. (2015). Partnerships with clinical settings: Roles and responsibilities of nurse educators. In M. H. Oermann (Ed.), *Teaching in nursing and role of the educator* (pp. 163–190). New York, NY: Springer Publishing.

Rowles, C. J. (2012). Strategies to promote critical thinking and active learning. In D. M. Billings & J. A. Halstead (Eds.), *Teaching in nursing: A guide for faculty* (pp. 258–284). St. Louis, MO: Elsevier Saunders.

Scheckel, M. (2012). Selecting learning experiences to achieve curriculum outcomes. In D. M. Billings & J. A. Halstead (Eds.), *Teaching in nursing: A guide for faculty* (pp. 170–187). St. Louis, MO: Elsevier Saunders.

Sopczyk, D. L. (2014). Technology in education. In S. B. Bastable (Ed.), *Nurse as educator: Principles of teaching and learning for nursing practice* (4th ed., pp. 559–600). Burlington, MA: Jones & Bartlett.

Stokes, L. G., & Kost, G. C. (2012). Teaching in the clinical setting. In D. M. Billings & J. A. Halstead (Eds.), *Teaching in nursing: A guide for faculty* (pp. 311–334). St. Louis, MO: Elsevier Saunders.

Walker, R., Henderson, A., Cooke, M., & Creedy, D. (2010). Impact of a learning circle intervention across academic and service contexts on developing a learning culture. *Nurse Educator Today, 31*(4), 378–382. doi:10.1016/j.nedt.2010.07.010

Ward-Smith, P., Peterson, J., & Schmer, C. (2010). Students' perceptions of group projects. *Nurse Educator, 35*(2), 79–82. doi:10.1097/NNE.0b013e3181ced87e

Woodley, L. K. (2015). Clinical teaching in nursing. In M. H. Oermann (Ed.), *Teaching in nursing and role of the educator* (pp. 141–161). New York, NY: Springer Publishing.

Wright, J. M., Heathcote, K., & Wibberley, C. (2014). Fact or fiction: Exploring the use of real stories in place of vignettes in interviews with informal carers. *Nurse Researcher, 21*(4), 39–43.

Yuan, H. B., Williams, B. A., & Fang, J. B. (2011). The contribution of high-fidelity simulation to nursing students' confidence and competence: A systematic review. *International Nursing Review, 59*, 26–33.

Zwirn, E. E., & Muehlenkord, A. (2012). Creating interactive learning environments using media and digital media. In D. M. Billings & J. A. Halstead (Eds.), *Teaching in nursing: A guide for faculty* (pp. 369–385). St. Louis, MO: Elsevier Saunders.

Educational Technology

FRANCES H. CORNELIUS AND LINDA WILSON

The great aim of education is not knowledge but action.
—Herbert Spencer

This chapter addresses the Certified Nurse Educator Exam Content Area 1: Facilitate Learning (National League for Nursing [NLN], 2016, pp. 5–6).

- Content Area 1 is 22% of the examination
- It is estimated that there will be approximately 38 questions from Content Area 1

LEARNING OUTCOMES

- Analyze the nurse educator's role with respect to the use of educational technology to support learning
- Examine the importance of the appropriate integration of technology in a meaningful and relevant manner to support learning
- Describe how to devise strategies to integrate technology in a learning activity

As technology progresses, academic nurse educators must keep up with technological advancement. Although this may be challenging at times, as an academic nurse educator, it is important to be open-minded, eager to learn, and willing to look outside of nursing for innovative ideas to enhance the quality of nursing education. Professional and special-interest organizations offer opportunities to stay current and to network. Some organizations include:

- *Educause* (www.educause.edu)—This nonprofit association's mission is to advance higher education by promoting the intelligent use of information technology.
- *National Education Association* (*NEA*; www2.nea.org/he/techno.html)—This organization was founded in 1857 with the goal to "both elevate the character and advance the interests of teaching, promoting the cause of education in the

United States" (NEA, 2013, p. 1). The NEA higher education website offers a forum to discuss the role of technology in education as well as an opportunity to learn about new trends.

- *Society for Applied Learning Technologies* (*SALT*; www.salt.org)—SALT is a society oriented toward professionals whose work requires knowledge and communication in the field of instructional technology.

Additional resources include Innovate (www.innovateonline.info) or EmergingEdTech (www.emergingedtech.com), which provide the faculty an opportunity to stay current with new technologies and innovations.

TECHNOLOGY IN THE LEARNING ENVIRONMENT

The learning environment has morphed into an arena where learners are no longer passive recipients of information. Learning has become an interactive and social experience, resulting in richer, more meaningful experiences for learners and faculty alike. Whether in the traditional face-to-face classroom, the clinical setting, or a virtual/hybrid environment, new technologies, Web 2.0 tools and Web 3.0 functionality provide many opportunities to enhance learning far beyond the traditional "ivory towers." Brown (2006) states:

> One would also expect a form of spiral learning to evolve, initially rooted in one community but then branching out to encompass expanding interests and skills. The spiral would weave a tapestry between activities in the niche communities of interest and the core curriculum, with both serving to ground and complement the other. This new learning scape would be supported by an understanding of the interplay between the social and cognitive basis of learning, and enabled by the networked age of the 21st century. Such an educational experience would undoubtedly build a strong foundation for life-long learning in a world of accelerating change. (p. 29)

There are many opportunities to incorporate new technologies into learning. For example, as a result of emerging technologies, all courses can be "web-enhanced" and can support any curriculum. The Internet, video streaming, podcasting, and Web 2.0 tools can help to enhance any classroom activity. Some popular Web 2.0 tools include:

- *Wikis*—A wiki is a collection of web pages that may be edited by anyone.
- *Blogs*—Journal entries that are presented in reverse chronological order.
- *Social networking*—Websites that build relationships and connections/networks, strengthening learning communities.
- *Twitter.com*—A "microblog" that allows users to send short text messages, not exceeding 140 characters in length, to a personalized homepage.
- *Podcasting or video podcasting*—A method of distributing multimedia content (lectures, discussions, etc.) via the Internet for playback on mobile devices and personal computers. This can be accomplished using really simple syndication (RSS) feeds that are freely available on the Internet.

- *Social bookmarking or tagging*—An online service that allows resources to be categorized using user-defined keywords or tags. Principally, social bookmarking allows users to assemble and annotate (tag) preferred web links/resources, to share with others. This creates a vast repository of shared resources, organized in a meaningful manner.
- *Gaming*—Often referred to as *serious gaming*, the use of games for educational purposes is growing exponentially. Gaming can provide opportunities for authentic learning and can generate a "tremendous amount of transactional data that can reveal insights not only about student success or failure but also about student teamwork and collaboration preferences, learning styles, and a variety of other learning issues" (Epper, Derryberry, & Jackson, 2012, p. 2).

These technologies can provide considerable support in developing higher level thinking among learners. For example, Twitter could be used to continue the class discussion on a given topic.

> **Teaching Gem:** Blogging is a great method to use when a portion of learners are on service-learning trips; this will keep the learning community at home in touch with the travels and experiences of the others.

Metacognition—the practice of thinking about and reflecting on your learning—has been shown to benefit comprehension and retention. As a tool for students or professional colleagues to compare thoughts about a topic, Twitter can be a viable platform for metacognition, forcing users to be brief and to the point—an important skill in thinking clearly and communicating effectively (Educause Learning Initiative, 2016a, p. 2).

CRITICAL THINKING QUESTION

Can you use metacognition to decrease the number of words on each PowerPoint slide by 10%?

EVIDENCE-BASED TEACHING PRACTICE

Hsu and Hsieh (2014) studied undergraduate nursing students' ($N = 99$) demographics, learning involvement, and learning performance influence on metacognition in a blended learning environment (a course in class and online). The results from this cross-sectional, correlational study showed that online dialogues, the Case Analysis Self Evaluation Scale, and the Blended Learning Satisfaction Scale were significant independent predictors of metacognition.

Recently, there has been considerable discussion regarding the next generation of the web—Web 3.0—and particularly what this next step in the evolution of the Internet will offer education. A variety of predictions regarding anticipated functionalities of Web 3.0 are available. Web 3.0 is described as the "intelligent web or semantic web with technologies like big data, linked data, cloud computing, 3D visualization, augmented reality and more" (p. 8) further scaffolding the transition from passive to active learning (Dominic, Francis, & Pilomenraj, 2014). Google's chief executive officer, Eric Schmidt, believes that Web 3.0 will transform things in a big way (Yun, 2007). It will be characterized by the following:

- A series of combined applications that are very small will be "pieced" together and will run using data stored in the cloud.
- These applications will be very fast, will run on any device (mobile phone, computer, etc.), and will be highly customizable.
- Applications will be distributed "virally" from person to person via text, e-mail, and so on.

The core software technology in Web 3.0 will be artificial intelligence. In short, the software can intelligently learn and understand semantics, and this will result in a more customized, personalized web experience (Yun, 2007). This customization will permit users (educators and learners alike) to forge new linkages between components/features transforming content to build new knowledge, further enriching the learning experience.

Singh and Lal (2012) state that the tools and services that will be available in Web 3.0 "would foster a more open approach to learning" (p. 4). These tools include:

- *Intelligent Search Engines and Intelligent Tutoring Systems*—providing direct, highly personalized and customized information searching, instruction, and/ or feedback to learners.
- *3-D Wikis, 3-D Online Games, and 3-D Encyclopedias*—providing increased interaction with content through 3-D representation of content and the capability for 360° camera rotation, allowing the user to examine content from multiple perspectives or vantage points.
- *Semantic Digital Libraries, Semantic Blogs, and Semantic Forums and Community Portals*—connecting content and making distinctions/connections among words, symbols, and concepts resulting in richer and deeper learning experiences.
- *Virtual Worlds*—providing "an interactive simulated environment accessed by multiple users through an online interface" and available in a "wide variety of forms, including 3-D re-creations of museum and gallery spaces, computer programming tutorials, virtual libraries, and meeting spaces for online university courses" (Creative Commons, n.d., pp. 1, 11).
- *Microblogging*—"Microblogging is the practice of posting small pieces of digital content—which could be text, pictures, links, short videos, or other media—on the Internet" (Educause Learning Initiative, 2016b, p. 1).
- *Virtual Laboratories/Education Laboratories*—similar to the virtual worlds described earlier, virtual laboratories will provide a realistic 3-D laboratory experience for the learners.

Shift From Passive to Active Learning

Student engagement is critical to learning and is "positively related to academic outcomes" and "has a compensatory effect on first-year grades and persistence to the second year of college at the same institution" (Kuh, Cruce, Shoup, Kinzie, & Gonyea, 2008, p. 555). Further, students who have opportunities to engage in level-appropriate academic challenges, participate actively in collaborative learning, encounter enriching educational experiences, and have frequent interaction with faculty are more likely to be successful and persist (Canney, 2015; Indiana University Center for Postsecondary Research [IUCPR], 2013; Robinson & Hullinger, 2008). National Survey of Student Engagement reported that "when students are both challenged and provided the appropriate amount of support, they are motivated to reach their potential" and are "more likely to engage in a variety of effective educational practices," which include reflection, quantitative reasoning, collaborative learning, discussions with diverse others, and student–faculty interactions (National Survey of Student Engagement, 2015, p. 3).

Generally, there is consensus among educators that student engagement is essential; however, Kuh (2009) stresses that these efforts must be individualized, pointing out that some educators sometimes adopt a hegemonic, one-size-fits-all way of thinking. Student engagement is too important, as well as too complicated, for the educational community to allow this to happen. For example, as with other college experiences, engagement tends to have conditional effects, with students with certain characteristics benefiting from some types of activities more so than other students (p. 15).

Strategies to engage students in active learning include opportunities for students to interact with content, instructors, and other learners. Teaching/learning technologies have expanded capabilities to support this interaction. For example, clicker technology, also referred to as an *audience-response system* (ARS), can be used to engage the learner in the classroom and in online environments and has demonstrated positive impact on learning (Kay & LeSage, 2009). These can be actually distinct "stand-alone" devices distributed to the participants or these can be set up to invite participants to respond to questions using a mobile phone or laptop connected to the Internet.

- One method for incorporating this technology is to create some preclass questions that the learners can respond to using the clicker technology, and then, following the lecture, the same questions are presented as postclass questions to see whether there is an increase in correct responses, thereby demonstrating learner comprehension of the content presented.
- Another method is to pose questions to which there may be differing opinions. Learners can respond anonymously and "the stage is set to support and deepen engagement and articulation as students try to mount arguments for their position" (Brown, 2006, p. 29).

In another example, students can be asked to create content using a variety of freely available tools and resources that not only permit student "authoring" of content but also support collaborative learning. These include tools like PlayPosit (www.playposit.com), Screencastomatic (screencast-o-matic.com), and Padlet (padlet.com). Students can use these tools to create reports, group presentations, and more.

EVIDENCE-BASED TEACHING PRACTICE

Tar-Ching, Loney, Elias, Ali, and Adam (2016) studied ARS's ability to obtain student consensus on presented issues in a modified three-stage Delphi process. The modified Delphi process included (a) agreeing on the topic/s of interest for which consensus is sought, (b) identifying key stakeholders whose opinions are required, and (c) assembling the stakeholders for a 1-day event. The ARS provided immediate feedback and students could consider the group view before moving forward in the process. This study resulted in expediting the Delphi method by decreasing the time needed to arrive at consensus.

To support academic nurse educators with the use of technology, a university can

- Provide access to new learning technologies.
- Offer faculty training to support the integration of new technologies into teaching.
- Establish web-based resource centers, such as Drexel University's Virtual Nursing Faculty Resource Center (Hasson, Cornelius, & Suplee, 2008).
  - The purpose of this type of resource center is to provide web-based support.
  - "This resource center can serve as a 'one-stop shopping' area for all faculty to access not only resources but also tutorials to support 'just-in-time' training needs" (Hasson et al., 2008, p. 23).
- Provide library liaisons and instructional designers to work with teaching faculty to "develop courses and/or class assignments, interactive teaching models, learning objects, and tutorials that introduce information literacy concepts, resources, and tools" (Donald, 2009, p. 2).

INFORMATICS IN THE LEARNING ENVIRONMENT

The NLN (2008) "advocates for support of faculty development initiatives and innovative educational programs that address informatics preparation. This call for reform is relevant to all prelicensure and graduate nursing education programs as the informatics revolution will impact all of nursing practice" (p. 1; see Exhibit 4.1).

EXHIBIT 4.1

Faculty Development

For Nurse Educators
- Participate in faculty development programs to achieve competency in informatics
- Designate an informatics champion in every school of nursing to (a) help faculty distinguish between using instructional technologies to teach versus

(continued)

EXHIBIT 4.1

Faculty Development (*continued*)

using informatics to guide, document, analyze, and inform nursing practice, and (b) translate state-of-the-art practices in technology and informatics that need to be integrated in the curriculum

- Incorporate informatics in the curriculum
- Incorporate American Nurses Association (ANA)-recognized standard nursing language and terminology into content (ANA, 2000)
- Identify clinical informatics exemplars, those drawn from clinical agencies and the community or from other nursing education programs, to serve as examples for the integration of informatics into the curriculum
- Achieve competency through participation in faculty development programs
- Partner with clinicians and informatics specialists at clinical agencies to help faculty and learners develop competence in informatics
- Collaborate with clinical agencies to ensure that learners have hands-on experience with informatics tools
- Collaborate with clinical agencies to demonstrate transformations in clinical practice produced by informatics
- Establish criteria to evaluate informatics goals for faculty

For Deans/Directors/Chairs
- Provide leadership in planning for necessary information technology (IT) infrastructure that will ensure education that prepares graduates for 21st-century practice roles and responsibilities
- Allocate sufficient resources to support IT initiatives
- Ensure that all faculty members have competence in computer literacy, information literacy, and informatics
- Provide opportunities for faculty development in informatics
- Urge clinical agencies to provide hands-on informatics experiences for learners
- Encourage nurse-managed clinics to incorporate clinical informatics exemplars that have transformed nursing practice to provide safe, quality care
- Advocate that all learners graduate with up-to-date knowledge and skills in each of the three critical areas: computer literacy, information literacy, and informatics
- Establish criteria to evaluate outcomes related to achieving informatics goals

For the NLN
- Disseminate this position statement widely
- Seek external funding and allocate internal resources to convene a think tank to reach a consensus on definitions of informatics, competencies for faculty and learners, and program outcomes that include informatics
- Participate actively in organizations that focus on education in nursing informatics to ensure that recommendations from those organizations are congruent with the NLN's positions on the curriculum
- Use the Educational Technology and Information Management Advisory Council (ETIMAC) and its task groups to (a) develop programs for faculty, showcasing exemplar programs and (b) disseminate outcomes from the think tank
- Encourage and facilitate accrediting bodies, regulatory agencies, and certifying bodies to reach a consensus on definitions related to informatics and minimal informatics competencies for practice in the 21st century (NLN, 2001, 2006)

Key driving forces in this process include:

- Reports and recommendations from the Institute of Medicine (IOM)
- Creation of the Office of the National Coordinator of Health Information Technology and its federal mandates
- The Technology Informatics Guiding Educational Reform (TIGER) Initiative
- The Robert Wood Johnson Foundation–funded Quality and Safety Education for Nurses (QSEN) Initiative (NLN, 2008)

The TIGER Initiative

The TIGER Initiative is a consortium of more than 40 nursing professional organizations that "aims to enable practicing nurses and nursing students to fully engage in the unfolding digital era of health care" (TIGER, 2016, p. 3). TIGER recommendations for schools of nursing include:

- Adopt informatics competencies for all levels of nursing education (undergraduate/graduate) and practice (generalist/specialist)
- Encourage faculty to participate in development programs in informatics
- Develop a task force or committee at each school to examine the integration of informatics throughout the curriculum
- Encourage the Health Services Resources Administration's (HRSA) Division of Nursing to continue and expand its support for informatics specialty programs and faculty development
- Measure changes from baseline in informatics knowledge among nursing educators and learners and among the full range of clinicians seeking continuing education
- Collaborate with industry and service partners to support faculty creativity in the design, acceptance, and adoption of informatics technology
- "Develop strategies to recruit, retain, and educate current and future nurses in the areas of informatics education, practice, and research" (NLN, 2008, p. 3)

Informatics Competencies

Specific informatics competencies include, but are not limited to, computer literacy or computer skills, information literacy or the ability to retrieve information, and general informatics skills. These skills include the ability to use informatics strategies and system applications to manage data and information and the ability to process the data retrieved (Saba & Calderone, 2010; Saba & McCormick, 2006). Informatics competencies for nurses are typically organized according to three proficiency levels:

1. Beginner, entry, or user level
2. Intermediate or modifier level
3. Advanced or innovator level of competency (Saba & Calderone, 2010; Saba & McCormick, 2006)

Informatics requires competency in three areas:

1. Technical competency
2. Utility competency
3. Leadership competency (Kaminski, 2007)

In 2008, the NLN issued a statement with recommendations for schools of nursing to prepare learners for practice in the dynamic health care arena. These recommendations are listed in Exhibit 4.2.

Rapidly advancing computer information technology mandates that the nurse educator not only acquire skills associated with teaching/learning technologies but also attain and maintain competencies related to the technology nursing graduates will be required to utilize in the workplace. These include lifelong learning skills, computer and information literacy, informatics and technology competency (Button, Harrington, & Belan, 2014; Rajalahti, Heinonen, & Saranto, 2014).

EXHIBIT 4.2	
Recommendations for Nursing Educational Units	
Technical competencies	Technical competencies are related to the actual psychomotor use of computers and other technological equipment. Specific nursing informatics competencies include the ability to use selected applications in a comfortable and knowledgeable way. It is important for nurses to feel confident in their use of computers and software in the practice setting, and especially at the bedside, to be able to attend to the client while using these devices.
Utility competencies	Utility competencies are the process of using computers and other technological equipment within nursing practice, education, research, and administration. Specific nursing informatics competencies include the process of applying evidence-based practice, critical thinking, and accountability to the use of selected applications in a comfortable and knowledgeable way.
Leadership competencies	Leadership competencies are related to the ethical and management issues of using computers and other technological equipment within nursing practice, education, research, and administration. Specific nursing informatics competencies include the process of applying accountability, client privacy and confidentiality, and quality assurance in documentation to the use of selected applications in a comfortable and knowledgeable way.

MOBILE LEARNING

The mobile device has emerged as a ubiquitous and powerful tool that can support learning in the mobile environment. Key trends include:

- Smartphone ownership by 68% of all adults in the United States in 2015. A higher percentage of younger adults own smartphones—86% of those aged 18–29 and 83% of those aged 30–49 (Anderson, 2015).
- Ownership of tablets/e-readers among American adults rose from 33% to 45% between 2012 and 2015 (Anderson, 2015).
- Postsecondary learners value technology—particularly mobile technology—in education (Derryberry, 2011).

These devices have become smaller and faster and have the capacity to contain a vast library of resources to support learning. The advent of "cloud" computing has further expanded these capabilities. There are a large variety of mobile devices that share several common characteristics:

- Highly portable (smartphone, reader, iPad, etc.)
- Internet capable
- Able to display rich content (images/videos)
- Delivery of "chunks" of information; just-in-time information
- Highly customizable (productivity tools, resources, references, decision support tools, etc.)
- Storage capacity (data)
- Autonomous ("stand-alone" devices)
- Mobility of devices supports contextual learning through use of Quick Response codes and the Global Positioning System

Mobile devices can be used to support learning in any setting and with a variety of activities. For example:

- Classroom: The electronic resources on these devices can be used in activities such as
  - Gaming activities (e.g., Jeopardy) to review class content and stimulate learners in the classroom
  - Modeling strategies to bring new evidence into practice

- Lab/Clinical: The electronic resources on these devices may be used to
  - Reference step-by-step instructions for a nursing procedure, such as nasogastric tube insertion or tracheostomy care
  - Model point-of-care/point-of-need information access such as drug compatibility/interactions

E-BOOKS

E-books have become a growth industry. In 2011, more e-books were sold than traditional books (Minzesheimer, 2012). E-book sales revenue in the United States from 2008 to 2014 rose from $63.9 million to $3.5 billion (Statista, Inc., 2016a, 2016b). Industry experts maintain that this trend will persist and is forecasted to reach $8.7 billion in 2018. The growth is also impacting higher education as well but not at such speed. Surprisingly, despite the lower cost and convenience, e-book purchases by college-age learners increased modestly from 12% in October 2010 to 26% in 2012 (Greenfield, 2013; NACS OnCampus Research, 2011, 2013).

E-books are gaining popularity over print for a variety of reasons.

- Ease of access and use
- Additional features and functionalities not available in the "hard copy" format
- Portability
- Cost
- Environmental factors (paperless, minimal environmental footprint)
- Interactivity (with the content)

E-books offer the following important features that support and enrich the learning experience. These include:

- Embedded links
- Note-taking capability
- Social interactivity with peers and faculty
- Video, audio enhancements to content
- Bookmarking and highlighting content

Another important aspect is that e-books can easily accommodate different learning styles by providing electronic reader functionalities as well as enhanced visual images or videos for the visual learner. Some people, especially millennials, simply prefer learning materials in electronic format. In addition, the use of e-books provides improved accessibility for those students who require accommodations and meets the requirements for compliance with Section 504 of the Rehabilitation Act of 1973 and Title III of the Americans with Disabilities Act. (More information about generational learner differences can be found in Chapter 9.)

CASE STUDIES

CASE STUDY 4.1

A new academic nurse educator is assigned to teach two sections of a medical–surgical nursing course. One of the sections of the course will have traditional, 4-year undergraduate nursing learners, whereas the other section will have accelerated undergraduate nursing learners. While planning the course and the use of technology, what types of technology could you use if you were teaching this course? Would you use the same types of technology for both sections of the course? Would you use different types of technology for each section?

CASE STUDY 4.2

A nurse educator is clinically teaching a group of nursing learners on a medical–surgical unit within a busy urban hospital. The nurse educator wants to make the most of the learning opportunities for the learners and thus plans to fully integrate mobile technology into the day's experience. Discuss how the nurse educator can leverage the "teachable moments" encountered at the bedside with the learners.

PRACTICE QUESTIONS

1. Informatics competencies require the educator to have competency in all areas except:
    A. Technical
    B. Utility
    C. Leadership
    D. Management

2. Which of the following statements regarding serious gaming is true?
    A. Needs to be done independently to be effective
    B. Provides opportunities for research
    C. Has minimal effect on learning but increases socialization
    D. Provides a method to assess learning

3. For which of the following activities can a mobile device be utilized to support learning? (Select all that apply.)
    A. Gaming activities
    B. Answer selection on a graded quiz
    C. Medication reference
    D. Reference books

4. What is the practice of posting small pieces of digital content—which could be text, pictures, links, short videos, or other media—on the Internet called?
    A. Semantic blog
    B. Virtual memos
    C. Microblogging
    D. Micromemos

5. What are some of the important features that e-books offer?
    A. Embedded links
    B. Individualism
    C. Book pages
    D. Index

6. The essential informatics competencies required by nurse educators can be categorized into all of the following EXCEPT:

A. Technical

B. Procedural

C. Utility

D. Leadership

7. A wiki is:

A. Journal entries that are presented in reverse chronological order

B. Community sites that build relationships and connections/networks

C. A collection of web pages that may be edited only by those invited

D. A method of distributing videos and web content

8. The TIGER initiative focused on the development of what?

A. Informatics competencies for nurse educators

B. Informatics competencies for all levels of nursing education

C. Informatics competencies for the clinical setting

D. Informatics competencies for electronic medical record managers

9. Social bookmarking is:

A. Categorizing resources using user-defined keywords or tags

B. Sharing websites with others at a conference

C. A method to distribute multimedia content

D. Recording short video and audio clips for education

10. Which of the following is an example of a microblog?

A. Instagram.com

B. Pinterest.com

C. Facebook.com

D. Twitter.com

REFERENCES

American Nurses Association. (2000). *Scope and standards of practice for nursing professional development*. Washington, DC: Author.

Anderson, M. (2015). Technology device ownership: 2015, Pew Research Center Internet, Science & Tech. Retrieved from http://www.pewinternet.org/2015/10/29/technology-device-ownership-2015

Brown, J. S. (2006). *New learning environments for the 21st century*. Forum for the Future of Higher Education's 2005 Aspen Symposium. Retrieved from http://www.johnseelybrown.com/newlearning.pdf

Button, D., Harrington, A., & Belan, I. (2014). E-learning & information communication technology (ICT) in nursing education: A review of the literature. *Nurse Education Today*, 34(10), 1311–1323.

Canney, C. (2015). *Elements that affect student engagement in online graduate courses* (Thesis). Available from ProQuest Dissertations & Theses Global (1682465830). (Order No. 3702588)

Creative Commons. (n.d.). What is a virtual world? Retrieved from http://www .virtualworldsreview.com/info/whatis.shtml

Derryberry, A. (2011, April 26). Dispatch from the digital frontier: Insights from and about Generation Z. *Learning Solutions Magazine, 1.* Retrieved from http://www .learningsolutionsmag.com/articles/672/dispatch-from-the-digital-frontier-insights -from-and-about-generation-z

Dominic, M., Francis, S., & Pilomenraj, A. (2014). E-learning in web 3.0. *International Journal of Modern Education and Computer Science, 2*(2), 8–14. doi:10.5815/ijmecs.2014.02.02

Donald, J. W. (2009). Using technology to support faculty and enhance coursework in academic institutions. *Texas Library Journal, 85*(4), 129–131.

Educause Learning Initiative. (2016a). 7 Things you should know about . . . Twitter. Retrieved from www.educause.edu/ir/library/pdf/ELI7027.pdf

Educause Learning Initiative. (2016b). 7 Things you should know about . . . Microblogging. Retrieved from http://net.educause.edu/ir/library/pdf/ELI7051.pdf

Epper, R. M., Derryberry, A., & Jackson, S. (2012). *Game-based learning: Developing an institutional strategy (Research Bulletin).* Louisville, CO: EDUCAUSE Center for Applied Research. Retrieved from http://www.educause.edu/ecar

Greenfield, J. (2013) Students still not taking to e-textbooks, new data show. *Digital Publishing News for the 21st Century.* Retrieved from http://www.digitalbookworld.com/2013/ students-still-not-taking-to-e-textbooks-new-data-show

Hasson, C., Cornelius, F., & Suplee, P. D. (2008). A technology driven nursing faculty resource center. *Nurse Educator, 23*(1), 22–25.

Hsu, L., & Hsieh, S. (2014). Factors affecting metacognition of undergraduate nursing students in a blended learning environment. *International Journal of Nursing Practice, 20*(3), 233–241. doi:10.1111/ijn.12131

Indiana University Center for Postsecondary Research. (2013). National survey of student engagement benchmarks of effective educational practice. Retrieved from http://nsse .iub.edu/pdf/nsse_benchmarks.pdf

Kaminski, J. (2007). Nursing informatics competencies: Self-assessment. Retrieved from http://www.nursing-informatics.com/niassess/index.html

Kay, R. H., & LeSage, A. (2009). Examining the benefits and challenges of using audience response systems: A review of the literature. *Computers & Education, 53*(3), 819–827. doi:10.1016/j.compedu.2009.05.001

Kuh, G. D. (2009). The national survey of student engagement: Conceptual and empirical foundations. *New Directions for Institutional Research, 141,* 5–20. Retrieved from http:// onlinelibrary.wiley.com/doi/10.1002/ir.283/abstract

Kuh, G. D., Cruce, T. M., Shoup, R., Kinzie, J., & Gonyea, R. M. (2008). Unmasking the effects of student engagement on first-year college grades and persistence. *Journal of Higher Education, 79*(5), 540–563. Retrieved from http://muse.jhu.edu/article/248905

Minzesheimer, B. (2012, January). E-books sales surge after holidays. *USA Today.* Retrieved from http://www.usatoday.com/life/books/news/story/2012-01-09/ebooks -sales-surge/52458672/1

NACS OnCampus Research 2011. (2011). Update: Electronic book and eReader device report March 2011. Retrieved from http://www.nacs.org/LinkClick.aspx?fileticket=uIf2No XApKQ%3D&tabid=2471&mid=3210

NACS OnCampus Research 2013. (2013). Student watch: Behaviour and trends of student consumers. Retrieved from http://www.nacs.org/email/html/OnCampusResearch/ SPR-080-03-12_Client%20Newsletter.pdf

National Education Association. (2013). Higher education faculty and staff. Retrieved from www2.nea.org/he/techno.html

National League for Nursing. (2001). *Position statement: Lifelong learning for nursing faculty.* Washington, DC: NLN Press. Retrieved from http://www.nln.org/docs/default -source/about/archived-position-statements/lifelong-learning-for-nursing-faculty -pdf.pdf?sfvrsn=8

National League for Nursing. (2006). Position statement: Mentoring of nurse faculty. *Nursing Education Perspectives, 27*(2), 110–113.

National League for Nursing. (2008). Position statement: Preparing the next generation of nurses to practice in a technology-rich environment: An informatics agenda. Washington, DC: NLN Press. Retrieved from http://www.nln.org/docs/default-source/professional-development-programs/preparing-the-next-generation-of-nurses.pdf?sfvrsn=6

National League for Nursing. (2016). Certified nurse educator (CNE) 2016 candidate handbook. Retrieved from http://www.nln.org/docs/default-source/professional-development-programs/certified-nurse-educator-(cne)-examination-candidate-handbook.pdf?sfvrsn=2

National Survey of Student Engagement. (2015). *Engagement insights: Survey findings on the quality of undergraduate education: Annual results 2015.* Bloomington: Indiana University Center for Postsecondary Research.

Rajalahti, E., Heinonen, J., & Saranto, K. (2014). Developing nurse educators' computer skills towards proficiency in nursing informatics. *Informatics for Health & Social Care, 39*(1), 47–66.

Robinson, C. C., & Hullinger, H. (2008). New benchmarks in higher education: Student engagement in online learning. *Journal of Education for Business, 84*(2), 101–108.

Saba, V. K., & Calderone, T. L. (2010). What nurse educators need to know about the TIGER initiative. *Nurse Educator, 35*(2), 56–60.

Saba, V. K., & McCormick, K. A. (2006). *Essentials of nursing informatics* (4th ed.). New York, NY: McGraw-Hill.

Singh, R., & Lal, M. (2012). Web 3.0 in education & research. *BVICAM's International Journal of Information Technology, 3*(2). Retrieved from http://www.bvicam.ac.in/bijit/Downloads/pdf/issue6/02.pdf

Statista, Inc. (2016a). Trade e-book sales revenue in United States from 2008–2014 (in million U.S. dollars). Retrieved from http://www.statista.com/statistics/278235/e-book-sales-revenue-in-the-us

Statista, Inc. (2016b). Revenue from e-book sales in the United States from 2008 to 2018 (in billion U.S. dollars). Retrieved from http://www.statista.com/statistics/190800/ebook-sales-revenue-forecast-for-the-us-market

Tar-Ching, A., Loney, T. J., Elias, A., Ali, S., & Adam, B. (2016). Use of an audience response system to maximise response rates and expedite a modified Delphi process for consensus on occupational health. *Journal of Occupational Medicine & Toxicology, 11*, 1–6. doi: 10.1186/s12995-016-0098-5

Technology Informatics Guiding Education Reform. (2016). The TIGER initiative: Evidence and informatics transforming nursing: 3-year action steps toward a 10-year vision. Retrieved from http://www.aacn.nche.edu/education-resources/TIGER.pdf

Yun, C. (2007). Eric Schmidt, Web 2.0 vs. Web 3.0. Retrieved from http://youtu.be/T0QJmmdw3b0

5

Online Learning

FRANCES H. CORNELIUS AND LINDA WILSON

Education is not the filling of a pail, but the lighting of a fire.
—William Butler Yeats

This chapter addresses the Certified Nurse Educator Exam Content Area 1: Facilitate Learning (National League for Nursing [NLN], 2016, pp. 5–6).

- Content Area 1 is 22% of the examination
- It is estimated that there will be approximately 38 questions from Content Area 1

LEARNING OUTCOMES

- Analyze nurse educators' role in an online learning environment to support learning
- Examine the importance of the appropriate integration of technology in a meaningful and relevant manner to support online learning
- Describe how to devise strategies to integrate technology in an online learning activity

As described in Chapter 4, there has been a significant transformation of the learning environment primarily because of the wide array of technological advancements currently available. This transformation has served as a catalyst in the shift away from traditional teaching paradigms. Learners are no longer passive recipients of information; the learning that takes place is deeper. As discussed in the previous chapter, new technologies and Web 2.0 tools provide many opportunities to engage students in active learning. The online learning environment is growing exponentially. Industry experts believe that this trend is likely to continue, citing the following facts:

- In the United States, the number of learners taking at least one online course increased from 5.6 million in the fall of 2009 to 6.1 million in the fall of 2010, an increase of approximately 560,000 learners (Allen & Seaman, 2011; Terantino & Agbehonou, 2012).

- Thirty-one percent of all higher education learners now take at least one course online (Allen & Seaman, 2011).
- Although the overall higher education learner population is only growing at a rate of 1% per year, the growth rate for online enrollments is 10% (Allen & Seaman, 2011).

ONLINE TEACHING VERSUS TRADITIONAL CLASSROOM TEACHING

Although there are some important differences, there are many similarities between online teaching and traditional classroom teaching. Both traditional and online courses use lectures, class discussions, readings and assignments, group activities, projects, and other activities. The difference lies in how these activities are delivered in the online environment. For example, let's look at class lectures (a stalwart standard in education). In the online learning environment, a "lecture" can be delivered in the following ways:

- Written text
- PowerPoint slides
- Audio only
- Voice-over PowerPoint slides
- Video
- Podcast
- Live (using a synchronous meeting room)

Strategies/techniques to deliver content in an online course are similar to those of the traditional face-to-face (F2F) classroom. However, with the use of available technologies, these activities can be enhanced with rich media and high levels of interaction and feedback. Some strategies include:

- Problem-based learning
- Self-directed learning
- Just-in-time learning
- Case-based learning
- Self-assessment
- Feedback
- Journals and portfolios
- Instructor feedback

In an online teaching environment, course content for learners can be presented or enhanced through the use of the following:

- Outside reading
- Links to websites
- Visual materials
- Audio and video recordings
- Links or folders that contain your own personal lectures, notes, and papers

The ability to have access to so many different materials is an advantage for nurse educators engaged in distance education because the opportunities for enriching the learning experience are limitless. Table 5.1 provides some examples of how traditional classroom activities can be transitioned into online learning activities.

In an online course, lectures are already completed before the learners get to class. So, an instructor spends more time engaged in discussions, feedback, and supervising activities/assignments. Keep in mind that in the online course, the instructor can put many more activities and assignments into each unit, and consequently, there is more to discuss and supervise. In addition, frequent constructive and meaningful feedback ensure that students remain engaged and on task (Bonnel & Boehm, 2011).

The benefits to online learning are well documented in the literature. The online learning environment increases the student's control over the content, as well as the time and place learning occurs—creating a more individualized, learner-centered experience. The online learning environment also provides more opportunity for students to be more engaged and to interact with faculty, peers, and content (Robinson & Hullinger, 2008). Furthermore, it can help students gain knowledge and skills more quickly than traditional instructor-led methods (Cook, 2007; Ilkay & Zeynep, 2014; McGarry, Theobald, Lewis, & Coyer, 2015).

TABLE 5.1
Comparison of Traditional F2F and Online Classroom Activities

ACTIVITY	ONLINE ACTIVITY	COMMENTS
Class lecture—traditional with faculty at the podium	Asynchronous, prerecorded lectures that can be viewed independently by learners at any time Opportunity for faculty to tweak or rerecord improvements Opportunity for learners to go back as many times as they want to listen to the prerecorded lecture	Accomplishes the same goal but an online activity provides more learner control; more easily viewed again for review and clarification. Learners can view lectures in their own time. Lectures can be saved to different formats so that they are portable (mp3 and mp4 files). Learners can e-mail questions to presenters or post them to a discussion forum.
Class discussion	Synchronous class discussion using virtual meeting rooms such as WebCT, Adobe Connect, Eluminate, or Zoom	A virtual meeting room provides a venue for dynamic, interactive class meetings. This is a great option for individual, group, or outside speaker presentations and Q&A sessions. Encourages introverted learners to actively participate in discussions. Benefit is that discussions are in "real time" so that the faculty can get a sense of how the learners think "on their feet" and can articulate thoughts and ideas clearly. Use of webcam allows learners to see the instructor, which can make visual learners more comfortable.

(continued)

TABLE 5.1
Comparison of Traditional F2F and Online Classroom Activities (*continued*)

ACTIVITY	ONLINE ACTIVITY	COMMENTS
Class discussion (*continued*)	Discussion board (text-based, asynchronous)	Great venue for learners to have discussions about various topics, readings, and assignments. One benefit is the asynchronous mode allows learners to participate at their convenience, around their schedule. Learners have a good opportunity to reflect and formulate a more powerful response to questions and have time to bring in the literature to support their position.
	Voice discussion board (audio based, asynchronous)	Provides opportunity to actually hear verbal comments from learners and instructors as well as the tone/verbal inflections of the speaker. Helps the auditory learner grasp important concepts.
Class debate	Discussion board/voice discussion board	A debate on a discussion board can be asynchronous to allow learners to respond at their convenience and have more time to reflect on their answers so as to respond in a more substantive way.
	Live debate in synchronous class meeting rooms	Benefit is that synchronous debate allows the faculty to get a sense of the learner's ability to construct a persuasive argument and articulate thoughts and ideas clearly.
Group work— small breakout groups during class to respond to questions	Synchronous class meeting using breakout rooms	This is a great way to manage group activities in online courses. Groups can work together in the synchronous classroom. Faculty can move from room to room to assist as needed. Benefit of using these small-group activities during synchronous class meetings is that it is an effective way the faculty can provide the structure to help build learner connections with the learning community.

(continued)

TABLE 5.1
Comparison of Traditional F2F and Online Classroom Activities (*continued*)

ACTIVITY	ONLINE ACTIVITY	COMMENTS
Group projects—learner teams work on projects outside the class	Group projects—using dedicated synchronous learner meeting rooms, wikis, and group discussion boards	This is another great idea. The learners can meet outside of "class" in the learner meeting rooms to work on a project during a time that is convenient for the members of small groups.
Group presentations in class	Group presentations in a synchronous classroom	There really isn't much difference in the group presentations in class versus the one in a synchronous class meeting room. Learners can use PowerPoint slides, handouts, etc., in both settings. Learners can be viewed through a webcam in a synchronous classroom so that other learners can see their expressions, etc.
Tests/quizes—traditional F2F	Online quizzes and tests using Blackboard and additional test security options (i.e., Remote Proctor, ProctorU) or live proctors	Live proctors can assist with test security and ensure that the learner is actually the one taking the examination. If quizzes are taken online, it is important to time them and randomize the questions. If desired, the online quizzes can be set up to provide immediate feedback to the learner. If the test is "high stakes," it is a good idea to give learners only the score until after the test is closed. If correct answers are given prior to closing of the test, the learners will share the correct answers.
Similar to the traditional F2F classroom, questions can be discussed in depth to drill down into deeper understanding regarding the rationale for why a particular answer was correct. The discussion can be engaging to get them to think critically about what the question demands truly, and why the correct answer is the "best" answer.		
Case study—presentations with questions about the case	Case studies posted on discussion board, learners respond to questions through discussion board (asynchronous)	This can be accomplished by either a lone learner or multiple learners in breakout groups to compile a case study or build upon each other ideas. Case studies presented in this way provide the learners time to look up information in reference books/articles so that they can build their understanding at their own pace.
	Synchronous class meetings in which learners present case studies and engage in real-time in-depth discussion	Benefit is that synchronous presentation allows the faculty to get a sense of the learners' understanding as well as their ability to think "on their feet" and articulate thoughts and ideas clearly.

Courses can be fully online, hybrid, or web facilitated, depending on how much of the course is delivered online.

In general, courses that deliver less than 30% of content online are considered web facilitated. A *web-facilitated* course usually delivers course materials, such as the syllabus, assignments, or readings, via an online course management system. Courses that provide a substantial amount of the content online (between 30% and 79%) are considered to be *blended* or *hybrid*. This type of course frequently uses online discussions in place of F2F meetings. A course that provides 80% or more content online or has no F2F meetings is considered to be an *online* course (Allen & Seaman, 2011). Online courses can be delivered using a variety of software applications. Some of these include:

- *Learning management systems (LMS):* An LMS may be a commercial product or an open-source system. It is defined as an "information system that administers instructor-led and e-learning courses and keeps track of student progress" (Learning management system, n.d.). Some examples of an LMS include the following:
  - Commercial LMS
    - Blackboard (www.blackboard.com)
    - eLeaP (www.eleapsoftware.com)
    - Desire2Learn (1999) (www.desire2learn.com/clients/higherEducation)
  - Open-source LMS
    - Moodle (moodle.org/sites)
    - Sakai (sakaiproject.org/organization-list)
    - Canvas by Instructure (www.instructure.com)
- *Content management system (CMS):* "An application (more likely web-based), that provides capabilities for multiple users with different permission levels to manage (all or a section of) content, data or information of a website project, or Internet/intranet application. Managing content refers to creating, editing, archiving, publishing, collaborating on, reporting, distributing website content, data and information" (Kohan, 2010). Examples of a CMS are:
  - WordPress (wordpress.org)
  - Drupal (drupal.org)
  - Joomla! (www.joomla.org)
  - ExpressionEngine (ellislab.com/expressionengine)
  - TextPattern (textpattern.com)

EVIDENCE-BASED TEACHING PRACTICE

Price, Whitlatch, Jane, Burdi, and Peacock (2016) discuss improvement in online teaching by providing faculty with an online teaching workshop. Results were positive from this pilot study, which used faculty ($N = 11$) and RN to BSN student ($N = 6$) focus groups.

BENCHMARKS AND QUALITY MEASURES FOR ONLINE TEACHING

The Institute for Higher Education Policy (IHEP) has identified 24 benchmarks as essential to ensuring excellence in Internet-based distance learning. These benchmarks include seven areas of quality measures presently used on college and university campuses nationwide (Phipps & Merisotis, 2000). These benchmark areas are:

1. Institutional support
2. Course development
3. Teaching/learning
4. Course structure
5. Student support
6. Faculty support
7. Evaluation and assessment

For a complete list of the 24 benchmarks, refer to Table 5.2.

TABLE 5.2
Benchmarks That Are Essential for Quality Internet-Based Distance Education

Educational organization support	The educational organization has a technological system that has protections build in to maintain student and faculty privacy. The technology is effective and there are back-ups in case of system failure.
Course Use of Technology	The course is designed at the appropriate level of the students and the course student learning outcomes are clear. The technology needs for the course are understood by students and assist the students to reach the course goals.
Using Technology in the Teaching/Learning Process	Students feel connected in the course through peer and faculty responses. They use a variety of online methods to learn and those methods are explained to them adequately.
Course Development	Before students enroll in an online course they understand the expectations and resources needed to be successful.
Technical Support	Students are able to access the technology department when needed and they have their questions answered well and in a timely manner.
Faculty Professional Development	Faculty professional development in online teaching is ongoing and accessible.
Course Evaluation	Online courses should be evaluated for effectiveness. Were the students able to complete the SLOs? Was there rigor in the courses? Were students satisfied and would they recommend taking another online course?

Adapted from Phipps and Merisotis (2000).

In addition to the 24 benchmarks identified by the IHEP (Phipps & Merisotis, 2000), there are many other quality resources/measures available to help the nurse educator ensure quality online course delivery. Quality Matters™ (QM) is an organization that provides quality assurance regarding the course design. The QM approach is designed to be a collegial, faculty-centered, peer-review process to evaluate the design of online and blended courses through the use of eight general standards and 43 specific standards (Table 5.3; QM, 2016). The full rubric provides a point value for each standard to aid in scoring for peer review. Additional information can be obtained at the QM website (www.qualitymatters.org).

The following key points are to be kept in mind:

- Course organization style can drive instructional intensity for the learners and the instructor and can affect the quality of the learning experience.
- Course structure generally refers to the organization of the course content and logical flow of the content.
- Course structure is particularly important in an online course because, for the most part, learners are working independently going through the course content.
- Learner satisfaction with a course is closely related to how well the course is organized.
- A well-organized course is like a well-constructed house—all the pieces fit and work together.

The key benefit of good course structure is that it gives the learner a sense of how the learning process will unfold. Elements that provide the structure are as follows:

- Course schedule
- Course syllabus
- Overview of how the course content is organized
- Statement in the course introduction providing information to the learner regarding how the course is structured
- A "getting started" module

TABLE 5.3
Quality Matters™ Standards From the QM *Higher Education Rubric*, Fifth Edition

Course overview and introduction	1.1 Instructions make clear how to get started and where to find various course components.
	1.2 Learners are introduced to the purpose and structure of the course.
	1.3 Etiquette expectations (sometimes called netiquette) for online discussions, e-mail, and other forms of communication are clearly stated.
	1.4 Course and/or institutional policies with which the student is expected to comply are clearly stated, or a link to current policies is provided.
	1.5 Minimum technology requirements are clearly stated and instructions for use provided.

(continued)

TABLE 5.3
Quality Matters™ Standards From the QM *Higher Education Rubric*, Fifth Edition (*continued*)

	1.6 Prerequisite knowledge in the discipline and/or any required competencies are clearly stated. 1.7 Minimum technical skills expected of the learner are clearly stated. 1.8 The self-introduction by the instructor is appropriate and available online. 1.9 Learners are asked to introduce themselves to the class.
Learning objectives (competencies)	2.1 The course learning objectives, or course/program competencies, describe outcomes that are measurable. 2.2 The module/unit learning objectives or competencies describe outcomes that are measurable and consistent with the course-level objectives or competencies. 2.3 All learning objectives or competencies are stated clearly and written from the learner's perspective. 2.4 The relationship between learning objectives or competencies and course activities is clearly stated. 2.5 The learning objectives or competencies are suited to the level of the course.
Assessment and measurement	3.1 The assessments measure the stated learning objectives or competencies. 3.2 The course grading policy is stated clearly. 3.3 Specific and descriptive criteria are provided for the evaluation of learners' work and are tied to the course grading policy. 3.4 The assessment instruments selected are sequenced, varied, and suited to the learner work being assessed. 3.5 The course provides learners with multiple opportunities to track their learning progress.
Instructional materials	4.1 The instructional materials contribute to the achievement of the stated course and module/unit learning objectives or competencies. 4.2 Both the purpose of instructional materials and how the materials are to be used for learning activities are clearly explained. 4.3 All instructional materials used in the course are appropriately cited. 4.4 The instructional materials are current. 4.5 A variety of instructional materials is used in the course. 4.6 The distinction between required and optional materials is clearly explained.
Learner interaction and engagement	5.1 The learning activities promote the achievement of the stated learning objectives or competencies. 5.2 Learning activities provide opportunities for interaction that support active learning. 5.3 The instructor's plan for classroom response time and feedback on assignments is clearly stated. 5.4 The requirements for learner interaction are clearly stated.

(*continued*)

TABLE 5.3
Quality Matters™ Standards From the QM *Higher Education Rubric*, Fifth Edition (*continued*)

Course technology	6.1 The tools used in the course support the learning objectives or competencies. 6.2 Course tools promote learner engagement and active learning. 6.3 Technologies required in the course are readily obtainable. 6.4 The course technologies are current. 6.5 Links are provided to privacy policies for all external tools required in the course.
Learner support	7.1 The course instructions articulate or link to a clear description of the technical support offered and how to obtain it. 7.2 Course instructions articulate or link to the institution's accessibility policies and services. 7.3 Course instructions articulate or link to an explanation of how the institution's academic support services and resources can help learners succeed in the course and how learners can obtain them. 7.4 Course instructions articulate or link to an explanation of how the institution's student services and resources can help learners succeed and how learners can obtain them.
Accessibility	8.1 Course navigation facilitates ease of use. 8.2 Information is provided about the accessibility of all technologies required in the course. 8.3 The course provides alternative means of access to course materials in formats that meet the needs of diverse learners. 8.4 The course design facilitates readability.

Note: The use of this 2014 Quality Matters™ rubric document is restricted to institutions that subscribe to the Quality Matters™ program and may not be copied or duplicated without written permission of MarylandOnline© 2016 MarylandOnline, Inc. www.qualitymatters.org.

Source: QM (2014).

Course structure presents course content in a logical manner, permitting learners to focus on learning rather than spending time trying to find information within the course. Content can be distributed by the week or by modules. It is advisable to use the same format of presentation for each week/module.

Another key consideration is *alignment*. It is important that course and module/unit level learning objectives are aligned with course materials and learning activities and directly support the assessments for the course. When these elements are aligned students are able to see how learning activities and materials connect with their assignments and, as a result, have a better learning experience. Conversely, this also helps the instructor see how course outcomes are being met and can more easily identify areas in which the course can be improved (Carnegie Mellon University, n.d.; Matuga, 2006).

Creating a quality online learning experience requires "more than simply uploading materials from a preexisting face-to-face class onto a web-based course management system . . . course design must begin with a foundation of measurable competencies, essential outcomes, and evidence-based practice" accompanied with educational materials that "not only actively engage and resonate with the learner but also encourage him or her to seek mentorship and the support of his or her peers" (Hoffmann, Klein, & Rosenzweig, 2016, p. 4). This includes the use of multiple interactive and engaging learning activities that "accommodate the multiple learning styles, skills, and experiences of the adult learners" (p. 4).

ROLE OF NURSE EDUCATORS

In the online environment, more so than in the traditional classroom environment, it is essential that the nurse educator role shifts to a facilitator role rather than one of deliverer of content. Qualities of a successful online instructor include content knowledge, teaching commitment, communication ability, time management, flexibility, and tolerance for ambiguity (Bigatel, Ragan, Kennan, May, & Redmond, 2012; Hathaway, 2013; Varvel, 2007).

Smith (2005) identifies 51 competencies (Exhibit 5.1) needed by online instructors. These competencies correspond with the 24 benchmarks for excellence in the IHEP discussed earlier in this chapter.

There are other perspectives regarding the essential competencies of online educators, and for the most part, all are in agreement. Some, such as Varvel's (2007), are more detailed, but all agree that the online educator must possess these competencies. Varvel (2007) identifies seven roles that comprise master online teacher competencies, and within each role, there are numerous specific criteria:

1. *Administrative Roles (Systems, Ethical, and Legal Issues):* "The competent instructor has an understanding of and belief in the administrative system under which he or she is employed" (p. 8).

EXHIBIT 5.1

Competencies for Online Instruction

- Become an online coach and assist students to learn in a non-threatening environment
- Help students to understand the course requirements without panicking them at the beginning of the course. Having an organized syllabus assist this process
- Review the grading criteria and the assignment expectations with the students
- If a student falls off the course radar reach out to them and assist them to get back into the fold
- Use case studies when appropriate
- Contact formative and summative evaluations in an ongoing fashion
- Provide timely and constant feedback
- Encourage students to critically think about assignments and to understand the culture of the leaning organization
- Keep the course exciting
- Help students to stay on task with discussions
- Make sure all the students participate
- Provide access to web resources
- Use humor appropriately and learn along with your students!

Adapted from Smith (2005).

2. *Personal Roles (Personal Qualities and Characteristics):* "The competent instructor possesses certain personal attributes that enhance his or her ability to instruct within any given educational paradigm" (p. 9).

3. *Technological Roles (Technology Knowledge and Abilities):* "The competent instructor is knowledgeable about the technologies used in the virtual classroom and can make effective use of those technologies" (p. 11).

4. *Instructional Design Roles (Instructional Design Processes, Knowledge, and Abilities):* "The competent instructor can judge the appropriateness and adequacy of materials and technology used in a course for the given audience, and can make materials and technology adjustments due to shifting audience needs and abilities" (p. 14).

5. *Pedagogical Roles (Teaching Processes, Knowledge, and Abilities):* "The competent instructor must be well versed and capable in the instruction of a high quality and effective educational experience for all participants" (p. 16).

6. *Assessment Roles (Assessing Student Learning and Abilities):* "The competent instructor is aware of online assessment issues and can effectively assess students using a variety of techniques in the online classroom that are designed not just to determine student progress but to aid in student learning" (p. 24).

7. *Social Processes and Presence (Social Roles):* "The competent instructor recognizes that a social aspect to education exists. The instructor will effectively incorporate that aspect into the teaching and learning process with the intent of creating a learning community" (p. 27).

Cook and Dupras (2004) point out that the educator should attend to the following principles when delivering online content:

- "Learners should be active contributors to the educational process
- Learning should closely relate to understanding and solving real-life problems
- Learners' current knowledge and experience need to be taken into account
- Learners should use self-direction in their learning
- Learners should be given opportunities and support for practice, accompanied by self-assessment and constructive feedback from teachers and peers
- Learners should be given opportunities to reflect on their practice" (p. 704)

CRITICAL THINKING QUESTION

What teaching activities can be used to decrease the amount of responses that nurse educators need to make to each learner on discussion boards?

Ragan (2012) identifies 10 principles of effective online teaching. These include the following:

1. *Show Up and Teach:* "Students in an online course rely on the instructor to follow the established course schedule and to deliver the course within the scheduled time frame. The online instructor is expected to make schedule adjustments as needed to manage special circumstances" (p. 6).

2. *Practice Proactive Course Management Strategies:* "These strategies include, but are not limited to, monitoring assignment submissions, communicating and reminding students of missed and/or upcoming deadlines, and making course progress adjustments where and when necessary" (p. 7).

3. *Establish Patterns of Course Activities:* "Although the online classroom environment provides tremendous flexibility of time and place of study, establishing and communicating a course pace and pattern of work can aid both instructor and student and alleviate confusion about course operation" (p. 9).

4. *Plan for the Unplanned:* "It is important that the instructor is visible and active in the online classroom. If an instructor will be unable to log into the course for more than four business days (e.g., during professional travel), the instructor is asked to give one week's notice to the students" (p. 11).

5. *Response Requested and Expected:* "Timely instructor feedback is essential for the online learners in order to manage their learning experience. Instructors are expected to provide feedback to student inquiries within one business day" (p. 13).

6. *Think Before You Write:* "Feedback on assignments is most helpful to students when clear and concise language is used to explain the degree to which relevant course outcomes have been met" (p. 15).

7. *Help Maintain Forward Progress:* "Students in the online classroom rely on the timely return of assignment and exam grades in order to maintain progress in their studies" (p. 17).

8. *Safe and Secure:* "It is highly recommended that all course-related communication between the instructor and the student occur within institutionally supported and maintained communication systems. Preferably these communications will occur within or be managed by the learning management system" (p. 19).

9. *Quality Counts:* "High-quality course content is essential for a successful learning experience. For this reason, instructors should monitor and address dimensions of the course that may impact course integrity, including inaccurate course content, editing errors, confusing information and instructions, broken links, and other course design issues" (p. 21).

10. *(Double) Click a Mile on My Connection:* "The online instructor needs immediate and reliable access to the same technology as is required for student participation. Online course delivery requires access to high-speed Internet access (DSL, cable modem, or satellite). The online instructor is also expected to experience each functional dimension of the online course in order to assess systems' functionality and performance" (p. 23).

Becoming skilled in online instruction is an iterative process. Jacobs (2015) offers some advice to the online instructor.

The mechanics of preparing and teaching online courses is a constant learning process. There are new techniques developed every day to support instructors and students in online courses. This is what makes this particular aspect of academia exciting and challenging. The successful online instructor must be aware and comfortable with new innovative techniques designed to improve the operation of online courses. To benefit from these techniques, it is also important to understand the factors that affect student ability. One such factor would be the creation of a learning community fostered by a sense of social connectedness. It is equally important to understand the various factors that affect student satisfaction with an online course. The challenges can seem overwhelming at times. The key is to always maintain a sense of humor about the process (Jacobs, 2015).

> **EVIDENCE-BASED TEACHING PRACTICE**
>
> McCutcheon, Lohan, Traynor, and Martin (2015) studied the use of hybrid teaching's effect on clinical skill development through a literature search yielding 19 published papers. Findings focused on four areas: performance/clinical skill, knowledge, self-efficacy/clinical confidence, and user experience/satisfaction and the study concluded that online development of clinical skills was no less effective than traditional learning methods.

COMMUNICATION

In an online learning environment, timely communication is essential. Fortunately, the instructor and learners can interact and communicate with each other, often in more substantive ways than traditionally afforded in the F2F classroom. Within the LMS, the instructor and learners can use built-in tools such as the following:

- Announcements (instructor only)—an easy way to disseminate course update information and remind learners of upcoming events and due dates
- Discussion board/voice board—can provide a centralized asynchronous message board to keep the lines of communication open among all class members
- E-mail/voicemail
- CMS/LMS instant messages
- Wikis and blogs—offer more robust authoring and collaborative capabilities, which can be effective in engaging students in active learning
- Synchronous class meeting rooms—virtual meeting rooms where attendees are present in "real time" although geographically dispersed (at remote locations)

Communication is essential when building a learning community within the online learning environment. The nurse educator must take a leadership role in "setting the stage" for expectations related to communication—either verbal or written—often referred to as *netiquette*. Ormrod (2011) identifies key features of learning communities in educational settings:

- All learners are active participants.
- Discussion and collaboration are common key elements.
- Diversity in learner interests and progress is expected and respected.
- Learners and teachers coordinate in helping one another learn; no one has exclusive responsibility for teaching others.
- Everyone is a potential resource for others; different individuals serve as resources for different topics and tasks.
- The teacher provides guidance and direction for activities, but learners also contribute.

- Constructive questioning and critiquing of one another's work is practiced.
- Process is emphasized as much as product.

Finally, the *most important* point regarding communication in the online learning environment is timeliness. Timely response to learners' questions or posts is *absolutely essential*.

BENEFITS OF THE ONLINE LEARNING ENVIRONMENT

There are many benefits associated with the online learning environment. These include the following:

- Online courses can be packed with study material.

  > **Teaching Gem:** Establish in the syllabus how often you will answer e-mails and questions and if they will be answered on the weekends so learners know what to expect regarding the nurse educator's response time.

  * Instructors have limited contact hours each week in an on-campus class and, as a result, have to pick and choose their activities to fit the time.
  * In an online course, instructors are not bound by the limits of these contact hours and can provide additional materials, videos, demonstrations, discussions, and assignments that are not limited to 3 or 4 hours of "contact" with the course content each week.
  * However, instructors must consider ways to make the learning environment rich and not overload the course too much.
- Flexibility
  * The asynchronous nature of the majority of the course provides learners with great flexibility for participation
  * The time flexibility also applies to instructors
  * Classes can be conducted at any time of the day or night on any days of the week
- There are opportunities for higher level learning. Specifically, Web 2.0 tools:
  * Increase social engagement to enrich learning
  * Promote engagement and learning
  * Use of these technologies resulted in higher order thinking, metacognitive awareness, team work/collaboration, improved affect toward school/learning, and ownership of learning (Chittleborough, Maybery, Patrick, & Reupert, 2009)
- There are increased opportunities for dialogue and questions.
  * Instructors can ask questions at any time during the course and have learners respond in a variety of ways, including discussion boards and e-mails
  * The online discussion may have deeper meaning and learners have time to reflect on their responses

* A typically "quiet" learner has an opportunity to participate fully
* Learners can ask questions any time by e-mail or by posting a question on a Q&A discussion forum
* Online course materials are reusable.
    * Instructors can reuse all or parts of their courses, including pithy comments and interesting discussions. (Although instructors might *think* that they are giving the same lecture from term to term in an on-campus course, they really *are* giving the same lecture in an online course, if they so choose.)
    * This gives instructors the opportunity to keep all the components that work well and modify the questionable ones.

COPYRIGHT LAW AND FAIR USE IN ONLINE LEARNING ENVIRONMENTS

The nurse educator who teaches in the online learning environment must have knowledge of copyright laws as these relate to academic use and the online learning environment. There are several laws that affect the use of materials for academic purposes. These include the following:

* The copyright laws
* Fair use
* The Technology, Education and Copyright Harmonization Act (TEACH Act) ("TEACH," 2006)

Copyright Laws

* "A form of protection provided by the laws of the United States (title 17, U. S. Code) to the authors of 'original works of authorship,' including literary, dramatic, musical, artistic, and certain other intellectual works
* Protects both published and unpublished works
* Protects exclusive rights of authors but authorizes others to do the following:
    * Reproduce the work in copies or phonorecords
    * Prepare derivative works based upon the work
    * Distribute copies or phonorecords of the work to the public by sale or other transfer of ownership, or by rental, lease, or lending
    * Perform the work publicly, in the case of literary, musical, dramatic, and choreographic works, pantomimes, and motion pictures and other audiovisual works
    * Display the work publicly, in the case of literary, musical, dramatic, and choreographic works, pantomimes, and pictorial, graphic, or sculptural works, including the individual images of a motion picture or other audiovisual work
    * Perform the work publicly (in the case of sound recordings) by means of a digital audio transmission" (U.S. Copyright Office, 2012a, p. 1)

Refer to Exhibit 5.2 for more information regarding what materials are protected under the copyright laws and what materials are not.

EXHIBIT 5.2

Works Protected and Works Not Protected Under Copyright Laws

What Works Are Protected?

Copyright protects "original works of authorship" that are fixed in a tangible
   form of expression.
The fixation need not be directly perceptible so long as it may be communicated
   with the aid of a machine or device. Copyrightable works include the following
   areas:

- Literary works
- Musical works, including any accompanying words
- Dramatic works, including any accompanying music
- Pantomimes and choreographic works
- Pictorial, graphic, and sculptural works
- Motion pictures and other audiovisual works
- Sound recordings
- Architectural works

These areas should be viewed broadly. For example, computer programs
   and most "compilations" may be registered as "literary works"; maps and
   architectural plans may be registered as "pictorial, graphic, and sculptural
   works."

What Is Not Protected by Copyright?

Several areas of material are generally not eligible for federal copyright
   protection. These include among others:

- Works that have not been fixed in a tangible form of expression (e.g.,
   choreographic works that have not been notated or recorded, or
   improvisational speeches or performances that have not been written or
   recorded)
- Titles, names, short phrases, and slogans; familiar symbols or designs; mere
   variations of typographic ornamentation, lettering, or coloring; mere listings
   of ingredients or contents ideas, procedures, methods, systems, processes,
   concepts, principles, discoveries, or devices, as distinguished from a
   description, explanation, or illustration
- Works consisting entirely of information that is common property and
   containing no original authorship (e.g., standard calendars, height and
   weight charts, tape measures and rulers, and lists or tables taken from public
   documents or other common sources)

Source: U.S. Copyright Office (2012a).

Fair Use

"Section 107 under the copyright laws identifies four factors to be considered in
determining whether or not a particular use is fair.

1. The purpose and character of the use, including whether such use is of commercial nature or is for nonprofit educational purposes
2. The nature of the copyrighted work

3. The amount and substantiality of the portion used in relation to the copyrighted work as a whole

4. The effect of the use upon the potential market for, or value of, the copyrighted work" (United States Copyright Office, 2012b, p. 2)

The TEACH Act (Technology, Education and Copyright Harmonization Act of 2002)

- "Facilitates and enables the performance and display of copyrighted materials for distance education by accredited, non-profit educational institutions (and some government entities) that meet the TEACH Act's qualifying requirements.

- Its primary purpose is to balance the needs of distance learners and educators with the rights of copyright holders.

- The TEACH Act applies to distance education that includes the participation of any enrolled student, on or off campus" (Copyright Clearance Center, 2011, p. 1).

Crews (2010) provided a clear review and update regarding the TEACH Act and identified the following responsibilities of an instructor:

1. Select materials that are *allowed* by the TEACH Act (see Exhibit 5.3).

2. Instructor oversight: "An instructor seeking to use materials under the protection of the new statute must adhere to the following requirements:

   * The performance or display 'is made by, at the direction of, or under the actual supervision of an instructor.'

   * The materials are transmitted 'as an integral part of a class session offered as a regular part of the systematic mediated instructional activities' of the educational institution.

   * The copyrighted materials are 'directly related and of material assistance to the teaching content of the transmission.'

   * The requirements share a common objective: 'to assure that the instructor is ultimately in charge of the uses of copyrighted works and that the materials serve educational pursuits and are not for entertainment or any other purpose' (Crews, 2010, p. 5).

   * The "use of the materials is integral to the course and under the instructor's supervision" (Crews, 2010, p. 5).

   * Precludes "an instructor from including, in a digital transmission, copies of materials that are specifically marketed for and meant to be purchased by students outside of the classroom in the traditional teaching model" (Crews, 2010, p. 5). Specifically, instructors are prohibited from scanning textbook content for distribution to students—circumventing the required purchase of a textbook.

EXHIBIT 5.3

The TEACH Act: Description of Works Allowed and Excluded

Works explicitly allowed:

- Performances of nondramatic literary works
- Performances of nondramatic musical works
- Performances of any other work, including dramatic works and audiovisual works, but only in "reasonable and limited portions"
- Displays of any work "in an amount comparable to that which is typically displayed in the course of a live classroom session"

Works explicitly excluded:

- Works that are marketed "primarily for performance or display as part of mediated instructional activities transmitted via digital networks"
- Performances or displays given by means of copies "not lawfully made and acquired" under the U.S. Copyright ActU.S. Copyright Act, if the educational institution "knew or had reason to believe" that they were not lawfully made and acquired

Adapted from Crews (2010).

Refer to Exhibit 5.4 for specific guidelines related to roles, rules, and responsibilities for academic institutions associated with the TEACH Act.

EXHIBIT 5.4

The TEACH Act: New Roles, Rules, and Responsibilities for Academic Institutions

A Brief Guide to the TEACH Act

Signed by President George W. Bush on November 2, 2002, the Technology, Education, and Copyright Harmonization (TEACH) Act is the product of discussion and negotiation among academic institutions, publishers, library organizations and Congress. It offers many improvements over previous regulations, specifically sections 110(2) and 112(f) of the U.S. Copyright Act. The following overview of the TEACH Act seeks to balance the perspectives of both copyright owners and content users, and provide guidance for today's academic institutions.

Although copyright law generally treats digital and nondigital copyright-protected works in a similar manner, special digital uses, such as online distance learning and course management systems, require special attention. Some of the special copyright requirements of online distance learning are specifically addressed by the TEACH Act.

The TEACH Act facilitates and enables the performance and display of copyrighted materials for distance education by accredited, nonprofit educational institutions (and some government entities) that meet the TEACH Act's qualifying requirements. Its primary purpose is to balance the needs of distance learners and educators with the rights of copyright holders. The TEACH Act applies to distance education that includes the participation of any enrolled student, on or off campus.

(continued)

EXHIBIT 5.4

The TEACH Act: New Roles, Rules, and Responsibilities for Academic Institutions (*continued*)

Under the TEACH Act:

- Instructors may use a wider range of works in distance learning environments.
- Students may participate in distance learning sessions from virtually any location.
- Participants enjoy greater latitude when it comes to storing, copying and digitizing materials.

TEACH Act Requirements

In exchange for unprecedented access to copyright protected material for distance education, the TEACH Act requires that the academic institution meet specific requirements for copyright compliance and education. For the full list of requirements, refer to the TEACH Act at www.copyright.gov/legislation/archive.
In order for the use of copyrighted materials in distance education to qualify for the TEACH Act exemptions, the following criteria must be met:
The institution must be an accredited, nonprofit educational institution.

- The use must be part of mediated instructional activities.
- The use must be limited to a specific number of students enrolled in a specific class.
- The use must either be for "live" or asynchronous class sessions.
- The use must not include the transmission of textbook materials, materials "typically purchased or acquired by students," or works developed specifically for online uses.
- The institution must have developed and publicized its copyright policies, specifically informing students that course content may be covered by copyright, and include a notice of copyright on the online materials.
- The institution must implement some technological measures to ensure compliance with these policies, beyond merely assigning a password. Ensuring compliance through technological means may include user and location authentication through Internet protocol (IP) checking, content timeouts, print-disabling, cut and paste disabling, etc.

What the TEACH Act Does Not Allow

The new exemptions under the TEACH Act specifically do not extend to:

- Electronic reserves, coursepacks (electronic or paper).
- Commercial document delivery.
- Textbooks or other digital content provided under license from the author, publisher, aggregator or other entity.
- Conversion of materials from analog to digital formats, except when the converted material is used solely for authorized transmissions and when a digital version of a work is unavailable or protected by technological measures.

It is also important to note that the TEACH Act does not supersede fair use or existing digital license agreements.
Ultimately, it is up to each academic institution to decide whether to take advantage of the new copyright exemptions under the TEACH Act. This decision should consider both the extent of the institution's distance education programs and its ability to meet the education, compliance and technological requirements of the TEACH Act.

LEARNER ASSESSMENT IN THE ONLINE LEARNING ENVIRONMENT

Test security is always a concern in both the traditional and online classroom. A concern expressed frequently by educators is that it is hard to monitor students in the online environment to ensure they are not cheating on tests. There are several techniques to use to prevent, or at least minimize, cheating.

- Proactive measures:
  - Education regarding academic integrity—some organizations provide mandatory training for all students to heighten awareness and understanding
  - Clear statements in student handbooks
- Low-tech measures:
  - Signature of integrity—required for all assignments and tests—is accompanied by a statement that attests to the originality of the document (Exhibit 5.5)
- High-tech measures:
  - Originality verification
    - Turnitin
    - iThenticate
    - WriteCheck
  - Proctoring resources
    - ProctorU
    - Remote proctor

These tools and strategies can be effective deterrents, but it is important to note that it is not possible to prevent or detect all incidents of cheating. The most important proactive measure that an educator can take is to convey the expectation of academic integrity and endeavor to create a culture of ethics.

EXHIBIT 5.5

Intellectual Honesty Certification Statement

I certify that this assignment is presented as entirely my own intellectual work. Any words and/or ideas from other sources (e.g., printed publications, Internet sites, electronic media, other individuals, groups, or organizations) have been properly indicated using the appropriate scholarly citation style required by the department or college.

I have not submitted this assignment in its entirety to satisfy the requirements of any other course. Any parts of this assignment from other courses have been discussed thoroughly with the faculty member before this submission so that there is an understanding that I have used some of this work in a prior assignment.

Student's Signature: _____

Course Submitted: _____

Term: _____

Date: _____

Source: Gambescia (2010). Reprinted with permission.

SUMMARY

Online teaching requires different competencies than the traditional classroom. The online learning environment is growing exponentially and this trend is likely to continue at a tremendous pace. As more and more educational programs are delivered online, the ability to teach online is an essential competency for the contemporary nurse educator. Brinthaupt, Fisher, Gardner, Raffo, and Woodard (2011) point out that online teachers can use a variety of approaches to foster student engagement, stimulate intellectual development, and build rapport with students. Recognizing the potential for individual variation in teaching well online suggests that there are no essential tools or techniques that all teachers should use. Rather, what is essential is a specific pedagogical attitude that reflects a high level of commitment to and investment in students. How these elements are operationalized into teaching practice is up to the individual teacher.

CASE STUDIES

CASE STUDY 5.1

A nurse educator at a small midwestern hospital has just joined a regional consortium of health care systems that have formed the alliance to address mutual interests and share costs. One priority area that has been identified is that of ongoing staff education and in-service updates. The nurse educator has been asked to develop a series of online courses that can be distributed to all partner-organization employees starting with one on the Health Insurance Portability and Accountability Act. Describe an approach to the design and implementation of this online course. How will the course be structured? How will the content be delivered?

CASE STUDY 5.2

A nurse educator has taught a very popular course in the traditional F2F classroom. Within this course, she uses a variety of interactive classroom strategies designed to engage the students in active learning—including small-group work, debates, case studies, guest speakers, and student-led panel discussions. The dean wants this educator to take the course online. Discuss the strategies that would be used to transfer the course to the online learning environment while still maintaining these highly interactive learning activities.

PRACTICE QUESTIONS

1. Generally, online courses provide students with:
   A. Less control over the content
   B. Less control over the time and place learning occurs
   C. An individualized, learner-centered learning experience
   D. More opportunities to interact with classmates

2. An online instructor provides a written transcript for a video that he is including in his course. The instructor is incorporating which of the following quality design standards identified by Quality Matters™ (2016)?

A. Course technology

B. Accessibility

C. Learner interaction and engagement

D. Learner support

3. In an online course, which of the following will provide one-on-one interaction with the faculty?

A. Asynchronous office hours

B. Synchronous office hours

C. Discussion board

D. Practice meet

4. Within an online course, the term *alignment* refers to:

A. The structure of the course content and navigation

B. Adherence to accessibility requirements

C. How course content links with established practice standards

D. How learning outcomes are linked with course materials and assessments

5. In an online course, which of the following will provided one-on-one interaction with the faculty?

A. Asynchronous office hours

B. Synchronous office hours

C. Discussion board

D. Practice meet

6. Designing an online course to be usable by all people to the greatest extent possible is called:

A. Usable design

B. Accessible design

C. Universal design

D. Versatile design

7. Ensuring learners can perform requirements with a minimal amount of effort and achieve the course goals is called:

A. Learnability and efficiency

B. Consistency and effectiveness

C. Efficiency and effectiveness

D. Usability and efficiency

8. Ensuring that learning objectives are aligned with course materials and learning activities that directly support the assessments for the course is called:

A. Curriculum

B. Synchronous

C. Alignment

D. Coordination

9. Providing alternative means of access to course materials in formats that meet the needs of diverse learners is called:

A. Support

B. Accessibility

C. Interaction

D. Engagement

10. Courses that deliver less than 30% of content online are considered:

A. Blended

B. Hybrid

C. Web-facilitated

D. Dual

REFERENCES

Allen, I. E., & Seaman, J. (2011). Going the distance: Online education in the United States, 2011. *Babson Survey Research Group and Quahog Research Group, LLC*. Retrieved from http://www.onlinelearningsurvey.com/reports/goingthedistance.pdf

Bigatel, P. M., Ragan, L. C., Kennan, S., May, J., & Redmond, B. F. (2012). The identification of competencies for online teaching success. *Journal of Asynchronous Learning Networks, 16*(1), 59–77.

Brinthaupt, T., Fisher, L., Gardner, J., Raffo, D., & Woodard, J. (2011). What the best online teachers should do. *Journal of Online Learning and Teaching, 7*(4). Retrieved from http://jolt.merlot.org/vol7no4/brinthaupt_1211.htm

Bonnel, W., & Boehm, H. (2011). Improving feedback to students online: Teaching tips from experienced faculty. *Journal of Continuing Education in Nursing, 42*(11), 503–509.

Carnegie Mellon University. (n.d.). Why should assessments, learning objectives, and instructional strategies be aligned? Retrieved from http://www.cmu.edu/teaching/assessment/basics/alignment.html

Chittleborough, P., Maybery, D., Patrick, K., & Reupert, A. (2009). The importance of being human: Instructors' personal presence in distance programs. *International Journal of Teaching & Learning in Higher Education, 21*(1), 47–56. Retrieved from http://files.eric.ed.gov/fulltext/EJ896241.pdf

Cook, D. A. (2007). Web-based learning: Pros, cons and controversies. *Clinical Medicine, 7*(1), 37–42. Retrieved from http://www.clinmed.rcpjournal.org/content/7/1/37.full.pdf+html

Cook, D. A., & Dupras, D. M. (2004). A practical guide to developing effective web-based learning. *Journal of General Internal Medicine, 19*(6), 698–707. Retrieved from http://www.ncbi.nlm.nih.gov/pmc/articles/PMC1492389/pdf/jgi_30029.pdf

Copyright Clearance Center. (2011). The TEACH Act: New roles, rules and responsibilities for academic institutions. Retrieved from http://www.copyright.com/wp-content/uploads/2015/04/CR-Teach-Act.pdf

Crews, K. (2010). Copyright law and distance education: Overview of the TEACH Act. Retrieved from http://www.ala.org/advocacy/copyright/teachact/distanceeducation#newc

Gambescia, S. (2010). *Intellectual honesty certification*. Philadelphia, PA: Drexel University College of Nursing and Health Professions. Retrieved from http://www.pages.drexel.edu/~cnhp/blackboard/ihcertification.html

Hathaway, K. L. (2013). An application of the seven principles of good practice to online courses. *Research in Higher Education Journal, 22*, 1–13. Retrieved from http://www.aabri.com/manuscripts/131676.pdf

Hoffmann, R. L., Klein, S. J., & Rosenzweig, M. Q. (2016). Creating quality online materials for specialty nurse practitioner content: Filling a need for the graduate nurse practitioner. *Journal of Cancer Education*. doi:10.1007/s13187-015-0980-3

Ilkay, A. O., & Zeynep, C. O. (2014). Impacts of e-learning in nursing education: In the light of recent studies. *World Academy of Science, Engineering and Technology International Journal of Social Behavioural, Education, Economic and Management Engineering, 8*(5), 1285–1287.

Jacobs, P. (2015). Suggestions for a smooth running online course. *Research in Higher Education Journal, 29*, 1–8.

Kohan, B. (2010). What is a content management system (CMS)? Views about enterprise web application development research and reports. Retrieved from http://www.comentum.com/what-is-cms-content-management-system.html

Learning management system. (n.d.). In *PC Mag.com encyclopedia*. Retrieved from http://www.pcmag.com/encyclopedia

Matuga, J. M. (2006). The role of assessment and evaluation in context: Pedagogical alignment, constraints, and affordances in online courses. In D. Williams, M. Hricko & S. Howell (Eds.), *Online assessment, measurement and evaluation: Emerging practices* (pp. 316–330). Hershey, PA: Idea Group Publishing. doi:10.4018/978-1-59140-747-8.ch019

McCutcheon, K., Lohan, M., Traynor, M., & Martin, D. (2015). A systematic review evaluating the impact of online or blended learning vs. face-to-face learning of clinical skills in undergraduate nurse education. *Journal of Advanced Nursing, 71*(2), 255–270. doi:10.1111/jan.12509

McGarry, B. J., Theobald, K., Lewis, P. A., & Coyer, F. (2015). Flexible learning design in curriculum delivery promotes student engagement and develops metacognitive learners: An integrated review. *Nurse Education Today, 35*(9), 966. doi:10.1016/j.nedt.2015.06.009

National League for Nursing. (2016). Certified nurse educator (CNE) 2016 candidate handbook. Retrieved from http://www.nln.org/docs/default-source/professional-development-programs/certified-nurse-educator-(cne)-examination-candidate-handbook.pdf?sfvrsn=2

Ormrod, J. E. (2011). *Human learning* (6th ed.). Upper Saddle River, NJ: Prentice Hall.

Phipps, R., & Merisotis, J. (2000). *Quality on the line: Benchmarks for success in Internet-based distance education*. Washington, DC: The Institute for Higher Education Policy. Retrieved from http://www.ihep.org/assets/files/publications/m-r/QualityOnTheLine.pdf

Price, J. M., Whitlatch, J., Jane, M. C., Burdi, M., & Peacock, J. (2016). Improving online teaching by using established best classroom teaching practices. *Journal of Continuing Education in Nursing, 47*(5), 222–227. doi:10.3928/00220124-20160419-08

Quality Matters™. (2014). *Higher education rubric* (5th ed.). Baltimore, MD: Author. Retrieved from www.qualitymatters.org/rubric

Quality Matters™. (2016). What is the QM Program? Retrieved from http://www.qmprogram.org

Ragan, L. (2012). 10 principles of effective online teaching: Best practices in distance education. *Magna Publications*. Retrieved from https://www.mnsu.edu/cetl/teachingwithtechnology/tech_resources_pdf/Ten%20Principles%20of%20Effective%20Online%20Teaching.pdf. Reprinted by permission of the author.

Robinson, C. C., & Hullinger, H. (2008). New benchmarks in higher education: Student engagement in online learning. *Journal of Education for Business, 84*(2), 101–108.

Smith, T. C. (2005). Fifty-one competencies for online instruction. *Journal of Educators Online, 2*(2), 1–18.

TEACH Act—A Distance educator's update. (2006). *Distance Education Report, 10*(23), 5–8.

Terantino, J. M., & Agbehonou, E. (2012). Comparing faculty perceptions of an online development course: Addressing faculty needs for online teaching. *Online Journal of Distance Learning Administration, XIV*(II). Retrieved from http://www.westga.edu/~distance/ojdla/summer152/terantino_agbehonou152.html

U.S. Copyright Office. (2012a). Copyright basics. Retrieved from http://www.copyright .gov/circs/circ01.pdf

U.S. Copyright Office. (2012b). U.S. Copyright Office fair use index. Retrieved from http:// www.copyright.gov/fls/fl102.html

Varvel, V. E. (2007). Master online teacher competencies. *Online Journal of Distance Learning Administration, X*(I). Retrieved from http://www.westga.edu/~distance/ojdla/ spring101/varvel101.htm

Skills Laboratory Learning

CAROL OKUPNIAK AND M. ANNIE MULLER

When you know better, you do better.
—Maya Angelou

This chapter addresses the Certified Nurse Educator Exam Content Area 1: Facilitate Learning (National League for Nursing [NLN], 2016, p. 5).

- Content Area 1 is 22% of the examination
- It is estimated that there will be approximately 33 questions from Content Area 1

LEARNING OUTCOMES

- Define skills laboratory learning
- Develop practice and testing environment for fundamental and advanced nursing skills
- Understand how to rehearse clinical skills safely before learners take care of real patients
- Prepare and organize a skills laboratory
- Compare skills lab training methods to determine proficiency
- Understand laboratory time in relation to clinical expectations of the nursing programs
- Determine learner competencies in the skills laboratory

In the skills laboratory, nurse educators create an atmosphere in which learners acquire new skills in a supportive, caring, and nonthreatening environment. A well-designed nursing skills laboratory should closely reflect the clinical environment where learners will care for their patients. The skills laboratory is a place where learners can practice the principles and technical skills necessary for safe patient care. Learners should be given the opportunity in a nursing skills laboratory to practice until proficient. The skills laboratory is an area where learners are taught through activities that support multiple learning styles. Learners are also taught the principles of evidence-based practice (EBP) as it applies to nursing skills. The learning that takes place in the skills laboratory will be transferred to the clinical setting and will be the foundation on which professional practice is built.

LEARNING IN THE LABORATORY

Learning in the laboratory can best be described as experiential because nurse educators incorporate both patient information and critical thinking skills into practice, including the following:

- Creating new knowledge through the transformation of experience
- Incorporating new experiences into the learner's existing cognitive framework
- Helping learners develop critical thinking and problem-solving skills
- Creating a learning environment in the laboratory in which skills are not only demonstrated, but new behaviors are learned
- Evaluate the effectiveness of deliberate practice on learning skills
- Reviewing previously taught skills using reflection, scenario-based learning, and return demonstration (Lisko & O'Dell, 2012)
- Integrating experiential learning theory and nursing education
- Learn communication skills to demonstrate proficiency in caring for vulnerable populations (Booth, 2014)

The clinical learning environment (CLE) is one of the best places for students to practice the psychomotor skills needed in professional nursing. Nursing students are often very concerned about mastering skills to gain confidence in their roles. Examples of common psychomotor skills for nursing learners, from beginning to advanced, are outlined in Table 6.1.

EVIDENCE-BASED TEACHING PRACTICE

Oetker-Black and Kreye (2015) evaluated the Clinical Skills Self-Efficacy Scale using nursing students ($N = 287$) to better understand the Scale's item analysis, reliability, and validity. Two factors had accounted for 57% of total variance and there was also evidence of construct validity. The authors suggest that there is a relationship between increased self-efficacy and the successful transferal of clinical skills learned in a simulated laboratory to the clinical setting; further studies are warranted.

TABLE 6.1 **Common Psychomotor Skills**	

Beginning Skills	• Assessment
	    ◦ Head-to-toe established routine
	    ◦ Normal versus abnormal
	    ◦ Essential equipment needed for
	        – Vital signs
	        – Neurological evaluations
	• Medication administration
	    ◦ Students rate their skills of pharmacology and medication calculation as limited and teaching different methods of math calculation may be beneficial (Stolic, 2014)

Advanced Skills	• Application of patient assessment with medication administration • When to refuse to administer an ordered medication • Appropriate steps to take when medications are not given

SKILLS LABORATORY LEARNING ACTIVITIES

The basic principles of skills learning are as follows:

- Learn the steps of skills
- Provide a full explanatory demonstration by faculty
- An evidence-based skills video should be viewed prior to demonstration
- Progress from simple to complex skills (McNiesh, Benner, & Chesla, 2011)
- Understand the scientific basis for the skill
- Use current evidence-based skills
- Ensure a safe environment during the implementation of the skill
- Safety includes the following:
  - Safety for simulated patient, learner, and faculty
  - Equipment safety
  - No distractions
    - No talking
    - Simulating visitors/providers should not move about room
    - Mobile devices are used for reference purposes only
- Use multimedia to teach nursing skills
- Use computer programs
- Record skills on video when possible
- Learn management systems to embed video, animation, and so on
- Use virtual reality simulators (Virtual IV Trainer is an example)
- Utilize deliberate practice until proficient

> ### DELIBERATE PRACTICE
>
> *Deliberate practice* refers to an effort to improve a skill or task with repeated practice, usually with a mentor who offers feedback. Increasing the complexity of the skill is an integral component of deliberate practice (Duvivier et al., 2011).

- Rapid cycle deliberate practice has learners' repeat required skills until proficient, reducing the amount of time it takes to learn a skill (Kutzin & Janicke, 2015)

Nursing Student Portfolios Should Include Clinical Skill Achievement

- Portfolios can be hard copy or electronic
- Compilation of skills learned giving a detailed picture of a learner's achievements, strengths and weaknesses, career objectives, and professional goals (Byrne et al., 2007)
- Documentation of competency
- Verification by faculty
- Used in conjunction with résumé for job search

> ### CRITICAL THINKING QUESTION
>
> What pieces of learners' portfolios can nurse educators encourage them to collect to enhance their chances of employment postgraduation?

Practice Computer Documentation

- Informatics
- Computerized medication administration record (MAR)
  - Scan bar codes
  - Scan quick response (QR) codes—this technology is newer than bar code scans and holds more information than a bar code (Figure 6.1)

Practice the Skill of Delegation

- Critical thinking related to delegation
  - Responsibility and accountability
- Rules for delegating skills or tasks to unlicensed assistive personnel (UAP)
- State requirements governing delegation to UAP or licensed practical nurses (LPNs)

> **Teaching Gem:** Learners may be more successful in learning a skill if they understand the physiological concept behind the task and if the skill is embedded in a case study.

FIGURE 6.1 An optically readable quick response (QR) two-dimensional bar code.

EQUIPMENT NEEDED TO ENSURE LEARNING OUTCOMES

Both learners and nurse educators need to know the safe operation of all laboratory equipment. The purchase and maintenance of equipment must be an ongoing, thoughtful process for program directors and nurse educators. Equipment is often referred to using the following terms:

- Low fidelity—technical skills performance—anatomical models
- Midfidelity—limited computer operations—heart and lung sounds
- High fidelity—complex computer systems with ability to change physiology (Brydges, Carnahan, Rose, Rose, & Dubrowski, 2012)

Some basic tenets of equipment use and maintenance are listed in the following:

- Safety of all equipment must be established prior to use
- Equipment similar to what the learner will experience in a clinical environment should be used
- Faculty may need additional education and training to use new equipment
- Invite a guest lecturer or representative of the technology company to demonstrate the equipment to learners

- Allow learners time to practice with equipment before testing their knowledge
- Make sure all equipment is functioning as desired prior to using for skills. Someone should be identified as a technological resource to troubleshoot technical malfunctions if needed

Equipment Learners Will Need

Learners are instructed to purchase equipment to be used in both the skills laboratory and their clinical practice. Some programs have the learners purchase a tote bag of equipment that will be needed, whereas other programs ask the learners to purchase separate items such as:

- Watch with a second hand (water resistant is preferred)
- Mobile device used to reference skills, medications, lab values, patient education material, evidence-based practice (EBP) guidelines, and so forth, per institution policy
- Stethoscope (must include bell-listening device)
- Pen light
- Name tag
- Ink pen (black only)

LABORATORY ATTIRE, APPEARANCE, AND BEHAVIOR

Because the skills laboratory is a simulation of a clinical setting, most nurse educators believe that laboratory attire should be professional (Clavelle, Goodwin, & Tivis, 2013) and include the following:

- Laboratory coat
- Street clothes if they reflect professional attire, or student uniform if appropriate
  - Skirts or dresses must be long enough to accommodate bending, twisting, or squatting
- Shoes need to be flat and comfortable

Personal Appearance

- No artificial nails
- No nail polish
- No false eyelashes
- Moderate makeup
- Hair secured to nape of neck or put up
- No excessive perfume
- No dangling jewelry (safety hazard)
- No piercings
- No visible tattoos

Behavior

Nursing learners are asked to adhere to the code of conduct that is determined by the institution and is recorded for their reference in the organization's student handbook or program guide. The two overriding themes of behavior for a skills laboratory are:

1. Academic honesty
2. Professional behavior (Moked & Drach-Zahavy, 2016)

EVALUATION AND REMEDIATION

Evaluating the skills acquired by the learner is a time-consuming and important task for the nurse educator, which commonly includes the following components:

- Skills checklists
  * Clarify and justify those skills required to be competent
  * Prepare a review of each skill when completed and discuss with student
- Importance of modeling experts who perform skills or tasks flawlessly (D. Cooper & Higgins, 2014)
- Agency-based policy and procedure manual
  * Pass or fail skill evaluation with explanation of errors
  * Able to perform with or without assistance from the faculty
  * If with assistance or with questions from faculty, determine how much facilitation should be offered by faculty
- Allow to repeat skill at a later date after remediation
  * Educator may want to have a different or additional laboratory faculty member evaluate a repeated skill
- Evaluate learner ability to practice safely in a clinical environment
  * Evaluate a chosen practice skill
  * Determine how well the skills are developed:
    - Is there need for improvement (Price, 2012)?
    - Is the learner competent to complete the skill in any clinical setting (Wilson, 2012)?
- Evaluate using all learning domains—cognitive, psychomotor, and affective (Florin, Ehrenberg, Wallin, & Gustavsson, 2012)

EVIDENCE-BASED TEACHING PRACTICE

Houghton, Casey, Shaw, and Murphy (2013) examined factors that impact on students' (N = 43) implementation of clinical skills in the practice setting using a multiple case study design. Factors that could facilitate and hinder students using their clinical skills were identified. Facilitating factors included provision of learning opportunities, staff support and supervision, and student confidence. Hindering factors were gaps in how skills were taught in the higher education institutions and the clinical setting, as well as missed learning opportunities.

Remediation

- Required by faculty for improved performance
- Open skills practice
  - Learners require open laboratory practice time
  - Improves learners' skills, judgment, and clinical knowledge (Lynn & Twigg, 2011)
  - Learners may wish to learn a skill practiced at their clinical site (Herrman, 2015)
- Student-centered approach
  - Individualized instruction (Lynn & Twigg, 2011)
  - Peer tutoring (Loke & Chow, 2007)
  - Evaluate improvement

INTEGRATING RESEARCH IN THE SKILLS LABORATORY

The skills laboratory is a great place to support nursing research by demonstrating how research is translated into practice and by developing the thinking process needed for professional practice after graduation (Florin et al., 2012).

- Incorporate EBP into nursing research courses (Leach, Hofmeyer, & Bobridge, 2016)
- Increase EBP for skill development
- Understand the need for EBP skills and incorporate objective structural clinical examination skills in the lab
  - Method of evaluating critical clinical skills and competency
  - Include communication skills with all diverse cultures (Oranye, Ahmad, Ahmad, & Bakar, 2012)
- Example of EBP in skills lab learning

EVIDENCE-BASED TEACHING PRACTICE

Fennessey and Wittmann-Price (2011) did a concept analysis on the incongruence between what skills learners are taught in the skills laboratory for physical assessment of patients and what they actually use in the clinical area when caring for patients. The analysis found that many skills taught are not actually used.

- J. R. Cooper, Martin, Fisher, Marks, and Harrington (2013) used a peer-to-peer communication exercise in the skills lab to enhance confidence and improve therapeutic communication before students report to the patient care environment
- Morris and Mynard (2010) reported students' improvement in skills and intelligence when permitted to use a mobile device to access evidence and clinical practice guidelines in a clinical setting

NURSING SKILLS LABORATORY MANAGEMENT

Points to verify and consider:

- Supplies and equipment meet the curricular needs
- Adequate space is given for student practice and testing
- Students and faculty are provided orientation to laboratory equipment and laboratory policy
- Faculty role in the skills laboratory is defined
- Laboratory design is learner centered
- Opportunity for remediation and skills practice
- Revenue available for disposable supplies, equipment maintenance, and upgrades
- Laboratory staff management
- Faculty are consistent in demonstration of skills taught
- Support skills based on EBP
- Clinical facilities collaborate to assist with the computer learning objectives
- Faculty training to ensure competency with equipment and with any new equipment obtained

Also note that in today's technological world, skills can be viewed and performed in the virtual world. As this technology emerges, faculty will need to embrace its usage where appropriate.

CASE STUDIES

CASE STUDY 6.1

A learner in the skills laboratory is having trouble donning sterile gloves because of excessively sweaty hands. As a nurse educator how would you handle this situation?
- Is it a functional issue? Larger gloves, different types of gloves, and small amount of powder on hands?
- Is it a psychological issue? Anxiety? Send to student services, provide relaxation techniques?
- Is it a physiological issue? Endocrine, allergy?

CASE STUDY 6.2

A learner has to care for a transgender patient for the first time. The learner has been raised in a very strict religious home and is having difficulties understanding how to approach the patient. How would you instruct the learner to meet and care for this patient?

PRACTICE QUESTIONS

1. A nurse educator who is assigned to an open skills lab observes a learner practicing Foley catheter insertion with a step out of the proper sequence. When the nurse educator corrects the learner, the learner responds, "This is how I was taught the skill during clinical skills lab." How should the nurse educator address this issue with the faculty?

   A. Tell the learner that he or she may have heard the information incorrectly and demonstrate the correct sequence

   B. Look up the skills checklist used in the clinical skills lab for Foley catheter insertion

   C. Speak to the faculty member directly to ascertain what is being taught in the skills lab

   D. Report this information to the dean/director of the nursing program

2. What is the best way to teach a senior-level learner the proper technique to administer a medication delivered by intravenous (IV) push in the nursing skills lab?

   A. Ensure a working IV arm is available with the proper simulated medication vial and the correct needle and syringe

   B. Use a midfidelity manikin with a working IV attached

   C. Have the learner verbalize the proper sequence of IV push medication administration

   D. Have an injection pad available and a simulated vial of the prescribed medication

3. Which of the following methods develops critical thinking skills in the clinical skills laboratory environment?

   A. Learners are able to choose the correct supplies from a variety of needles and syringes when practicing intramuscular (IM) injections

   B. Learners gather all necessary supplies and equipment prior to performing tracheotomy care and suctioning

   C. Learners are given a medical record and history from a simulated patient and need to administer medication

   D. Learners are required to teach a nursing skill to their peers in the clinical skills laboratory

4. The nurse educator asks a learner to describe a health assessment. The learner describes his understanding of how an assessment is performed when he makes which of the following statements?

   A. Components used in an assessment are based on the independent judgment of the nurse

   B. Routinely, the nurse will always do an in-depth full-body assessment

   C. In-depth assessments are always referred to as head-to-toe assessments

   D. Prior to a nurse's assessment, an advanced practice nurse should do a full screening of all body systems

5. A learner is assigned to perform a task during a clinical experience. Which of the following would be a responsibility of the learner?

   A. Perform the task with the staff nurse present

   B. Perform only those tasks that the learner has been deemed competent to perform

   C. Have the instructor present during the task to be sure the learner doesn't make any mistakes

   D. Only perform the task after observing the staff several times

6. The first line of defense against infection is intact skin. Which statement made by the learner indicates a need for further teaching?

   A. "Hand washing is to prevent infection through contact transmission"

   B. "It's okay to use antibacterial gel instead of soap and water in some instances"

   C. "It isn't necessary to wash your hands prior to patient care as long as you wash them before you leave the room"

   D. "You should always wash your hands prior to and after using gloves"

7. The nursing learner has been assigned a patient in isolation and realizes this patient is in respiratory isolation. Which of the following indicates that the learner correctly understands the need for self-protection with personal protective equipment (PPE)?

   A. Regular PPE is hanging on the door and can be used by anyone entering the room

   B. Respiratory isolation requires a specialized protective mask before entering the room

   C. Anyone can use any available mask for protection

   D. Patients are not contagious unless they are actively coughing while you are in the room

8. A learner comes to the laboratory without a laboratory coat and is unprepared to practice the skill for the day. The nurse educator should first:

   A. Send the learner home

   B. Have the learner make up the day later that week

   C. Discuss the behavior with the learner

   D. Write the learner a disciplinary warning

9. Which of the following is an example of peer-to-peer review in the skills lab?

   A. Senior students practicing urinary catheterization repeatedly until proficient

   B. Freshman students comparing websites on EBP on their mobile devices

   C. Junior students learning how to speak empathetically by example from the senior students

   D. Observing faculty experts demonstrating complex skills in a simulated clinical environment

10. When a learner is faced with caring for a transgender patient, what would be the best way for the learner to address this patient?

    A. Tell the patient you will care for him or her regardless of what the patient's preferences are

    B. Ask someone else to care for the patient

    C. Ask the patient politely how he or she would prefer to be addressed

    D. Offer the patient psychiatric counseling for gender confusion

REFERENCES

Booth, J. (2014). Viewpoint: Treating transgender patients with respect. *American Nurse Today, 9*(8), 1–3.

Brydges, R., Carnahan, H., Rose, D., Rose, L., & Dubrowski, A. (2012). Coordinating progressive levels of simulation fidelity to maximize educational benefit. *Academic Medicine, 85*(5), 806–812.

Byrne, M., Delarose, T., King, C. A., Leske, J., Sapnas, K. G., & Schroeter, K. (2007). Continued professional competence and portfolios. *Journal of Trauma Nursing, 14*(1), 24–31.

Clavelle, J. T., Goodwin, M., & Tivis, L. J. (2013). Nursing professional attire. *Journal of Nursing Administration, 43*(3), 172–177. doi:10.1097/NNA.0b013e318283dc78

Cooper, D., & Higgins, S. (2014). The effectiveness of online instructional videos in the acquisition and demonstration of cognitive, affective and psychomotor rehabilitation skills. *British Journal of Educational Technology, 46*(4), 768–799.

Cooper, J. R., Martin, T., Fisher, W., Marks, J., & Harrington, M. (2013). Peer-to-peer teaching: Improving communication techniques for students in an accelerated nursing program. *Nursing Education Perspectives, 34*(5), 349.

Duvivier, R. J., Van Dalen, J., Muijtjens, A. M., Moulaert, V., Van der Vleuten, C., & Scherpbier, A. (2011). The role of deliberate practice in the acquisition of clinical skills. *BMC Medical Education, 11*, 101.

Fennessey, A., & Wittmann-Price, R. A. (2011). Physical assessment: A continuing need for clarification. *Nursing Forum, 46*(1), 45–50.

Florin, J., Ehrenberg, A., Wallin, L., & Gustavsson, P. (2012). Educational support for research utilization and capability beliefs regarding evidence-based practice skills: A national survey of senior nursing students. *Journal of Advanced Nursing, 68*(4), 888–897.

Herrman, J. (2015). Creative lab skills. In J. Herrman (Ed.), *Creative teaching strategies for the nurse educator* (2nd ed., pp. 175–176). Philadelphia, PA: F. A. Davis.

Houghton, C. E., Casey, D., Shaw, D., & Murphy, K. (2013). Students' experiences of implementing clinical skills in the real world of practice. *Journal of Clinical Nursing, 22*(13-14), 1961–1969.

Kutzin, J. M., & Janicke, P. (2015). Incorporating rapid cycle deliberate practice into nursing staff continuing professional development. *Journal of Continuing Education in Nursing, 46*(7), 299–301. doi:10.3928/00220124-20150619-14

Leach, M. J., Hofmeyer, A., & Bobridge, A. (2016). The impact of research education on student nurse attitude, skill and uptake of evidence-based practice: A descriptive longitudinal survey. *Journal of Clinical Nursing, 25*(1/2), 194–203. doi:10.1111/jocn.13103

Lisko, A., & O'Dell, B. (2012). Integration of theory and practice: Experiential learning theory and nursing education. *Nursing Education Perspectives, 32*(2), 106–108.

Loke, A. J., & Chow, F. (2007). Learning partnership—The experience of peer tutoring among nursing students: A qualitative study. *International Journal of Nursing Students, 44*(2), 237–244.

Lynn, M. C., & Twigg, R. D. (2011). A new approach to clinical remediation. *Journal of Nursing Education, 50*(3), 172–175.

McNiesh, S., Benner, P., & Chesla, C. (2011). Learning formative skills of nursing practice in an accelerated program. *Qualitative Health Research, 21*(1), 51–61.

Moked, Z., & Drach-Zahavy, A. (2016). Clinical supervision and nursing students' professional competence: Support-seeking behaviour and the attachment styles of students and mentors. *Journal of Advanced Nursing, 72*(2), 316–327. doi:10.1111/jan.12838

Morris, J., & Maynard, V. (2010). Pilot study to test the use of a mobile device in the clinical setting to access evidence-based practice resources. *Worldviews on Evidence-Based Nursing, 7*(4), 205–213.

National League for Nursing. (2016). Certified nurse educator (CNE) 2016 candidate handbook. Retrieved from http://www.nln.org/docs/default-source/professionaldevelopment -programs/certified-nurse-educator-%28cne%29-examination-candidate-handbook .pdf?sfvrsn=2

Oetker-Black, S. L., & Kreye, J. (2015). Global psychometric evaluation of the clinical skills self-efficacy scale in Moshi, Tanzania. *Nursing Education Perspectives, 36*(3), 163–166. doi:10.5480/13-1256

Oranye, N. O., Ahmad, C., Ahmad, N., & Bakar, R. A. (2012). Assessing nursing clinical skills competence through objective structural clinical examination (OSCE) for open distance learning students in open university Malaysia. *Contemporary Nurse: A Journal for the Australian Nursing Profession, 41*(2), 233–241.

Price, B. (2012). Skill analysis part 2: Evaluating a practice skill. *Nursing Standard, 26*(18), 51–57.

Stolic, S. (2014). Educational strategies aimed at improving student nurse's medication calculation skills: A review of the research literature. *Nurse Education in Practice, 14*(5), 491–503. doi:10.1016/j.nepr.2014.05.010

Wilson, C. (2012). Clinical competence of nursing students. *Australian Nursing Journal, 19*(7), 34.

7

Facilitating Learning in the Clinical Setting

MARYLOU K. McHUGH AND TRACY P. GEORGE

Live as if you were to die tomorrow. Learn as if you were to live forever.

—Mahatma Gandhi

This chapter addresses the Certified Nurse Educator Exam Content Area 1: Facilitate Learning (National League for Nursing [NLN], 2016b, p. 5).

- Content Area 1 is 22% of the examination
- It is estimated that there will be approximately 33 questions from Content Area 1

LEARNING OUTCOMES

- Discuss the goals of clinical education
- Explain the different types of clinical learning activities
- Describe the purpose of pre- and postclinical conference
- Analyze evaluation methods appropriate to measuring clinical outcomes of learners

Clinical education is a "core component of nursing education" (Dahlke, O'Connor, Hannesson, & Cheetham, 2016, p. 145). Clinical education is more than just being a proficient practitioner; it is synthesizing nursing and educational knowledge to guide learners. The clinical learning environment (CLE) allows students to integrate nursing theory into practice, develop critical thinking skills, and mature into their professional identity as a nurse (O'Mara, McDonald, Gillespie, Brown, & Miles, 2014).

Appropriate CLEs need to be planned throughout the curriculum and should grow in skill and complexity. The CLE must be congruent with the desired course, curriculum, and program outcomes (Billings & Halstead, 2016). The CLE provides practical implementation of the didactic content that has been taught.

When selecting the CLE, the clinical nurse educator should consider:

- The ability of the site to meet the course outcomes
- The level of the learner
- Whether the clinical nurse educator is permitted to schedule learning activities at the site
- The availability of appropriate role models at the site
- The location and type of facility
- Orientation and agency requirements
- Presence of a positive relationship among staff, learners, and clinical nurse educators
- The ability of learners to participate in interprofessional clinical activities (Gaberson, Oermann, & Shellenbarger, 2015)

The learning outcomes of clinical nursing education are to assist learners to:

1. Apply theoretical learning to patient care situations using critical thinking skills to recognize and resolve patient care problems and use the nursing process to design therapeutic nursing interventions and evaluate their effectiveness.
2. Develop communication skills when working with patients, their families, and other health care providers.
3. Demonstrate skill in the safe use of therapeutic nursing interventions when providing care to patients.
4. Evaluate and utilize evidence-based practices and research findings in designing patient care.
5. Evince caring behaviors in nursing actions.
6. Recognize and respect the varied beliefs, values, and customs of individual patients inherent in an increasingly diverse population.
7. Consider the ethical implication of clinical decision making and nursing actions.
8. Gain a perspective of the contextual environment of health care delivery.
9. Develop a beginning mastery of technology as it is utilized in patient care settings.
10. Experience the various roles of the nurse within the health care delivery system.
11. Develop the skills necessary to continuously update knowledge in the practice nursing (O'Connor, 2015).

SELECTING APPROPRIATE CLEs THROUGHOUT THE CURRICULUM

CLEs usually include acute care hospitals, outpatient clinics and other community-based sites, and simulation laboratories (Flott & Linden, 2016). Nursing practice is shifting from acute care to community-based settings, so rotations in community health settings, such as ambulatory care, hospice, summer camps, occupational locations, long-term care, and homeless shelters, are being utilized more frequently (Billings & Halstead, 2016).

Normally, clinical groups in acute settings consist of eight to 10 learners (Scholtz, 2007). The number of learners that can be supervised in an acute or nonacute setting is usually dictated by the state board of nursing in which the educational program resides. Some clinical agencies may also dictate the number of students they can accommodate in certain clinical settings.

According to McNelis et al. (2014), nurse educators may need to optimize the CLE so that students obtain experiences that foster critical thinking skills, patient safety, and quality care. In a multi-methods study of 30 final-semester nursing students and six faculty members from three different sites on the CLE, four themes emerged:

1. Missing opportunities for learning in a clinical setting
2. Getting the work done as the measure of learning
3. Failing to enact situation-specific pedagogies to foster clinical learning
4. Failing to engage as part of the team (McNelis et al., 2014)

One approach is to provide students the opportunity to work with interprofessional team members. Turner (2015) developed an interprofessional clinical experience in a medical–surgical course, in which each of the nursing students collaborated with respiratory therapists, physical therapists, and emergency medical technicians, with positive feedback from students.

In certain areas of the United States, there is a shortage of clinical sites resulting from competition from multiple nursing programs. Andresen and Levin (2014) developed alternative clinical learning activities, including simulation, service-learning experiences, and collaborative learning activities, which were developed to meet the course objectives. In addition to increasing the enrolment capacity of students, there was an improved quality and variety of clinical experiences, while maintaining high student satisfaction.

To ensure that the goals are met, Infante (1975) suggested that the essential elements of any CLE should include:

- Opportunity for patient contact
- Objectives for activities
- Competent guidance
- Individuation of activities
- Practice for skill learning, both motor and intellectual
- Encouragement of critical thinking
- Opportunity for problem solving
- Opportunity for observation
- Opportunity for experimentation
- Development of professional judgment or decision making
- Encouragement of creative abilities
- Provision for the transfer of knowledge
- Participation in integrative activities
- Utilization of the team concept

CHOOSING AND EVALUATING THE CLE

Faculty choose and evaluate the clinical area carefully in order to meet the goals of the curriculum. Chan (2002) identified six attributes that the clinical area should offer students:

- Individualization—Students can make decisions and are treated differently according to their ability or interest.
- Innovation—The faculty is able to plan new and interesting learning techniques and activities.
- Satisfaction—Students enjoy the clinical placement and leave with a sense of satisfaction.
- Involvement—Students can participate actively and attentively in the learning activities.
- Personalization—Students have opportunities to interact with clinicians who are concerned with the students' welfare.
- Task orientation—Assignments are clear and meet the learning objectives for the day.

EVIDENCE-BASED TEACHING PRACTICE

Newton, Jolly, Ockerby, and Cross (2012) concluded that developing sustainable approaches to enhance the CLE experience for student nurses is an international concern. They found that students in a clinical preceptorship partnership model responded more positively to their experience.

ATTRIBUTES OF CLINICAL EDUCATORS

Gaberson and colleagues (2015) state that an effective clinical educator needs to:

- Be familiar with the practice area
- Exhibit clinical competence
- Effectively teach students in the clinical area
- Relate well to students
- Demonstrate enthusiasm
- Act as a role model
- Provide feedback on student performance
- Be available to students in the clinical area when needed

Hanson and Stenvig (2008) developed a list of attributes needed for nurse educators to be successful clinical instructors. These include the following:

- Educator knowledge attributes
  - Knowledge of theory and clinical practice
  - Knowledge of the facility
  - Knowledge of the learner

- Educator interpersonal presentation attributes
  - Positive educator attitude
  - Encouraging demeanor
  - Organizational skill
  - Serve as a primary resource
  - Available and approachable
- Learning activities attributes
  - Managing paperwork
  - Keeping learners challenged
  - Postconference planning
  - Firm knowledge of the technology or computer charting system used by the facility

Kan and Stabler-Haas (2014) state that learners will expect that clinical nurse educators have attributes that can be expressed with the acronym CAP:

- C = Consistent
- A = Approachable
- P = Proficient

Professional relationships with staff are very important for the learning experience. Clinical nurse educators need to focus on education and stay clear of unit conflicts. Professional role modeling is essential for the role of clinical nurse educator. Remembering at all times that you are a "guest" is helpful (Kan & Stabler-Haas, 2014).

EVIDENCE-BASED TEACHING PRACTICE

In a study of undergraduate students (N = 165) using Carl Rogers' Person-Centered Model, realness was the attribute that was most likely to facilitate positive interpersonal relationships with students. Nurse educators who are genuine may be better able to motivate students, develop positive relationships with students, and encourage positive attitudes about the course (Bryan, Lindo, Anderson-Johnson, & Weaver, 2015).

PART-TIME CLINICAL EDUCATORS

Nursing programs frequently utilize part-time clinical faculty members. Although clinical nurse educators may not be as visible as classroom nurse educators, their role is vital in the education of nursing students. Transitioning from a staff nurse position to the role of the clinical nurse educator can be challenging. In a study of 10 clinical nurse educators, Clark (2013) identified five themes relevant for nurses' socialization to the role of clinical nurse educator:

- Beginning the role
- Employing strategies to survive in the role
- Coming to a turning point in the role

- Sustaining success in the role
- Finding fulfilment in the role

Many of the part-time clinical educators are new to their role. In a study of 15 clinical educators and 17 preceptors, investigators identified the need for additional support and mentoring in the area of teaching (Dahlke et al., 2016). It may be difficulty to provide face-to-face orientation sessions because of the work schedules of the full-time and part-time nurse educators. In a study of 17 part-time nurse educators, the learning management system (LMS) was used to provide an online orientation to the role of the clinical educator (Fura & Symanski, 2014).

The retention of part-time clinical faculty is necessary for consistency and the achievement of student learning outcomes. In a national web-based survey ($N = 533$), part-time nursing faculty reported that enjoyment of teaching, pay and benefits, support, and being a valued member of the program were reasons they continued in their role (Carlson, 2015). Conflicts with a job and family responsibilities, low pay, and a heavy workload were cited as reasons not to continue working as a clinical nurse educator.

PRECEPTING

> **Teaching Gem:** For high-acuity patients, learners can be assigned to teams to increase safe supervision.

Precepting is a term used to describe the pairing of learners with experienced nurses to collaborate on the delivery of care. Many educational units use this model in their senior nursing courses, advanced nursing curricula, and on dedicated educational units (DEUs). When precepting a nursing student, frequent and specific feedback is necessary and the preceptor needs to report any issues to the faculty member (Ingwerson, 2014).

Assets of precepted experiences include:

- Flexibile hours (learners may be able to work evenings, nights, and weekends if they follow their preceptor's schedule)
- Role modeling (preceptors show learners not only how to provide nursing care but how nurses think and act)
- Clinical advancement (precepting contributes to the expectations of advancing on a clinical ladder track; Woolsey & Bracy, 2012)
- Preceptors may be better able to determine appropriate assignments for students because of the close one-to-one working relationship that is established (Haitana & Bland, 2011)
- Socialization into the role of nursing is facilitated by a preceptor's mentorship and a close working relationship

EVIDENCE-BASED TEACHING PRACTICE

Nurse preceptors are an effective way to bridge the academic and clinical settings. In a qualitative study of 26 nurse preceptors, three themes emerged: need for engagement in the educational process, desire for recognition for their efforts, and that the qualities of students influence the preceptors' experiences (Raines, 2012).

Disadvantages of using a preceptorship model include:

- Lack of time for staff nurses to teach (Carlson, Pilhammar, & Wann-Hansson, 2010)
- Understanding that developing a personal friendship may not serve the preceptor well when evaluations need to be completed (Kan & Stabler-Haas, 2014)
- Preceptors need to be chosen carefully and should want to be involved in nursing education
- Preceptors need to be educated about precepting activities as well as about evaluation principles because often they are asked to evaluate the learner

DEDICATED EDUCATIONAL UNITS

DEUs are nursing units in which the staff nurses actually become the clinical instructors for the learners. They are similar to precepting learners but foster an entire unit in which all or most of the nurses are preceptors. The staff nurses work closely with clinical nurse educators and have been educated in instructing learners. DEUs are being actively studied and the preliminary results are favorable for the learners and for patient care safety.

DEUs are increasing in popularity for several reasons. They

- Increase patient safety
- Assist with the nurse educator shortage
- Promote learner attainment of competencies in a one-on-one situation
- Assist staff nurses to fulfill the teaching portion of their professional roles (Mulready-Shick, Kafel, Banister, & Mylott, 2009)

EVIDENCE-BASED TEACHING PRACTICE

In a mixed-methods study, nurses reported that students received better clinical experiences on DEUs. The nurses on the DEUs also felt that they had better work–life satisfaction and professional development (Nishioka, Coe, Hanita, & Moscato, 2014a).

Students on DEUs reported a high-quality clinical experience as a result of having the same mentor throughout the rotation; they also had the opportunity to practice teamwork, communication, and time-management skills. According to the students, DEUs were more welcoming to students, and the care provided to patients was higher in quality (Nishioka, Coe, Hanita, & Moscato, 2014b).

LEARNING ACTIVITIES FOR THE CLINICAL SETTING

One of the goals of the clinical instructor is to assist learners as they reflect on their practice (Baker, 1996). A reflective learning practice includes:

- A sense of inner discomfort triggered by a live experience
- Identification or clarification of the concern makes the nature of the problem or issue more evident

- Openness to new information from internal and external sources, along with the ability to observe and take information from a variety of perspectives; there is a willingness to forego a quick resolution concerning a problem
- Resolution occurs through insight, whereby the learner feels he or she has changed or learned something that is personally significant
- A change is experienced in self as a result of internalization of a new perspective
- A decision is made whether to act on the outcome of the reflective process by determining whether the insight can be operationalized (p. 20)

There is a whole set of strategies available for the clinical nurse educator, that is different from those available to the classroom nurse educator. Table 7.1 presents selected clinical teaching and supervision activities, along with some clinical tips for implementing these activities.

TABLE 7.1
Clinical Teaching

LEARNING ACTIVITIES	TIPS FOR IMPLEMENTING ACTIVITIES
Demonstration	The instructor demonstrates physical skills as well as reasoning skills, and can encourage the learner to be attentive to his or her own mental work.
War stories/personal experiences	War stories describe particularly memorable events in a nurse's past practice, which now serve as a paradigm for the learners' current practice.
Questioning	This is a constant in clinical practice. A form of Socratic questioning will stimulate the students to think the problem though and will elicit formative evaluation.
Listening	Clinical nurse educators must pay careful attention to what the learners are saying in the clinical area. Paraphrase the learners' comments to ensure clear communication.
SUPERVISION OF LEARNER PERFORMANCE OF TECHNICAL SKILLS	
Process of skill mastery	Learners are at very low levels of skill mastery and will need to go through the sequential steps for all procedures. For information on this process, see Benner (1982).
How to let go	Clinical nurse educators need to allow the learners to work through their technical skills. Although taking over is a natural skill, do this only if it is absolutely necessary, then allow the learner to assume an assistant role. Process the experience with the learner. Allow learners to ask the patients what works best for them.
When to jump in	The clinical instructor should be prepared to intervene when the learner's actions, inaction, or ineptitude jeopardize patient safety. Be calm and assertive. Remember to help the learner work through the situation in a way that does not destroy self-esteem.

(continued)

TABLE 7.1
Clinical Teaching (*continued*)

LEARNING ACTIVITIES	TIPS FOR IMPLEMENTING ACTIVITIES
Ensuring that patient needs are met	Help learners set priorities so that all care is delivered in a timely manner. Keep the context of the whole situation in mind. The timing of all procedures, as well as the schedule, should be addressed. If the learner is caring for more than one patient, help the learner to set priorities. Make sure that the learner allows enough time for all activities.
PROMOTING THE INTEGRATION OF THEORY AND PRACTICE	
Case studies	If patients are not available to meet the clinical objectives, preparing case studies that include some of the prescribed outcome will assist the learner.
Seminars	Seminars based on patient problems that learners have encountered can be used to foster integration. Several learners who care for the same patient on different days can work as a group with patients.
Nursing rounds	Nursing rounds involve a group. They provide an opportunity for all learners to reflect on clinical events. Although background information and conclusions are discussed away from the bedside, the patient can add to the discussion by articulating his or her experience and expectations.
Written assignments	Major nursing care plans, care maps, synthesis papers, and journaling may be part of the clinical experience. Clinical and classroom nurse educators must collaborate so that learners are clear about the assignment.
DEVELOPING CRITICAL THINKING SKILLS AND REFLECTIVE PRACTICE	
Strategies for promoting critical thinking and reflective practice	Clinical instructors must use higher order cognitive questioning that includes "why" instead of "what." Debrief all of the experiences in postclinical conferences. Process recordings and self-evaluations to assist the learners to think at higher cognitive levels.

Learning activities used by effective clinical nurse educators include:

- Questioning
- Role-playing
- Interactive discussions (Kan & Stabler-Haas, 2014)

EVIDENCE-BASED TEACHING PRACTICE

Nafei, Markani, Motearafi, Moghadam, and Sakaei (2015) studied critical thinking skills in undergraduate students ($N = 24$). They found that the use of reflective journals significantly increased students' critical thinking skills when compared to a control group that did not use journaling.

"Ah ha" moments are especially important to focus on in the clinical domain. These moments occur when the learner successfully integrates the application of concepts. Many times, "ah ha" moments are a result of faculty's questioning, which produces critical thinking in the learner (Kan & Stabler-Haas, 2014).

EVIDENCE-BASED TEACHING PRACTICE

In a systematic review of 19 articles, McCutcheon, Lohan, Traynor, and Martin (2015) found that online learning was as effective as traditional teaching methods in teaching clinical skills in undergraduate students. However, there is a lack of evidence on the use of blended learning in the development of clinical skills in undergraduate nursing students.

MAKING LEARNER ASSIGNMENTS

All learners as well as clinical nurse educators should have an orientation to the unit on which students will be learning. Many times, meeting the nurse manager or director and understanding his or her expectations is a great way to start a clinical rotation. Some aspects that may be included in orientation are:

- Icebreakers and tours
- Defining and reviewing goals
- Understanding course requirements
- Evaluating math skills for medication calculations
- Reviewing the learners' responsibilities (Kan & Stabler-Haas, 2014)

CRITICAL THINKING QUESTION

Many nurse educators use scavenger hunts to familiarize the learners with the unit. What activity can be used to familiarize learners with interdisciplinary communication?

Patient assignments should assist the learner to tie the course's didactic content to practical applications. Factors to consider are:

- The skill level of the learner
- The acuity of the patient
- The number of learners in the clinical group
- The availability of patients whose conditions directly meet the objectives of the day

Types of assignments can also differ to meet the clinical objectives and include:

- *Dual assignments:* These should be used when the complexity of care is more than one learner can handle. The clinical nurse educator is responsible for making sure each student is clear about each learner's role in this situation.

- *Observational assignments:* These should be used to augment the learner's appreciation of the various procedures that patients experience but when there is no reason for the learner to practice these procedures. Faculty can send learners to observe the operating room, radiology or laboratory departments, clinics, and so.

When making clinical assignments, the following considerations may be useful (O'Connor, 2015):

1. Assess available clinical material
   - What experiences are available in the clinical setting?
   - What potential learning opportunities are presented in relation to specialty-specific theoretical content, skill development, and overriding curricular content (e.g., interpersonal communication, patient teaching, advocacy, and life span development)?
   - What anticipated patient events (e.g., absence from the unit for prolonged testing, imminent discharge) might interrupt or interfere with student learning?
   - Have staff voiced concerns or cautions regarding specific patient care assignments?

2. What are the curricular goals and related clinical outcomes for this experience?
   - What is the primary focus of learning for this clinical experience?
   - Can that focus be described as a larger concept of which the specific patient case at hand is an example?
   - What other learning can be extracted from the situation? Scan curricular goals and clinical objectives to identify two or three other objectives that might be addressed in the experience.
   - Does the student have sufficient background knowledge, either from previous courses or experiences or from the concurrent theoretical class, to deal with the situation? If not, can sufficient theory be provided to permit the student to function safely and effectively in an otherwise excellent learning situation?

3. What is the overall environment for learning?
   - Can connections be made between the proposed assignment and the previous experiences of the learner that will help to integrate the experiences?
   - What lessons might be drawn from the specific clinical setting that can be carried over into another setting (e.g., what information from the patient setting would be helpful to the nurse providing care for the patient in a community setting or to the nurse providing care for a nursing home resident admitted to the hospital for an episodic illness)?
   - What staffing issues need to be considered in making the assignment (e.g., short staffing because of illness or planned meetings) that may impact the learning experienced?

4. What do you, as the instructor, feel comfortable managing?
   - Where do you anticipate needing to spending the most time with specific students and/or specific patient care assignments?

* Does the overall assignment shortchange any students or create safety issues?

* What patient events can or might happen in the course of the clinical day? If one or more of these events were to occur, would this be manageable given the assignments planned for all students in the group?

5. What are the characteristics of the learner group and individual learners?

* What previous experiences have the students had that can be drawn on when managing the proposed clinical assignment?

* What is the performance level of individual students? Is each student capable of managing the proposed assignment?

* Has each student had opportunities to progress toward achieving clinical outcomes?

* What level of independent functioning has each student achieved? Will one or several students require more attention than others?

* What learning needs have individual students expressed? Are these addressed in the assignment?

* Have students voiced any specific needs or desires in relation to clinical assignments? Can these be accommodated?

* What is the level of student confidence? Anxiety?

* Can each student function safely? If not, what precautions must be taken as the student proceeds through the clinical day?

* Are there any special needs of patients that can be matched to a student's special abilities?

6. What backup plans are available?

* Can students be paired in providing care without diluting the experience?

* Can students be assigned multiple patients to provide opportunities to practice planning and priority setting when challenging clinical situations are not available?

* Are there any off-unit experiences available that address clinical objectives?

* Can students focus on a single skill set with multiple patients?

* Can case studies and "what if" scenarios be developed to use "down time" effectively (O'Connor, 2015)?

Alternative assignments need to be considered if the clinical site does not support the learners' needs because of lack of patients or an unplanned accreditation visit that curtails student activity in some places. Alternative assignments should meet the course outcomes. Alternative assignments can also be used for makeup days for learners who are absent from clinical assignments. Some alternative assignments may be:

• Observational experiences if they are congruent with the course outcomes

• Case studies about patients who manifest conditions that are consistent with course content (O'Connor, 2015)

LEGAL CONSIDERATIONS OF CLINICAL EDUCATION

Understanding the legal ramifications of clinical instruction is important. Many novice nurse educators say that the learner *"is working under my license."* This is not accurate; the only person who can be working under a license is the person to whom the license is issued. Some guidelines to remember for legal considerations are as follows:

> **Teaching Gem:** Unfolding case studies, books are excellent mechanisms to promote critical thinking and can be used as an alternative assignment when a learner misses clinical instruction (Wittmann-Price & Cornelius, 2011, 2013; Wittmann-Price & Thompson, 2010).

- The staff nurse is ultimately responsible for the patient.
- The nurse educator needs to supervise new procedures.
- Staff nurses, if they choose, can supervise learners.
- Clinical nurse educators should be familiar with the student handbook of the educational unit on which they are working because it outlines what is "unsafe practice."
- Clinical nurse educators should be familiar with the nursing educational program's evaluation forms and program goals.
- Clinical nurse educators should know their learners and the learners' capabilities in order to properly supervise them.

Confidentiality is another issue when teaching in the clinical domain. Learners need to maintain competence in understanding the Health Insurance Portability and Accountability Act (HIPAA), and no patient care issues can be discussed outside the clinical unit's realm (Kan & Stabler-Haas, 2014). Additional precaution must be taken when using mobile electronic devices (MEDs) as reference portals. Devices that are Internet accessible can be a threat to patient confidentiality if used wrongly (Wittmann-Price, Kennedy, & Godwin, 2012).

Nursing students should not share information from the clinical setting on social media. There is a risk of breach of confidentiality when nursing students make posts on social media about a patient (Westrick, 2016). As a result of professional boundaries, students should not become "friends" on social media with patients (Ashton, 2016). It is important to remind nursing students that they should be careful about what they post on social media. Posts can be scrutinized by potential employers or by the nursing program.

PRE- AND POSTCLINICAL CONFERENCES

The clinical day requires thought and preparation for the learners to successfully apply to patient care the knowledge that they have learned in the classroom. The clinical nurse educator needs to reserve space that is accessible and private to facilitate pre- and postclinical conferences. The preclinical conference is a time to review the clinical outcomes, the kinds of the patients the learners will care for, the degree of the preparation the learners have done, and any procedures that may be part of the day. Whether this is done in a formal setting with all learners present or done informally and individually with each learner depends on the level of the learner and the instructor's preference. The goal is to be sure that all learners are adequately prepared. The postclinical conference is a time for learners to process the day's experiences, to debrief, and reflect. According to O'Connor (2015), there are several purposes to postclinical conferences:

- Providing a time for students and instructor to pause and reflect on the day's events, their meaning, and the relation between what has been observed and experienced and what was taught in the classroom or discussed in assigned readings
- Contributing to the achievement of the course and to clinical outcomes by making explicit the connections between clinical activities and the goals for learning
- Examining commonalities and differences in patient responses to illness and its treatment within the clinical specialty
- Permitting students to vicariously share in their peers' experiences, broadening their exposure to the clinical situations they might encounter in practice
- Promoting affective learning through debriefing that allows students to express feelings and attitudes about the experiences they encountered during the day's activities
- Providing students with the experience of the effective use of the group process (O'Connor, 2015).

REFLECTIVE TECHNIQUES AS PART OF THE CLINICAL POSTCONFERENCE

The NLN, in collaboration with the International Nursing Association for Clinical Simulation and Learning (INACSL), believes that "integrating debriefing across the curriculum not just in simulation has the potential to transform nursing education" (2015, p. 2). Critical reflection via debriefing can be a powerful method to guide a postconference discussion. It helps the student to:

- Examine information to see the whole of reality
- Promote "knowing how" and "knowing why" rather than "knowing what"
- Reframe the context of the a situation
- Attach meaning to information

A good debriefing is a theory driven with formal training and ongoing assessment competencies for faculty (NLN, 2015). Two of the most commonly used methods are:

Debriefing with good judgement (Rudolph, Simon, Dufresne, & Raemer, 2006) focuses on:

- Creating a context for adult learners (including the instructor) to learn important lessons that will help them move toward key objectives, determined either unilaterally by the instructor or collaboratively with the trainee and
- Widens to include not only the trainees' actions, but also the meaning-making systems of the trainees such as their frames, assumptions, and knowledge

Debriefing for meaningful learning (Dreifuerst, 2012) has six components.

- Engage (the participants)
- Explore (options reflecting-in-action)
- Explain (decisions, actions, and alternatives using deduction, induction, and analysis)
- Elaborate (thinking like a nurse and expanding analysis and inferential thinking)
- Evaluate (the experience reflecting-on-action
- Extend (inferential and analytic thinking, reflecting-beyond-action)

Students must feel safe. Faculty must correct errors in judgement while helping students feel valued. What is said in postconference must stay in postconference.

THE AFFECTIVE DOMAIN IN CLINICAL PRACTICE

The American Association of Colleges of Nursing (AACN; 2008) identified five core values that epitomize the caring, professional nurse.

1. *Altruism* is a concern for the welfare and well-being of others. In professional practice, altruism is reflected by the nurse's concern and advocacy for the welfare of patients, other nurses, and other health care providers.
2. *Autonomy* is the right of self-determination. Professional practice reflects autonomy when the nurse respects patients' rights to make decisions about their health care.
3. *Human dignity* is respect for the inherent worth and uniqueness of individuals and populations. In professional practice, concern for human dignity is reflected when the nurse values and respects all patients and colleagues.
4. *Integrity* is acting in accordance with an appropriate code of ethics and accepted standards of practice. Integrity is reflected in professional practice when the nurse is honest and provides care based on an ethical framework that is accepted within the profession.
5. *Social justice* is acting in accordance with fair treatment regardless of economic status, ethnicity, age, citizenship, disability, or sexual orientation.

These core values come into play in the clinical area; the clinical nurse educator must be alert to demonstrating how these values inform patient care. Opportunities to apply ethical principles are present in every clinical experience, but often learners need to be prompted to examine their performance and attitudes in light of these values.

STRATEGIES FOR EVALUATING LEARNING IN THE CLINICAL AREA

Although evaluation of learner performance in the clinical area is vital, the clinical nurse educator needs to remember that teaching is primary. Learners need clear definitions of safe and unsafe behaviors, and faculty need to give very specific rationales for their decision to give an unsatisfactory grade. On the other hand, the teacher should remember that often the first time a learner performs a procedure, he or she may need some coaching. There is a fine line between teaching and evaluating in the clinical area. Table 7.2 presents a variety of evaluation methods that are useful when evaluating learners' clinical performance, which include:

- Observation of learners as they perform in the clinical area
- Learners' written work that is used to reveal intellectual processes that guide learners' clinical performance
- Oral presentations
- Simulations
- Learner self-evaluation
- Testimonials/feedback from staff

Frequent feedback (daily if possible) is essential for learners to have the opportunity to improve on areas found to be deficient. Without positive and frequent feedback, the goal of the clinical experience can be lost. Remember, most clinical evaluations are done using a pass/fail mechanism; therefore, the formative evaluations done during the course inform the summative evaluation of pass/fail at the end of the course.

TABLE 7.2
Evaluation Methods

OBSERVATIONS OF LEARNERS AS THEY PERFORM IN CLINICAL SETTINGS	
Anecdotal notes	Data obtained through observation and recorded for later evaluation
Incident reports	Instances of unsafe behavior or unprofessional behavior; if no other instances of unsafe behavior occur, the event should be ignored, unless it is a sentinel event in the learner's final evaluation
Rating scales	Provide a summary of accumulated observations of the learner's clinical performance; these scales are usually based on the course objectives
External raters	A rating done by a person who has not seen the learner perform previously
Videotapes	Videotapes can be recorded in a simulated setting; they are also of value in distance learning settings
Skills checklist	Skills checklists are usually used in the college laboratory and detail the steps for a particular skill; they can be used for teaching as well as learning
EXAMPLES OF WRITTEN WORK THAT REVEAL THE INTELLECTUAL PROCESSES THAT GUIDE LEARNERS' CLINICAL PERFORMANCES	
Observation guides	These guides can be developed to assist the learners in observing an independent assignment or off-unit experience

(continued)

TABLE 7.2 Evaluation Methods (*continued*)	
Process recordings	Process recordings are used to capture interpersonal interactions between the learner and another person; they focus on communication skills
Nursing care plans and care maps	The major nursing care plan and care map details the application of the nursing process for all nursing diagnoses that the learner has identified for a selected patient

Oral presentations—Include communication with staff and instructors, active participation in pre- and postclinical conference, and formal presentations

Simulations—May also be used for evaluation and teaching; these standardize the stimuli to which learners respond and may be in the form of a case study, the use of manikins or models, or standardized patients

Self-evaluation—Often learners provide valuable insights for their instructors when they conduct a self-evaluation

Testimonial—Verbal comments from staff, patients and, in some cases, other learners may play a part in the evaluation process; however, the instructor should validate the observation for himself or herself

Clinical nurse educators often use a clinical evaluation form that ranks learner behavior in all three domains—cognitive, affective, and psychomotor. One of the more well-known ranking scales was devised by Bondy (1983), which rates learner performance as:

- Independent—indicating the learner is proficient and does not waste unnecessary time when completing patient care
- Supervised—the learner expends some extra energy and takes some extra time to complete care, but is safe
- Assisted—the learner needs frequent cues and expends unnecessary energy, but is safe most of the time
- Marginal—at this level, the learner is inefficient and not safe alone
- Dependent—the learner is unsafe and needs continuous verbal cues

Walsh, Jairath, Paterson, and Grandjean (2010) developed a clinical evaluation tool based on the Quality and Safety Education for Nurses (QSEN) that includes rating of the following:

- Provides patient-centered care (caring, spirituality, human dignity, and ethics)
- Exhibits teamwork and collaboration (communication and roles)
- Incorporates evidence-based practice (critical thinking)
- Promotes quality improvement (leadership, assessment)
- Promotes safety (skill)
- Uses informatics (decision making)

THE CLINICAL EVALUATION PROCESS

Clinical evaluation is a process by which judgments are made about learners' competencies in practice. This practice may involve care of patients, families, and communities; other types of learning activities in the clinical setting; simulation activities; performance of varied skills in the learning laboratories; or activities using multimedia (Gaberson et al., 2015).

In the clinical setting, learners are evaluated by the observation of the educator, rating scales, rubrics, skills checklists, journals, logs, and various other types of sources. The major thing to remember is that clinical evaluations should always be based on the objectives/outcomes for the course and the criteria need to be clearly defined.

There are a few principles to keep in mind regarding the clinical evaluation process

- Objectives/outcomes and expectations should be shared with the learner at the beginning of the course and referred to throughout the clinical experience.
- The objectives and criteria can be used in multiple settings, such as the clinical skills laboratory, simulation learning, and clinical experiences in the practice setting.
- In some nursing programs, the clinical evaluations are conducted at Midsemester or midrotation (formative evaluation) and at the end of the experience (summative evaluation). In other programs, daily or weekly evaluations are done after the clinical experience to show progress toward meeting objectives (formative evaluation) and are used to determine whether or not objectives have been achieved at the end of the experience (summative evaluation).
- The clinical grade may be assigned as pass/fail, satisfactory/unsatisfactory, or as a numerical grade in the course. In the course syllabus, nurse educators must document how the grade is calculated. Usually, the learner must achieve a passing or satisfactory grade in the clinical course to pass the nursing course; failure to achieve a satisfactory grade in clinical results in failure of the course in many nursing programs regardless of the grade achieved in the theoretical component of the course.
- The nurse educator should keep anecdotal notes throughout the clinical experience for each learner based on his or her performance for each experience within the confines of the objectives or outcomes. Anecdotal notes are not shared with the learner as they are strictly for the nurse educator's reference.
- If a learner is not doing well in any aspect of the clinical, course conferences should be held with the learner on a regular basis and a formal note, plan, or contract may need to be written that clearly outlines the expectations and what the learner needs to do to meet the objectives. The learner should sign the notes after such meetings.

Feedback is an important aspect of the clinical evaluation. Learners should receive feedback throughout the clinical experience regarding their performance in the clinical setting, areas of strengths, and areas that need improvement. As stated earlier, the learner is judged in the clinical setting by the nurse educator based on objectives, outcomes, competency achievement, and knowledge.

Gaberson et al. (2015) suggest the following principles regarding feedback in the clinical evaluation process:

- The feedback provided by the nurse educator should indicate specific areas of knowledge, competency, skill performance, critical thinking, and judgment that need further development or improvement.
- If the learner needs to improve performance in areas of psychomotor skills or use of technologies, the educator should explain where errors were made, demonstrate to the learner the correct procedure, then allow the learner the opportunity to practice the skill in the presence of the educator.
- Feedback should be given to the learner at the time of learning or as close to it as possible.
- The amount of feedback needed is dependent on the individual learner and the level of progression within the nursing program.
- Positive reinforcement is essential to promote learning in the clinical setting.

EVIDENCE-BASED TEACHING PRACTICE

Clinical nurse educators have an important role in clinical education. Higher self-efficacy levels of students ($N = 236$) were associated with faculty members who gave suggestions for improvement, provided feedback on strengths and weaknesses, observed students frequently, offered clear expectations, gave positive feedback, and offered constructive criticism (Rowbotham & Owen, 2015).

STRATEGIES FOR DEALING WITH UNSAFE OR UNSATISFACTORY LEARNER BEHAVIOR

Unfortunately, clinical nurse educators must deal with unsatisfactory and, at times, unsafe learner behavior. Unsatisfactory behavior by a learner can be exhibited in any of the three learning domains:

1. Cognitive—the learner is just not making the connection in applying theory to practice, demonstrated by thought processes that do not prioritize, delegate, or recognize significant patient care needs
2. Affective—the learner's behavior is unprofessional in appearance (per the student handbook) or there is a habit of tardiness or there are communication (verbally and nonverbally) issues
3. Psychomotor—the learner's behavior is not up to par when performing skills such as gloving, sterilizing, dressing changes, or other procedures

Unsafe behavior may include a sentinel event; this is an occurrence that poses a real risk to the physical or psychological safety of patients. Sometimes it is difficult to determine the difference between unsatisfactory or unsafe behavior. When behavior is unsafe, the clinical nurse educator has an obligation to step in and protect both the patient and the learner.

Documentation and remediation of unsatisfactory behavior is necessary. Many times, the learner can be sent back to the skills laboratory for remediation. Correction of the unsatisfactory behavior is usually expected within a specific time period. A mechanism for documenting the need for remediation is a "learning contract" that specifies the following:

- What behaviors need remediation
- How the remediation will be completed
- What the time frame is for remediation completion
- What consequences can be expected if remediation is not completed or the behavior is repeated

Another common unsatisfactory and potentially unsafe learner behavior is not being prepared for the clinical day. Although many educational units do not participate in "pick up" or recording information about the patient the day before clinical because of security and unit congestion issues, the learner is expected to know the basic information needed to participate in care. Many times, the nursing staff on the unit will also comment on an unprepared learner. The staff on a clinical unit who are familiar with learners are keen observers and can be an evaluative asset (Kan & Stabler-Haas, 2014).

FOSTERING DIVERSITY IN CLE

Minority nursing students may have higher attrition rates. One factor in attrition is not having a sense of "belonging," so it is important for clinical nurse educators to foster that sense of "belonging." Minority students may experience discrimination and bias by patients, nursing staff, other students, and clinical nurse educators. Discriminatory words by patients, nurses, other students, and faculty are hurtful to students, as are gestures, expressions, and certain tones of voice. Experiences in the clinical setting are important to professional integration and socialization of students (Graham, Phillips, Newman, & Atz, 2016). Instructors need to intervene when students are exposed to discriminatory actions by patients and/or nurses (Sedgwick, Oosterbroek, & Ponomar, 2014). Nurse educators need to create environments in which diversity is welcomed and fostered (National League for Nursing, 2016a).

CASE STUDY

CASE STUDY 7.1

A learner at the midpoint of the first senior semester is on an acute care CLE and is assigned three patients. The learner cannot prioritize care and spends an excessive amount of time and energy in organizing the day's tasks. The learner is provided with a formative evaluation and does not improve enough to be passed to the final semester. The learner seeks a grade appeal because the clinical nurse educator was unfair and assigned the learner patients who were more acutely ill than those assigned to other learners. The college's grade appeal committee upholds the clinical nurse faculty member's decision and the learner will have to repeat the course the following semester. What suggestions do you have that would increase the learner's chance of success and promote a fair evaluation process?

PRACTICE QUESTIONS

1. When choosing a clinical unit, the faculty member would consider all of the following environmental conditions EXCEPT:

   A. How actively the students are able to participate in the care of patients

   B. Whether or not new ideas may be implemented

   C. The ratio of staff nurses to patients

   D. Students are able to express their own ideas and opinions

2. When the student says _____, the clinical environment is considered to be a negative one.

   A. "The nurses on this unit consider my feelings and listen to me"

   B. "The nurse manager has decided that I should take a different patient"

   C. "My clinical faculty thinks of innovative activities for the students"

   D. "The nurses on this unit go out of the way to help the students"

3. When conducting a postconference, the faculty feels that the student is reflecting on practice when the student states:

   A. "I gave my patient time to consider her options for the day, but I should have been more directive"

   B. "Our textbook says that the correct dose for that drug is always the same no matter what"

   C. "The nurse manager says we should treat all the patients the same way because it indicates that we do not have favorites"

   D. "The patient was uncomfortable but the staff did not think I should move her"

4. Critical reflection via debriefing enables the faculty member to help the students in all ways EXCEPT:

   A. Examining information to see all of reality

   B. Promoting knowing what to knowing how

   C. Reframing the context of a situation

   D. Ignoring past learning

5. The clinical nurse educator realizes that dedicated educational units (DEUs) include which of the following qualities: (Select all that apply.)

   A. Promote quality care and patient safety

   B. Are confusing to students

   C. Allow students the chance for enhanced mentorship

   D. Permit students to practice with communication and teamwork

6. A clinical nurse educator is on a renal unit with senior-level students. There is a low patient census today. All of the following are alternatives that may be considered for students EXCEPT:

   A. Observational assignment that meets the course outcomes

   B. Dual assignments

   C. Case studies

   D. Cancellation of the clinical day

7. The clinical nurse educator receives a phone call from a family member that a student has posted information about a patient on social media. What is the most appropriate response?

A. This is a HIPAA violation and must be reported

B. HIPAA does not include social media

C. Maybe no one else will find out about this, so I will just keep it to myself

D. Have the student apologize to the patient

8. The students in the clinical group feel that postclinical conference is a "waste of time." How should the clinical nurse educator respond? (Select all that apply.)

A. We will start doing a shorter postclinical conference because it is not beneficial to you

B. Postclinical conference gives you a chance to reflect on your day

C. Postclinical conference allows you to learn from the instructor

D. Student-led postclinical conferences are not an option

9. During the first 2 weeks of the semester, the clinical nurse educator has noticed that one student has had difficulty with assessing patients in the clinical learning environment. What is the best response by the nurse educator?

A. I will wait until the student's summative evaluation to discuss this because the student may be nervous

B. I will provide feedback to the student after each clinical day and assess whether improvement occurs

C. I will keep careful notes on this and communicate with the course coordinator at the end of the course

D. I will wait until the midterm clinical evaluation to discuss this

10. The nurse educator in a women's health course has scheduled a clinical day in a women's homeless shelter. Another educator is concerned because it is not a traditional clinical setting and the shelter does not have a nurse. All of the following are appropriate responses EXCEPT:

A. The women at the homeless shelter have unmet health care needs, and I want the students to learn more about their experiences

B. I feel that the clinical setting meets the course learning outcomes objective related to health disparities

C. The hospital is having an accreditation visit and this is an alternative clinical site that fits well with my course

D. I will schedule a traditional clinical day because there are no nurses at the shelter

REFERENCES

American Association of Colleges of Nursing. (2008). *The essentials of baccalaureate education for professional nursing practice.* Washington, DC: Author. Retrieved from http://www.aacn.nche.edu/education-resources/BaccEssentials08.pdf

Andresen, K., & Levin, P. (2014). Enhancing quantity and quality of clinical experiences in a baccalaureate nursing program. *International Journal of Nursing Education Scholarship, 11*(1), 137–144. doi:10.1515/ijnes-2013-0053

Ashton, K. S. (2016). Teaching nursing students about terminating professional relationships, boundaries, and social media. *Nurse Education Today, 37*, 170–172. doi:10.1016/j. nedt.2015.11.007

Baker, C. (1996). Clinical education: A teaching strategy for critical thinking. *Journal of Nursing Education, 35*, 19–22.

Benner, P. (1982). From novice to expert. *American Journal of Nursing, 82*(3), 402–407.

Billings, D. M., & Halstead, J. A. (2016). *Teaching in nursing: A guide for faculty* (5th ed.). St. Louis, MO: Elsevier.

Bondy, K. (1983). Criterion-referenced definitions for rating scales in clinical evaluation. *Journal of Nursing Education, 122*(9), 376–382.

Bryan, V. D., Lindo, J., Anderson-Johnson, P., & Weaver, S. (2015). Using Carl Rogers' person-centered model to explain interpersonal relationships at a school of nursing. *Journal of Professional Nursing, 31*(2), 141–148. doi:10.1016/j .profnurs.2014.07.003

Carlson, E., Pilhammar, E., & Wann-Hansson, C. (2010). Time to precept: Supportive and limiting conditions for precepting nurses. *Journal of Advanced Nursing, 66*(2), 432–441. doi:10.1111/j.1365-2648.2009.05174.x

Carlson, J. S. (2015). Factors influencing retention among part-time clinical nursing faculty. *Nursing Education Perspectives, 36*(1), 42–45. doi:10.5480/13-1231

Chan, D. (2002). Development of the clinical learning environment inventory: Using the theoretical framework of learning environment studies to assess nursing students' perceptions of the hospital as a learning environment. *Journal of Nursing Education, 41*(2), 69–76.

Clark, C. L. (2013). A mixed-method study on the socialization process in clinical nursing faculty. *Nursing Education Perspectives, 34*(2), 106–110.

Dahlke, S., O'Connor, M., Hannesson, T., & Cheetham, K. (2016). Understanding clinical nursing education: An exploratory study. *Nurse Education in Practice, 17*, 145–152. doi:10.1016/j.nepr.2015.12.004

Dreifuerst, K. (2012). Using debriefing for meaningful learning to foster development of clinical reasoning in simulation. *Journal of Nursing Education, 61*(6), 326–333.

Flott, E. A., & Linden, L. (2016). The clinical learning environment in nursing education: A concept analysis. *Journal of Advanced Nursing, 72*(3), 501–513. doi: 10.1111/jan.12861

Fura, L. A., & Symanski, M. E. (2014). An online approach to orienting clinical nursing faculty in baccalaureate nursing education. *Nursing Education Perspectives, 35*(5), 324–326. doi:10.5480/12-868.1

Gaberson, K., Oermann, M. H., & Shellenbarger, T. (2015). *Clinical teaching strategies in nursing* (4th ed.). New York, NY: Springer Publishing.

Graham, C. L., Phillips, S. M., Newman, S. D., & Atz, T. W. (2016). Baccalaureate minority nursing students perceived barriers and facilitators to clinical education practices: An integrative review. *Nursing Education Perspectives, 37*(3), 130–137.

Haitana, J., & Bland, M. (2011). Building relationships: The key to preceptoring nursing students. *Nursing Praxis in New Zealand, 27*(1), 4–12.

Hanson, K., & Stenvig, T. E. (2008). The good clinical nursing educator and the baccalaureate nursing clinical experience: Attributes and praxis. *Journal of Nursing Education, 47*(1), 38–42.

Infante, M. S. (1975). *The clinical laboratory in nursing education*. New York, NY: Wiley.

Ingwerson, J. (2014). Tailoring the approach to precepting: Student nurse vs. new hire. *Oregon State Board of Nursing Sentinel, 33*(2), 11–13.

Kan, E. Z., & Stabler-Haas, S. (2014). *Fast facts for the clinical nursing instructor* (2nd ed.). New York, NY: Springer Publishing.

McCutcheon, K., Lohan, M., Traynor, M., & Martin, D. (2015). A systematic review evaluating the impact of online or blended learning vs. face-to-face learning of clinical skills in undergraduate nurse education. *Journal of Advanced Nursing, 71*(2), 255–270. doi:10.1111/jan.12509

McNelis, A. M., Ironside, P. M., Ebright, P. R., Dreifuerst, K. T., Zvonar, S. E., & Conner, S. C. (2014). Learning nursing practice: A multisite, multimethod investigation of clinical education. *Journal of Nursing Regulation, 4*(4), 30–35.

Mulready-Shick, J., Kafel, K. W., Banister, G., & Mylott, L. (2009). Enhancing quality and safety competency development at the unit level: An initial evaluation of student learning and clinical teaching on dedicated education units. *Journal of Nursing Education, 48*(12), 716–719. doi:10.3928/01484834-20091113-11

Nafei, A. R., Markani, A. K., Motearafi, H., Moghadam, Y. H., & Sakaei, S. H. (2015). The effect of reflecting journaling on nursing students' critical thinking in clinical activities. *Journal of Urmia Nursing & Midwifery Faculty, 13*(1), 19–26.

National League for Nursing. (2016a). Achieving diversity and meaningful inclusion in nursing education. Retrieved from http://www.nln.org/docs/default-source/about/vision-statement-achieving-diversity.pdf?sfvrsn=2

National League for Nursing. (2016b). Certified nurse educator (CNE) candidate handbook. Retrieved from http://www.nln.org/docs/default-source/professionaldevelopment-programs/certified-nurse-educator-%28cne%29-examination-candidate-handbook.pdf?sfvrsn=2

Newton, J. M., Jolly, B. C., Ockerby, J. M., & Cross, W. M. (2012). Student centredness in clinical learning: The influence of the clinical teacher. *Journal of Advanced Nursing, 68*(1), 2331–2340. doi:10.1111/j.1365-2648.2012.05946.x

Nishioka, V. M., Coe, M. T., Hanita, M., & Moscato, S. R. (2014a). Dedicated education unit: Nurse perspectives on their clinical teaching role. *Nursing Education Perspectives, 35*(5), 294–300. doi:10.5480/14-1381

Nishioka, V. M., Coe, M. T., Hanita, M., & Moscato, S. R. (2014b). Dedicated education unit: Student perspectives. *Nursing Education Perspectives, 35*(5), 301–307. doi:10.5480/14-1380

O'Connor, A. (2015). *Clinical instruction and evaluation: A teaching resource* (3rd ed.). Sudbury, MA: Jones & Bartlett.

O'Mara, L., McDonald, J., Gillespie, M., Brown, H., & Miles, L. (2014). Challenging clinical learning environments: Experiences of undergraduate nursing students. *Nurse Education in Practice, 14*(2), 208–213. doi:10.1016/j.nepr.2013.08.012

Raines, D. A. (2012). Nurse preceptors' views of precepting undergraduate nursing students. *Nursing Education Perspectives, 33*(2), 76–79. doi:10.5480/1536-5026-33.2.76

Rowbotham, M., & Owen, R. M. (2015). The effect of clinical nursing instructors on student self-efficacy. *Nurse Education in Practice, 15*(6), 561–566. doi:10.1016/j.nepr.2015.09.008

Rudolph, J., Simon, R., Dufresne, R., & Raemer, D. (2006). There's no such thing as "nonjudgmental" debriefing: A theory and method for debriefing with good judgment. *Simulation in Health Care, 1*(1), 49–55.

Scholtz, S. M. P. (2007). Management strategies in clinical care settings. In B. Moyer & R. A. Wittmann-Price (Eds.), *Nursing education: Foundations for practice excellence* (pp. 251–261). Philadelphia, PA: F. A. Davis.

Sedgwick, T., Oosterbroek, T., & Ponomar, V. (2014). 'It all depends': How minority nursing students experience belonging during clinical experiences. *Nursing Education Perspectives, 35*(2), 89–93. doi:10.5480/11-707.1

Turner, S. (2015). Interprofessional clinical assignments: A project in nursing education. *Creative Nursing, 21*(3), 156–160.

Walsh, T., Jairath, N., Paterson, M. A., & Grandjean, C. (2010). Quality and safety education for nurses clinical evaluation tool. *Journal of Nursing Education, 49*(9), 517–522.

Westrick, S. J. (2016). Nursing students' use of electronic and social media: Law, ethics, and e-professionalism. *Nursing Education Perspectives, 37*(1), 16–22. doi:10.5480/14-1358

Wittmann-Price, R. A., & Cornelius, F. (2011). *Maternal–child nursing test success: An unfolding case study review.* New York, NY: Springer Publishing.

Wittmann-Price, R. A., & Cornelius, F. (2013). *Nursing fundamentals: An unfolding case study review.* New York, NY: Springer Publishing.

Wittmann-Price, R. A., Kennedy, L., & Godwin, K. (2012). The use of personal phones by senior nursing students to access health care information during clinical education: Staff nurses' and students' perceptions. *Journal of Nursing Education, 51*(11), 642–646. doi:10.3928/01484834-20120914-04

Wittmann-Price, R. A., & Thompson, B. R. (Eds.). (2010). *NCLEX-RN® EXCEL: Test success through unfolding case study review.* New York, NY: Springer Publishing.

Woolsey, C., & Bracy, K. (2012). Building a clinical ladder for ambulatory care. *Nursing Economic$, 30*(1), 45–49.

Learning With Simulation

LINDA WILSON AND DORIE WEAVER

> *A mind is a simulation that simulates itself.*
> —Erol Ozan

This chapter addresses the Certified Nurse Educator Exam Content Area 1: Facilitate Learning (National League for Nursing [NLN], 2016, pp. 5–6).

- Content Area 1 is 22% of the examination
- It is estimated that there will be approximately 38 questions from Content Area 1

LEARNING OUTCOMES

- Discuss the role of simulation learning experiences in nursing education
- Describe the types of simulation and their use in nursing education
- Describe strategies to integrate simulation into the learning environment
- Discuss the importance of evaluation of simulated experiences
- Review the opportunities for certification in simulation

TYPES OF SIMULATION

Simulation Using the Human Patient Simulator

Human patient simulator (HPS) simulation includes the use of low-fidelity, midfidelity, and high-fidelity manikins. The fidelity of the manikin determines the complexity and realism of the manikin's capabilities. The high-fidelity manikin can cry, sweat,

Teaching Gem: Simulation is an effective teaching strategy in enhancing collaborative communication, mutual respect, problem solving, and shared decision making when conducted utilizing a team-based, interprofessional approach. Simulation can use individuals from various professions, such as medicine, pharmacy, case management, physical therapy, and nutrition.

seize, has pupils that react to light, has changeable heart sounds, has changeable lung sounds, can physiologically react to medication administration, and much more. There are several companies that produce and sell these manikins with varying fidelity. HPS simulation provides students opportunities to apply their skills and knowledge based on realistic clinical scenarios. HPS simulation allows students to practice in a safe and controlled environment where there is no threat for patient harm (Turrentine et al., 2016).

EVIDENCE-BASED TEACHING PRACTICE

Liaw, Siau, Zhou, and Lau (2014) carried out a prospective, quasi-experimental study to examine the effects of an interprofessional simulation-based communication education program on medical and nursing students' attitudes toward nurse–physician collaboration. The study included third-year nursing students ($N = 79$), and third- and fourth-year medical students ($N = 23$). The 14-item Jefferson Scale of Attitudes Toward Physician–Nurse Collaboration (JSATPNC) was given as pre- and posttests to determine the participants' attitudes toward physician–nurse collaboration. The JSATPNC has four subscales: shared educational and collaborative relationships, caring as opposed to curing, nurses' autonomy, and physician's authority. An internal consistency of Cronbach's alpha (0.85–0.87) was obtained in this study. Both nursing and medical participants demonstrated a significant improvement in posttest scores from baseline for their total score on attitudes toward nurse–physician collaboration.

Simulation Using Standardized Patients

A *standardized patient* (SP) is an actor who has been trained to portray a patient in a consistent manner in a specific scenario portraying a medical condition, a psychiatric disorder, an ethical situation, or any other health care situation (Onori, Pampaloni, & Multak, 2012). The SP simulation is an excellent method of simulation because the patients can portray real emotions, such as anxiety or depression, and can even cry on demand.

SPs can be hired to work in the simulation laboratory for specific simulation experiences. If an organization cannot afford to hire SPs, it can possibly contract with the drama department at their school, a drama club in their community, or they can even seek volunteers for patients.

Hybrid Simulation

Hybrid simulation is the term used for a simulation that uses a combination of HPS simulation and SP simulation. For example, a simulation scenario in which a baby manikin is being used as the patient and an SP is portraying the parent is considered to be a hybrid simulation.

Simulation Using Part-Task Trainers

Part-task trainers (PTT) are used to teach a specific skill or set of specific skills, usually related to clinical procedures. PTTs "range in complexity from a piece of fruit to teach injections to a torso to teach central line placement" (Arnold & Wittmann-Price, 2015, p. 170). Simulation using a PTT "usually does not include patient feedback or debriefing" (Arnold & Wittmann-Price, 2015, p. 170). Complex PTTs increase the fidelity of the learning experience by allowing the learner to use a combination of PTT in conjunction with a computer-based simulated environment (Galloway, 2009).

CRITICAL THINKING QUESTION

If there are no actors or actresses available in your educational system, what other resources could be used to incorporate SPs? Perhaps senior groups, other learners, and so forth?

SIMULATION CASE DEVELOPMENT

HPS Simulation Cases

> **Teaching Gem:** When selecting an actor for a standardized patient simulation, to be most effective it is most important to be most effective it is someone whom the learner does not know.

HPS simulation cases can be obtained in a variety of ways. They can be purchased as preprogramed scenarios from a manikin vendor. The faculty can also choose to create and program their own scenarios using the simulator software. Another easy way to run scenarios is to have a faculty member adjust the actions of the manikin while the scenario is taking place based on the actions of the simulation participants. See Exhibit 8.1 for a sample template HPS case development.

EXHIBIT 8.1

HPS Simulation Scenario Template

Authors:
Date/Time of Scenario:
Case Title:
Target Audience:
Primary Learning Objectives: key learning objectives of the scenario
Critical actions checklist: a list to ensure the educational/assessment goals are met.
Environment (if using as a simulation case)
    1. Room Setup
       a. Audio visual
       b. Other equipment
Actors
    1. Roles

For Instructor ONLY
Authors:
Case Title:

(continued)

EXHIBIT 8.1

HPS Simulation Scenario Template *(continued)*

CASE SUMMARY

SYNOPSIS OF CASE

SYNOPSIS OF HISTORY/SCENARIO BACKGROUND

SYNOPSIS OF PHYSICAL

For Participants

HISTORY

Onset of Symptoms:

Background Info:

Chief Complaint:

Past Medical History:

Past Surgical History:

Family Medical History:

Social History:

For Instructor ONLY

PHYSICAL EXAMINATION

Patient:
Age and Sex:
General Appearance:
Vital Signs:
Blood pressure:
Pulse:
Respiratory rate:
Temperature:

(continued)

EXHIBIT 8.1

HPS Simulation Scenario Template *(continued)*

Head:
Eyes:
Ears:
Mouth:
Neck:

Skin:
Chest:
Heart:

Abdomen:
Extremities:
Neurological:
Mental Status:

Learner Stimulus

Hospital

Admitting Form

Name:

Age:

Sex:

Method of transportation:

Person giving information:

Presenting Complaint:

Background:

Triage or Initial Vital Signs:

Blood pressure:
Pulse:
Respiratory rate:
Temperature:

CASE:

Critical Actions:

Additional documentation and supporting material for scenario: (i.e., Advanced Cardiac Life Support [ACLS] algorithm, APGAR scoring, etc.)

Developed by Carol Okupniak.
Reprinted with permission.

SP Simulation Cases

SP simulation cases are usually written by the faculty member who is planning and running the simulation experience. Because the SPs are actors, they need a very detailed script. The SP simulation case will include the following sections: patient name, timing for the simulation encounter, setting, overview of the scenario, instructions or door sign explaining the condition of the patient in the room, opening line, patient position and attire, challenge questions, questions that might be asked during the simulation and the specific answer required, evaluation criteria/checklist items, passing score, and type of feedback.

Prior to an SP simulation experience, the SPs will participate in training for the simulation experience (Onori et al., 2012; Wilson, 2015). The training will include the review of the SP case scenario or script, opportunity for questions and answers, demonstration of physical exam techniques if indicated, and role-play to practice the scenario.

See Exhibit 8.2 for a sample template of an SP simulation case development.

EXHIBIT 8.2

SP Simulation Case Template

Title of the Case:

Patient name: Mr./Mrs. Toni Smith

Length of time for the encounter (maximum time the student can be in the room—15 minutes/30 minutes/45 minutes):
Checklist time: 10 minutes
Feedback time: 10 minutes
Turnaround time: 5 minutes

Setting:

Overview of the scenario background for the patient:

Instructions/door sign: (Information for the student to see prior to the experience includes what is to be done during the experience and ends with how many minutes the student has to complete the experience.):

Mr./Mrs. Toni Smith came to the _____ for _____.
You have _____ minutes to _____.

Opening line (What you want the patient to say at the beginning of the experience.):

Patient position at start of the scenario (sitting on table/sitting in chair):

Patient dress at start of the scenario (regular clothes/patient gown):

(continued)

EXHIBIT 8.2

SP Simulation Case Template (*continued*)

Challenge question (The question that the patient is to ask the student during the experience, plus the answer to the question.):

Questions during the experience (training questions) (Identify questions that the learner may ask during the experience that *require a specific answer*—List the questions below *and* the answers to the questions. For all other questions, the patient can "use his or her own" information.):

Please delete/change/add to the list below

What is your age? Use your own

Are you married? Use your own

Occupation? Use your own

Have you ever had anything similar in the past? Yes. I was seen in the emergency department approximately 6 months ago with the same problem.

Have you ever used any recreational drugs? No

Have you ever been hospitalized? No, or use your own if necessary (e.g., due to scar).

Have you ever had surgery? No, or use your own if necessary (e.g., due to scar)

Have you ever been pregnant? Use your own

Do you have any chronic illnesses? I have diabetes

Are you taking any medications? Insulin 70/30

How is your father? Died a few years ago from a stroke

How is your mother? Alive, has a history of knee amputation, history of diabetes

(continued)

EXHIBIT 8.2

SP Simulation Case Template *(continued)*

How is/are your sibling(s)? Healthy

Past health history:

Immunizations up to date?

Diet activity/exercise:

Medications:
Prescription medications—
Over the counter medications—
Medication allergies—
Seasonal allergies—

Psychosocial history:

Passing score:

Checklist items (Items used to evaluate the student during the experience. Each
of these items will be marked one of the following: Done/Not Done/N/A):

Communication
1. Introduces self with name and title
2. Good eye contact (at least 50% of the time)
3. Was professional in manner
4. Speaks clearly in terms the patient can understand (three-strikes rule)
5. Active listener
6. Asked about
7. Asked about
8.
9.
10.

Physical Examination
1. Washes hands before the examination
2. Explained to me what he or she was doing with each step of the examination
3.
4.
5.
6.
7.
8.

(continued)

EXHIBIT 8.2

SP Simulation Case Template *(continued)*

    9.
    10.

    Patient Education
    1. Discussed the importance of
    2. Discussed the danger signs of
    3. Offered information or suggested some options for
    4.
    5.
    6.
    7.
    8.
    9.
    10.
                SP will also provide feedback—Interpersonal

Developed by Linda Wilson.

SIMULATION EVALUATION

HPS Simulation Evaluation

The evaluation for the HPS simulation usually includes an evaluation of a group as a team plus individual evaluations. The evaluation is usually developed in the form of a checklist to evaluate what the learner did or did not do during the simulation encounter. The checklist will usually include evaluation items on communication, physical examination, and patient teaching. The evaluation checklist can be as simple or complex as needed, based on the objectives of the simulation. The evaluation checklist is usually completed by the faculty member who is observing the simulation encounter.

Adamson, Kardong-Edgren, and Willhaus (2013) state simulation use continues to spiral upward as an effective pedagogical method across undergraduate nursing curricula. As a result of this significant surge, there is a substantial need for further development of reliable and valid measurement tools specifically designed to accurately assess student performance in the simulation environment. According to Stiller et al. (2015), it is imperative that careful consideration be given when selecting an instrument to ensure it is suitable to both the activity and the learner. "Evaluation instruments must match the scenario and be specific enough to identify the essential performance requirements in order to decrease subjectivity of the rater" (Stiller et al., 2015, p. 89).

It is equally important to continue building evidence for the use of stimulation to facilitate learning. Faculty should have an evaluation of the effectiveness of the actual simulation case created, students' subjective report of satisfaction and self-confidence levels pre- and postsimulation, and/or the educational practices at the end of the simulation. Several tools have been developed to obtain this data (Franklin, Burns, & Lee, 2014). Refer to the box titled "Evidence-Based Teaching Practice" (Franklin et al., 2014). In contrast to the skills/competencies checklist, these two scales would be completed by the student.

EVIDENCE-BASED TEACHING PRACTICE

Adamson and Kardong-Edgren (2012) psychometrically assessed three simulation evaluation instruments—the Lasater Clinical Judgment Rubric, Seattle University Evaluation, and the Creighton Simulation Evaluation Instrument—by having nurse educators (N = 29–38) assess videotaped scenarios with nursing learners. The Cronbach's alpha of all three instruments was 0.97, 0.97, and 0.98, respectively. This method is a reliable one to use to evaluate the instruments used in simulation experiences.

Franklin et al. (2014) conducted psychometric measures of the Student Satisfaction and Self-Confidence in Learning Scale, Simulation Design Scale, and Educational Practices in Simulation Scale on prelicensure nurses. All three scales were noted to have adequate reliability and validity to be used in education research.

SP Simulation Evaluation

The evaluation for the SP simulation is usually an evaluation of an individual who participated in the simulation with the SP. If there is more than one participant in the SP simulation, team evaluation can also be incorporated. The evaluation is usually developed in the form of a checklist to evaluate what the learner did or did not do during the simulation encounter (Saewert & Rockstraw, 2012). The checklist can include evaluation items on communication, physical examination, patient teaching, diagnosis, follow-up, and teamwork. The selection of evaluation items are also based on the level and type of health professions learner. The evaluation checklist can be as simple or complex as needed, based on the objectives for the simulation.

FEEDBACK

The "final phase in a SP simulation experience is the feedback" session (Onori et al., 2012, p. 26). Once the simulation encounter is done, and the evaluation checklist or postencounter documentation has been completed, the learner and the SP will meet for the feedback session. During the feedback session, the SP is no longer acting and the SP provides the learner with constructive feedback on how the learner made him or her feel as a patient, and any other specifics as determined by the faculty member prior to the encounter. The learners often comment that the feedback session is the most rewarding part of the SP simulation experience.

DEBRIEFING

Debriefing is an essential and vital learning component of simulation. It is a learning experience in which "reflective thinking on past actions" is used to "enhance student learning, clarify concepts, and acknowledge and support the student" (Morse, 2012, p. 58). Debriefing commonly takes place following an HPS simulation experience in a location near but separate from the simulation location. The time spent by the students, with faculty direction in a form of guided reflection, is the reason debriefing is a significant component of simulation. Debriefing affords the student an opportunity to analyze the events as they occurred. Students can examine the scenario from various perspectives, which will enhance their future clinical decision-making and problem-solving skills. Debriefing is critical to the learning experience (Shinnick, Woo, Hardwick, & Steadman, 2011) and it is imperative that the facilitator is adequately prepared to ensure a successful outcome.

Essentials for the debriefing facilitator include the following:

- Formal training in debriefing
- Being present to observe the scenario to be debriefed
- Select and use a specific model for debriefing
- Facilitate guided reflection

There are many different methods for debriefing, including the following:

- Case Study Review Debriefing (Overstreet, 2009)
- Plus/Delta Debriefing (Gardner, 2013)
- Advocacy Inquiry/Debriefing with Good Judgement (Rudolph, Simon, Rivard, Dufresne, & Raemer, 2007)
- Structured and Supported Debriefing
- Promoting Excellence and Reflective Learning in Simulation: PEARLS (Eppich & Cheng, 2015)
- Debriefing for Meaningful Learning: DML (Dreifuerst, 2015)
- 3-D Model of Debriefing: Defusing, Discovering, Deepening (Jigmont, 2011)

As faculty facilitators are developing their debriefing skills, they should identify which model of debriefing they find most effective. Some nursing programs may instead select a specific type of debriefing model and require that specific type of debriefing be used for all simulation activities in their program.

SIMULATION CERTIFICATIONS

Certified Healthcare Simulation Educator (CHSE)—The CHSE certification is offered by the Society for Simulation in Healthcare (SSH). Eligibility, benefits, application process, fees, and exam prep resources can be found on the SSH website at www.ssih.org/Certification.

Certified Healthcare Simulation Educator—Advanced (CHSE-A)—The CHSE-A certification is offered by the SSH. Eligibility, benefits, application process, fees, and portfolio requirements can be found on the SSH website at www.ssih.org/Certification.

Certified Healthcare Simulation Operations Specialist (CHSOS)—CHSOS certification is offered by the SSH. Eligibility, benefits, application process, fees, and exam prep resources can be found on the SSH website at www.ssih.org/Certification.

CASE STUDY

CASE STUDY 8.1

A simulation coordinator is orienting the nursing learners to the HPS for the first time. The simulation coordinator and the clinical nursing faculty members are in the simulation room with the learners. The learners start to practice vital signs on the HPS, and the clinical nursing instructor starts to tell them that they are taking the blood pressure incorrectly. How should the simulation coordinator respond to this? Is this the purpose of the orientation session? How can difficult situations in the orientation session be prevented?

PRACTICE QUESTIONS

1. When discussing HPS simulation, what does *HPS* stand for?
   A. Health care procedure simulation
   B. Human patient simulator
   C. Health care process simulator
   D. Human procedure simulation

2. What is a standardized patient?
   A. An actor trained to portray a patient
   B. A type of HPS manikin
   C. A computer program for health care diseases
   D. A virtual reality serious game

3. What attribute is not associated with *fidelity*?
   A. Realism
   B. Capabilities
   C. Complexity
   D. Risk-taking

4. What is the process by which the standardized patients (SPs) learn the simulation scenario?
   A. Simulation feedback
   B. Role-play
   C. Scenario review
   D. SP training

5. Possible resources for standardized patients include the following:
   A. Volunteers
   B. Faculty
   C. Students
   D. Immunosuppressed patients

6. Which of the following is an example of a part-task trainer (PTT)?

    A. Pelvis that can be used for Foley catheter insertion

    B. Pelvis that can birth a baby with complications such as bleeding

    C. An intravenous (IV) arm connected to a virtual patient

    D. Nasogastric insertion setup connected to a virtual patient

7. Following an standardized patient (SP) simulation experience the learner has the opportunity to meet with the SP one on one. What is this process called?

    A. Debriefing

    B. Evaluation

    C. Feedback

    D. Review

8. Which of the following is an example of complex a part-task trainer (PTT)?

    A. Patient torso with multiple lung sounds

    B. Laparoscopic trainer connected to virtual patient

    C. IV cushion with multiple injection sites

    D. Pelvis with male and female genitalia

9. Which of the following are essential for a debriefing facilitator?

    A. Has observed someone else debrief

    B. Received a report of how the scenario went

    C. Select and use a specific model for debriefing

    D. Be ready to explain better interventions than what was done

10. Where can a faculty obtain simulation scenarios for a human patient simulator (HPS) manikin?

    A. Free from a vendor

    B. Design their own

    C. Run the scenario on the fly

    D. Take it from medicine

REFERENCES

Adamson, K. A., & Kardong-Edgren, S. (2012). A method and resources for assessing the reliability of simulation evaluation instruments. *Nursing Education Perspectives, 33*(5), 334–339.

Adamson, K. A., Kardong-Edgren, S., & Willhaus, J. (2013). An updated review of published evaluation instruments. *Clinical Simulation in Nursing, 9*(9), e393–e400. doi:10.1016/j.ecns.2012.09.004

Arnold, D., & Wittman-Price, R. (2015). Part-task trainers. In L. Wilson & R. Wittmann-Price (Eds.), *Review manual for the certified healthcare simulation educator exam*. New York, NY: Springer Publishing.

Dreifuerst, K. T. (2015). Getting started with debriefing for meaningful learning. *Clinical Simulation in Nursing, 11*(5), 268–275.

Eppich, W., & Cheng, A. (2015). Promoting excellence and reflective learning in simulation (PEARLS). *Simulation in Healthcare, 10*, 106–115.

Franklin, A. E., Burns, P., & Lee, C. S. (2014). Psychometric testing on the NLN student satisfaction and self-confidence in learning, simulation design scale, and educational practices questionnaire using a sample of pre-licensure novice nurses. *Nurse Education Today, 34*(10), 1298–1304. doi:10.1016/j.nedt.2014.06.011

Galloway, S. J. (2009). Simulation techniques to bridge the gap between novice and competent healthcare professionals. *Online Journal of Nursing Issues in Nursing, 14*(2), 166–174. Retrieved from http://www.nursingworld.org/MainMenuCategories/ANAMarketplace/ANAPeriodicals/OJIN/TableofContents/Vol142009/No2May09/Simulation-Techniques.html?css=print

Gardner, R. (2013). Introduction to debriefing. *Seminars in Perinatology, 37*(3), 166–174. doi:10.1053/j.semperi.2013.02.008

Jigmont, J. J. (2011). The 3D model of debriefing: Defusing, discovering, and deepening. *Seminars in Perinatology, 35*(2), 52–58. doi:10.1053/j.semperi.2011.01.003

Liaw, S., Siau, C., Zhou, W. T., & Lau, T. C. (2014). Interprofessional simulation-based education program: A promising approach for changing stereotypes and improving attitudes towards nurse–physician collaboration. *Applied Nursing Research, 27*, 258–260.

Morse, C. J. (2012). Debriefing after simulated patient experiences. In L. Wilson & L. Rockstraw (Eds.), *Human simulation for nursing and health professions.* New York, NY: Springer Publishing.

National League for Nursing. (2016). Certified nurse educator (CNE) 2016 candidate handbook. Retrieved from http://www.nln.org/docs/default-source/professional-development-programs/certified-nurse-educator-(cne)-examination-candidate-handbook.pdf?sfvrsn=2

Onori, M., Pampaloni, F., & Multak, N. (2012). What is a standardized patient?. In L. Wilson & L. Rockstraw (Eds.), *Human simulation for nursing and health professions.* New York, NY: Springer Publishing.

Overstreet, M. L. (2009). *The current practice of nursing clinical simulation debriefing: A multiple case study* (Doctoral dissertation). University of Tennessee, Knoxville, TN. Retrieved from http://trace.tennessee.edu/utk_graddiss/627

Rudolph, J. W., Simon, R., Rivard, P., Dufresne, R. L., & Raemer, D. B. (2007). Debriefing with good judgement: Combining rigorous feedback with genuine inquiry. *Anesthesiology Clinics, 25*, 361–376.

Saewert, K., & Rockstraw, L. (2012). Development of evaluation measures for human simulation: The checklist. In L. Wilson & L. Rockstraw (Eds.), *Human simulation for nursing and health professions.* New York, NY: Springer Publishing.

Shinnick, M. A., Woo, M., Horwich, T. B., & Steadman, R. (2011). Debriefing: The most important component in simulation. *Clinical Simulation in Nursing, 7*(3), e105–e111. doi:10.1016/j.ecns.2010.11.005

Stiller, J. J., Nelson, K. A., Anderson, M., Ashe, M. J., Johnson, S. T., Sandhu, K., . . . LeFlore, J. (2015). Development of a valid and reliable evaluation instrument for undergraduate nursing students during simulation. *Journal of Nursing Education and Practice, 5*(7), 83–90.

Turrentine, F. E., Rose, K. M., Hanks, J. B., Lorntz, B., Owen, J. A., Brashers, V. L., & Ramsdale, E. E. (2016). Interprofessional training enhances collaboration between nursing and medical students: A pilot study. *Nurse Education Today, 40*, 33–38.

Wilson, L. (2015). Principles, practice and methodologies for SP simulation. In L. Wilson & R. Wittmann-Price (Eds.), *Review manual for the certified healthcare simulation educator exam.* New York, NY: Springer Publishing.

Facilitating Learner Development and Socialization

MARYANN GODSHALL

Be the change you want to see in the world.
—Mahatma Gandhi

This chapter addresses the Certified Nurse Educator Exam Content Area 2: Facilitate Learner Development and Socialization (National League for Nursing [NLN], 2016, p. 5).

- Content Area 2 is 14% of the examination
- It is estimated that there will be approximately 21 questions from Content Area 2

LEARNING OUTCOMES

- Discuss individual learning styles
- Explore the characteristics of the adult learner
- Understand academic dishonesty and incivility
- Recognize culturally diverse learners
- Identify those with learning disabilities
- Discuss socialization into nursing

Today, learners present educators with a wide variety of challenges in meeting their educational needs. An educator must take into account the learner's cultural, social, and economic background, as well as his or her individual learning style and cognitive ability. These challenges are increased by the need of faculty to incorporate diverse learning environments into teaching, including simulation experiences, online learning, and the integration of new technology into the classroom, including audience response systems (clickers), podcasts, blogs, and wiki pages. Added to this is the ever-present need to present information while making the learning environment interactive. This challenges even the most experienced nurse educator. Integrating all these elements while also incorporating basic education principles is important so that learners not only learn, but also are able to pass the National Council Licensure Examination (NCLEX®) when they graduate.

ASSESSING READINESS TO LEARN

Before learning can occur, one must determine whether learners are ready to receive the information to be learned (Table 9.1).

Readiness to learn occurs when the learner is receptive, willing, and able to participate in the learning process (Bastable, 2013). There are five major components to physical readiness that affect learning:

1. Measure of ability
2. Complexity of the task
3. Environmental effects
4. Learner's health status
5. Gender

INDIVIDUAL LEARNING STYLES

"Learning styles are cognitive, emotional, and physiological traits, as well as indicators of how learners perceive, interact, and respond to their learning environments" (Czepula et al., 2016, p. 1).

- Cassidy (2004) adds that the approach that learners take to different tasks is also important.

TABLE 9.1
Learner Readiness

TYPE OF READINESS	ATTRIBUTES TO ASSESS TO DETERMINE READINESS
P = Physical readiness	• Measure of ability • Complexity of the task • Environmental effects • Health status • Gender
E = Emotional readiness	• Anxiety level • Support system • Motivation • Risk-taking behavior • Developmental age
E = Experiential readiness	• Level of aspiration • Past coping mechanisms • Cultural background • Locus of control • Orientation
K = Knowledge readiness	• Present knowledge base • Cognitive ability • Learning disabilities • Learning styles

Adapted from Lichtenthal (1990) in Bastable (2013, p. 106). Reprinted with permission of Jones & Bartlett Learning.

- Simply put, a learning style is an approach to learning that works for the individual learner.
- Learners may have more than one learning style.
- Educators must first assist learners in identifying their learning style(s) if they do not already know them, and then present information in a manner consistent with the learners' learning styles. The four most common learning styles are defined by the acronym VARK, as described by Fleming and Mills (1992).
  - V = Visual
  - A = Auditory
  - R = Read/write
  - K = Kinesthetic

Visual (Spatial) Learners (V)

This type of learner learns best through what he or she sees.

- Pictures, diagrams, flow charts, timelines, maps, and demonstrations are more effective than texts or lectures.
- A good learning assignment for a visual learner might involve concept mapping.
- These learners like using computers and graphics. These learners could also be called graphic (G) learners, as this term also explains how they learn.
- It is important to note that they do not learn by viewing movies, videos, or PowerPoint presentations (Fleming, 2001).

> **EVIDENCE-BASED TEACHING PRACTICE**
>
> Johnston and colleagues (2015) found that students clearly knew their own learning style. In teaching anatomy and physiology nursing students student satisfaction was increased by introducing a range of activities and/or delivery methods that incorporate many learning styles rather than just the traditional rote learning previously relied upon. This use of varied learning styles led to a better learning environment and students had better course outcomes.

Aural, or Auditory, Learners (A)

Aural, or auditory, learners prefer to learn through what is heard or spoken.

- These learners learn best from lectures, tapes, tutorials, group discussions, speaking, web chats, e-mail, mobile phones, and talking things through out loud.
- By talking about a topic, these learners are able to process the given information (Fleming, 2001).

> **EVIDENCE-BASED TEACHING PRACTICE**
>
> Pellico, Duffy, Fennie, and Swan (2012) found that auditory training through music assisted learners to significantly increase their ability to ($p < .0001$) hear heart, lung, and bowel sounds correctly in a controlled study.

Learning by Reading or Writing (R)

These learners prefer to have the information to be learned displayed as words.

- These learners prefer text-based input and output in all of its forms.
- Many academics have a preference for this style of learning.
- People with this learning style are often fond of PowerPoint presentations, the Internet, lists, dictionaries, thesauri, quotations, and anything else featuring words (Fleming, 2001).

Kinesthetic or Active Learners (K)

Kinesthetic, or active, learners use their bodies and sense of touch to enhance learning while engaged in physical activity.

- They like to think about issues while working out or exercising.
- They like to participate, play games, role-play, act, and model experiences through practicing.
- Learning activities tailored to this style could include simulations or real-life experiences.
- Kinesthetic learners appreciate demonstrations, simulations, videos, and movies of "real things," as well as case studies, practice sessions, and applications (Fleming, 2001).
- Felder and Solomon (1998) refer to these learners as *active learners*.

Multimodal/Mixtures (M)

Multimodal learners are individuals who prefer to learn via two or more styles of learning or using a variety of methods.

- These individuals' preferred learning style may be context specific, or they might choose a single mode to suit a certain occasion or situation.
- These individuals like to gather information from each mode and thereby often gain a deeper and broader understanding of the topic (Fleming, 2001).

OTHER LEARNING STYLES

In addition to the aforementioned styles, there are other learning styles that include:

- Verbal (linguistic) learners
- Tactile learners
- Global learners
- Intuitive learners
- Sequential learners
- Reflective learners
- Analytical learners
- Accommodative learners
- Digital learners

Verbal (Linguistic) Learners

This learning style is an outgrowth of the auditory mode.

- Verbal learners get more value from words that are written or spoken.
- These learners enjoy talking through procedures using a simulator in clinical practice.
- These learners use recordings of content for repetition.
- These learners frequently write things down or use mnemonics to retain information.

Tactile Learners

Tactile learners remember what they touch and learn by touching or manipulating objects.

- These learners require movement.
- Tactile learners trace words and use letter tiles to help them learn to spell words.
- Tactile learners love Scrabble.
- Tactile learners often doodle, sketch, write, or conduct experiments (Mahoney, 2007).

Global Learners

Global learners make decisions based on their emotions and intuition.

- They are spontaneous and focus on creativity.
- A tidy environment is not important to global learners.
- These learners enjoy learning. They use humor, tell stories, and enjoy group work.
- Global learners like to participate in activities.
- These learners tend to absorb material randomly. They frequently do not see connections at first, but then suddenly "get it."
- Global learners are able to solve complex problems quickly or put things together in unique ways once they have grasped the big picture, but they may have difficulty explaining how they did it.
- These learners lack good sequential thinking abilities (Felder & Solomon, 1998; Mahoney, 2007).

Intuitive Learners

These learners like to discover the possibilities in relationships.

- Intuitive learners like solving problems using well-established methods and do not like complications or surprises.
- Intuitive learners do not like repetition.
- These learners tend to work faster and be more innovative than other learners.
- Intuitive learners hate courses that involve a lot of memorization or routine calculations and will easily become bored by them.

- Intuitive learners are prone to careless mistakes on tests because they are impatient with details and do not like repetition, such as checking math calculations (Felder & Solomon, 1998).

Sequential Learners

These learners prefer to gain understanding using linear steps.

- For sequential learners, steps follow one another logically and directly, in an assigned order.
- These learners focus on following a logical sequence to find solutions (Mahoney, 2007).
- Sequential learners do not like educators who jump from topic to topic or who skip steps.
- Sequential learners like outlines and prefer to follow a defined format (Felder & Solomon, 1998).

Reflective Learners

A reflective learner prefers to think about new material by reflecting quietly on it first.

- Reflective learners prefer to work alone, rather than with groups.
- These learners do not like classes that cover large amounts of material quickly.
- Reflective learners do not like to be asked simply to read and memorize material.
- These learners like to stop periodically to review what they have read and think of possible questions or applications.
- Reflective learners may find it helpful to write short summaries of readings or class notes in their own words to help them retain the material better (Felder & Solomon, 1998).

Analytical Learners

These learners base all of their decisions on logic.

- They plan and organize well. They focus on details and facts.
- They like a tidy, well-organized environment.
- They enjoy learning, take sequential steps, and follow "the rules."
- They like examples and clear goals (Mahoney, 2007).

Accommodative Learners

Accommodative learners like a combination of concrete experiences and active experimentation.

- They complete tasks and are less concerned about the theories supporting their actions.
- They are risk takers.

- They solve problems by trial and error.
- They are concerned with abstract concepts and assimilate abstract conceptualizations with reflective observations (Mahoney, 2007).

Digital (Online) Learners

With technological advances, the millennial students almost always uses technology, smartphones, and less frequently use traditional formats such as archives, newspapers, and other print sources (Orkiszewski, Pollitt, Leonard, & Hayes-Lane, 2016). Characteristics of these learners include:

- Focus on enthusiastic and collaborative learning
- Digital literacy
- Constant connection via hand-held digital devices

EVIDENCE-BASED TEACHING PRACTICE

Li, Wen-Pin, Chin-Fang, Shieh, and Yang (2014) studied learning styles in two different groups of nursing students (2-year [$N = 96$] and 5-year [$N = 189$] programs) and compared styles to academic achievement. The Myers-Briggs was used and compared to students' grade point average. The most common learning styles were introversion, sensing, thinking, and judging; and introversion, sensing, feeling, and judging and academic performance were significantly related to learning style ($p < .05$, $df = 15$).

ADULT LEARNERS

Adult learners display a variety of learning characteristics.

- Knowles, Houlton, and Swanson (2015) were among the first researchers to theorize how adults learn.
- The most common reason an adult enters any learning experience is to create change. This could encompass change in their:
  * Skills
  * Behavior
  * Knowledge level
  * Attitudes about things

    Barriers to adult learning include:

- Lack of time
- Lack of confidence
- Lack of information about opportunities to learn
- Scheduling problems
- Lack of motivation
- Red tape

It is important to incorporate adult learning principles into teaching to maximize learning potential for this population. Adult learners learn best when:

- Learning is related to an immediate need, problem, or deficit.
- Learning is voluntary and self-initiated.
- Learning is person centered and problem centered.
- Learning is self-controlled and self-directed.
- The role of the teacher is that of a facilitator.
- Information and assignments are pertinent.
- New material draws on past experiences and is related to something that the learner already knows.
- The learner's perception of threats to himself or herself is reduced to a minimum in the educational situation.
- Learners are able to participate actively in the learning process.
- Learners are able to learn in a group.
- The nature of the learning activity changes frequently.
- Learning is reinforced b†y application and prompt feedback (Knowles et al., 2015).

EVIDENCE-BASED TEACHING PRACTICE

Veteran learners are comfortable with the traditional classroom and well-defined goals and objectives. They may not embrace creativity and have varying degrees of comfort with technology (Blevins, 2014).

CULTURALLY DIVERSE LEARNERS

The culture of the individual encompasses an individual's values, attitudes, perceptions, interpersonal needs, roles, and cognitive styles (Tomey, 2008). It is important for faculty to recognize that cultural diversity can influence learning ability and needs when teaching nursing learners and when socializing them into the role of nurse. In addition, diversity may influence how nursing is perceived by individuals from diverse alternative cultural backgrounds. For example, a nurse who, in one culture, may be considered a "caring nurse" may be perceived by members of another culture as cold and aloof. Perceptions of individuals must be considered from each individual's cultural background.

The American Association of Colleges of Nursing (AACN) issued a position statement in 1997 stating that, because the U.S. population is so culturally diverse, cultural diversity training needs to be included in nursing education, and a greater number of culturally diverse learners should be recruited into nursing schools (AACN, 2016). Despite this position statement, minorities continue to be underrepresented in nursing and nursing programs (Burruss & Popkess, 2012). Moreover, culturally diverse learners face certain barriers that may impinge on their ability to achieve success in college. The most common of these barriers are:

- The lack of ethnically diverse faculty
- Finances
- Academic preparation (Burruss & Popkess, 2012)

Culturally diverse learners may also suffer from a lack of:

- Available role models
- Academic support
- Family support
- Peer support

The culture or customs of an individual learner may, at times, come into conflict with the values of the clinical environment, and his or her values system may be disrupted.

- A value represents a basic conviction about what is right, wrong, desirable, or just, and may support an individual's decision about how to act or perform in relation to what is perceived as preferable or valuable within the individual's culture.
- This can contribute to forming attitudes, which are similar to values, and are learned from the individual's parents, caregivers, and family.
- Teachers and peers may have a significant impact on one's actions.
- Some learners may experience a situation that differs from the values of their cultural tradition and usual behavior, thus causing them to experience cognitive dissonance.
- The inconsistencies revealed by cognitive dissonance are both uncomfortable and ambiguous for learners (Tomey, 2008).
- It is important, especially for nursing educators, to offer clear directions and rationales for decision making for culturally diverse learners to help alleviate any sense of dissonance they might experience.

A study by Amaro, Abriam-Yago, and Yoder (2006) interviewed ethnically diverse learners who had recently completed an associate or baccalaureate nursing program, and the study identified the major themes related to educational barriers:

- Personal needs (lack of finances, time issues, family responsibilities and obligations, and difficulties related to language and communication)
- Academic needs (large or heavy workload)
- Language needs (difficulty reading and understanding assignments, a prejudice resulting from their accents, and verbal communication barriers)
- Cultural needs (expectations related to assertiveness and cultural norms, lack of diverse role models, and difficulty with communication)

An important issue among culturally diverse learners is their level of knowledge of the English language, which, if inadequate, can be problematic. Barriers may also exist for English-as-a-second-language (ESL) learners in applying and gaining admission to nursing programs and in their ability to progress through the program, once accepted.

Suggestions for accommodating learners from culturally and linguistically diverse backgrounds include:

- Using nonstandardized and standardized methods of testing
- Dynamic assessments
- Nonverbal measures of ability

- Multiple methods of testing
- Testing in both the learner's native and second language
- The use of the Test of English as a Foreign Language (TOEFL) test (Overton, Fielding, & Simonsson, 2004)
- Hansen and Beaver (2012) discuss test development for ESL learners and provide the following tips:
  - Use short, simple sentences
  - Be direct when stating information
  - Use questions rather than statements that need completion
  - Highlight key words such as *most*, *least*, *best*
  - Use common vocabulary

CRITICAL THINKING QUESTION

As you teach your course each day what concepts do you teach that might be interpreted incorrectly by a culturally diverse learner and how might you remedy that situation?

The TOEFL Examination

The TOEFL examination measures a learner's potential ability to communicate in English in a college or university environment.

- The TOEFL score can be helpful in identifying learners who may be at risk for failure and/or may need additional support throughout a program (Educational Testing Services, 2016).
- It is important to use the TOEFL score as only one piece of admission criteria.
- Be aware that learners may be offended if they are asked to take a TOEFL examination if they have been living in the United States for many years.

Faculty commitment to the success of minority learners is crucial for the success of diverse learner populations. Minority learners need a strong learner–faculty relationship with a faculty member who is not responsible for assigning a grade to the learner.

- Learners need someone to talk to about their feelings and experiences as they move through the nursing program.
- Having a strong learner–faculty relationship will minimize learners' experiences with cognitive dissonance.
- Role models are ideal if appropriate faculty candidates are available.
- If no faculty role model is found, other faculty members must spend time with the learners to ensure their success (Burruss & Popkess, 2012).

Developing adequate support services for culturally diverse learners will increase their success in nursing or other academic programs. Reading, comprehension, and writing skills need to be developed in a nonthreatening manner to assist the diverse learner's academic success.

EVIDENCE-BASED TEACHING PRACTICE

In a study by Long (2015), she concluded that a 2-week medical service learning experience in Belize significantly improved self-efficacy, self-confidence, and self-awareness among associates degree in nursing students toward working with the Hispanic culture and developing cultural competence. All students agreed it was a valuable learning experience and they were extremely pleased with what they had learned and experienced.

LEARNING DISABILITIES

Learning disabilities are the most common type of learner limitation found on college campuses. Frequently, learners with a learning disability begin college before their disability has been detected.

- In nursing education, these disabilities are often noted when significant differences are noticed between a learner's classroom and clinical performance.

- Often, a learner may perform well in the clinical area, but may be unable to demonstrate the same ability, skills, and competency when taking tests in the classroom.

- These learners should be referred to the appropriate counselors for assistance (Frank, 2012).

Teaching Gem: Smith, Ooms, and Marks-Maron (2016) describe a teaching session about service users' experiences accessing and receiving health and social care that was designed and delivered by service users to first-year bachelor of science in nursing students. The aim was to enhance students' knowledge, skills, and confidence in caring for people with a learning disability. The session impacted students' knowledge and understanding of people with a learning disability. After the session, students reported that they felt more comfortable and confident interacting with people with a learning disability. In addition, they reflected on their feelings about caring for people with a learning disability.

Learners with documented disabilities are entitled to the same access to education as traditional learners. Academic services must be available to provide learners with reading, writing, and test-taking strategy support services.

The Elementary and Secondary Education Act

The Elementary and Secondary Education Act was passed in 1965 to "ensure equal educational opportunity for all children . . . and to close the achievement gap between poor and affluent children." This has since undergone changes and has most recently been enhanced by the No Child Left Behind Act (NCLB; U.S. Department of Education, 2016).

The NCLB Act

The NCLB is the most significant federal education policy in a generation. This Act calls on all educators to measure all learners' performances using a set of fixed indicators and it has tied federal monetary compensation to these performance outcomes.

It should be noted that although both these laws are aimed at elementary and secondary education, they cannot be ignored and will have tremendous impact when learners taught under the auspices of these Acts reach college. Educators should be prepared for challenges yet to be determined that may stem from these Acts, especially NCLB (U.S. Department of Education, 2016).

Characteristics of Learners With Learning Disabilities

- Trouble with basic reading skills
- Memory difficulties
- Trouble remembering details and sequencing
- Reading and spelling difficulties
- Poor handwriting
- Distractibility and difficulty concentrating
- History of poor academic performance
- Difficulty meeting deadlines
- Anxiety and low self-esteem
- Difficulty following verbal instructions
- Difficulty organizing ideas into writing
- Difficulty articulating ideas verbally
- Auditory processing deficits
- Time-management problems (Frank, 2012)

It is important for faculty to know that the nature of learning disabilities can be highly individualized and can be manifested differently through a variety of issues. Faculty should be aware that:

- These learners are usually of average or above average intelligence (Frank, 2012).
- Employing teaching strategies that match the learners' learning styles may enhance their chances of success and may serve to minimize their learning disability.
- The skilled educator should be aware and open to employing teaching strategies to assist learning-disabled learners to achieve.

Many colleges and universities have an office that coordinates the diagnosis of learning disabilities and the accommodation and provision of support services for learners who need them.

- If a learner agrees, a faculty member can be made aware of the learner's disability and a variety of accommodations can be made to meet his or her learning needs. One example involves giving the learner extra time to take an examination or allowing the learner to take an examination in another secured environment.

- It is not appropriate for the faculty to discuss a student's learning disability with other faculty members unless given permission to do so by the learner (Frank, 2012).

Nurse educators must also be familiar with the accommodations made by their state for learners with disabilities. The NCLEX has accommodations for students with documented learning disabilities.

- Accommodations must be made for students with learning disabilities in accordance with the Americans with Disabilities Act (National Council of State Boards of Nursing).
- It is important for educators to be aware of learners with physical disabilities, such as learners with a documented or apparent physical limitation, problems with substance abuse, chemical or alcohol impairments, and/or mental health problems (Frank, 2012).

LEARNER SOCIALIZATION

Socialization of learners is defined as a process of internalizing the norms, beliefs, and values of a professional culture to which one hopes to gain admission (Philipin, 1999).

- New nurses are instructed in ways and attitudes of the organization and gradually adopt the attitudes, values, and unspoken messages of the organization (Mooney, 2007).
- It is important to note that a lack of socialization to nursing has been associated with negative outcomes such as turnover, attrition from the profession, and decreased productivity (Nesler, Hanner, Melburg, & McGowan, 2001).

The transition from new graduate to professional nurse is challenging. In some cases, more than 50% of new nurses have left their position in the first year. One strategy that has been shown to yield positive results in facilitating new-graduate role transition is the nurse internship program. This reduced the rate of turnover in the first year after hire when compared with traditional orientation programs (Letourneau & Fater, 2015).

Kramer's (1974) work delineates four phases of what is described as "reality shock" when a new nurse or neophyte realizes that what he or she learned in school does not match what is experienced in actual clinical practice.

- The excitement of passing the licensure examination quickly fades as these new nurses struggle to move from the role of learner to the staff nurse role.
- This reality shock leads to stress, which can cause exacerbations of symptoms that affect one's health and cause a loss of time from work (Cherry & Jacob, 2005).

Kramer's four phases of reality shock are:

1. Honeymoon
2. Shock or rejection
3. Recovery
4. Resolution

Benner's Novice to Expert Theory

Benner (1984) discussed the same issue in her "from novice to expert nurses" theory. The phases outlined are:

1. Novice
2. Advanced beginner
3. Competent
4. Proficient
5. Expert

It is important to note that socialization takes place primarily through social interaction with people who are significant to an individual, usually a nursing school's faculty members (Barretti, 2004). In the hospital environment, the following contributed to the successful socialization of new nursing graduates as they developed self-confidence and high role satisfaction (Boyle, Popkess-Vawter, & Taunton, 1996):

- Positive precepting experiences
- Social support systems
- Assignment congruence

What nurse educators can do to enhance learner socialization into nursing is twofold:

- First, a nurse educator should be a great role model for the profession.
- Second, a nurse educator should prepare nursing students for the reality of the profession by integrating socialization principles into every nursing course in the curriculum.

Also important are mentorship and a supportive learning environment. Mentors need to be confident in their skills and teaching ability as well as knowing their learners. Mentors need to plan learning experiences and facilitate new-graduate nurses to respond to the unexpected in the clinical environment with ease and support (Vinales, 2015). This support and mentorship are crucial in helping the novice nurse acclimate to the new role and assisting them to grow.

Today's nursing educators are shaping tomorrow's nurses. What is paramount to the successful shaping of tomorrow's nursing staff is that nurse educators not only teach nursing content but also shape the learning environment where that content is taught, including the use of appropriate clinical experiences, so that learners are fully socialized to the reality of nursing and its role. Accomplishing this will serve to reduce the chance of negative experiences and reality shock on graduation.

EVIDENCE-BASED TEACHING PRACTICE

In a comparison of outcomes between associate- and baccalaureate-prepared nurses participating in a nurse residency program, both groups found job satisfaction greater at 1 month than at 1 year. All were less satisfied at 6 months, with satisfaction improving but not returning to baseline by the end of a year. The statistically significant difference between the two groups related to feelings of professional satisfaction and support. Baccalaureate-degree nurses (bachelor of science in nursing [BSN]) felt less supported by colleagues, preceptors, and supervisors than did associate-degree nurses. Baccalaureate-prepared new graduates were perceived as having "book knowledge" but as not having mastered the clinical technical skills prior to arriving on the job. In this setting, it is noted that preceptors serve a major role in socialization of the new nurse (Thomson, 2011).

ADDRESSING INCIVILITY

Incivility is defined as "speech or action that is discourteous, rude, or impolite" (Merriam-Webster's Online Dictionary, 2012).

- Incivility in the academic nursing environment may range from insulting remarks, verbal abuse, and talking when others are talking (Tiberius & Flak, 1999). Clark (2009) defines incivility as rude and disruptive behavior that, when left unaddressed, may spiral into aggressive or violent behavior.

A study by Clark and Springer (2007) outlines the learner behaviors most often reported as uncivil by both learners and faculty:

- Cheating on examinations or quizzes
- Using cell phones or pagers during class
- Holding distracting conversations
- Making sarcastic remarks or gestures
- Sleeping in class
- Using computers for purposes not related to the class
- Demanding makeup examinations, extensions, or other favors
- Making disapproving groans
- Dominating class discussions
- Refusing to answer direct questions

Incivility is a symptom of a larger problem of *academic dishonesty*, which is defined as the "intentional participation in deceptive practices regarding one's academic work or the work of another" (Kolanko et al., 2006, p. 1).

EVIDENCE-BASED TEACHING PRACTICE

Amos (2015) conducted a descriptive, quantitative study that examined perceived levels of workplace incivility among nursing faculty members. The sample consisted of 257 nursing faculty members employed at community colleges in North Carolina. The methodology included a nonexperimental, online survey. Data analysis included use of descriptive and inferential statistics. Findings revealed three themes: (a) the description of workplace incivility among nursing faculty aligned with Bandura's (1977) social learning theory and Andersson and Pearson's (1999) incivility spiral, (b) workplace incivility among nursing faculty existed in the community college setting, and (c) most demographic factors did not influence the extent to which faculty members perceived uncivil behaviors among their peers. However, there were four exceptions: hostility and full-time employment, hostility and salary range, privacy invasion and ethnicity, and uncivil behaviors and the number of years of full-time teaching. Implications for nursing education included turning conflict into problem solving and collaboration, and cultivating climates of civility and cultures of openness, inclusion, and social connectedness.

- As many as 70% to 95% of learners reported having engaged in practices of academic dishonesty.
- Some have suggested that the problem of academic dishonesty is a result of a deterioration in morals, as reported over the past decade by the Joseph Institute (Kolanko et al., 2006).

Learners described the following behaviors as *ineffective* for deterring cheating:

- Assigning specific topics for papers
- Putting numbers on test booklets
- Assigning seats for examinations
- Permitting only pencils to be brought into the examination room
- Not permitting anyone to leave during the course of the examination
- Leaving increased space between learners during an examination

Learners describe the following behaviors as *most effective* in deterring cheating:

- Having learners place their belongings in the front of the classroom
- Having a minimum of two proctors per examination to walk up and down the aisles during the examination
- Providing new examinations for each test
- Keeping each test in a locked cabinet with shredding conducted by full-time secretaries, not by student workers.

Kolanko et al. (2006) also noted that "faculty should include opportunities within the education process for the moral development of learners in addition to their theoretical and clinical development. Learners must understand what constitutes academic integrity. Unethical behavior is ultimately responsible for the deterioration of the very fabric of the nursing profession" (p. 35).

It is also important to note that incivility can flow from the faculty member to the learner. Faculty members must always be aware of their behavior and their position as role models for learners. Unfortunately, Clark (2006) found that it is not unusual for learners to perceive faculty members as uncivil. Her study found uncivil faculty behaviors to include:

- Making demeaning and belittling comments
- Treating learners unfairly
- Pressuring learners to conform to unreasonable faculty demands

Faculty members arriving unprepared or late for class can also be considered uncivil, and any of the characteristics identified as uncivil learner behaviors may also be applied to faculty. Three themes emerged from Clark's study related to learners' emotional responses to faculty incivility:

1. Traumatization
2. Powerlessness and helplessness
3. Anger

> **Teaching Gem:** One of the most common topics of discussion among new nursing educators today is the increasing incidence of student incivility or classroom management of incivility resulting from changes in social norms. When a faculty member receives an affectively charged statement from a student, the worst course of action is to respond with an affectively charged response. The key is to close the communication gap. The main objective when faced with incivility is to keep the student's ego and integrity intact. If a student is being uncivil, it is often because he or she feels that his or her ego is threatened. One of the best ways to protect ego is to give the student an opportunity to be self-correcting. Clements suggests using reflection, which is simply rephrasing a statement to get at the intended meaning. For example, the faculty member should state, "So, what I think you are telling me is . . ." Standards of conduct need to be explicit and communicated to students (Clements, 2012; Suplee, Lachman, Siebert, & Anselmi, 2008).

As these studies reveal, uncivil behavior is a double-edged sword that must be examined and remedied at both ends of the learning continuum.

INCIVILITY AND BULLYING IN THE WORKPLACE

The most common types of incivility are lateral (nurse to nurse) and hierarchical (nurse administrator to manager or nurse, nurse to learner, faculty to learner, and physician to nurse). In July 2008, The Joint Commission (TJC) issued a *Sentinel Event Alert* that discussed intimidating and disruptive behaviors that undermine a culture of safety. In January 2009, TJC implemented leadership standards that require hospital leaders to create and maintain a culture of safety and quality. TJC further noted that bullying is a contributor to medical errors, avoidable adverse patient outcomes, increased cost of care, as well as professional attrition.

Types of abuse include verbal abuse, nonverbal abuse, sexual harassment, passive-aggressive behaviors, and bullying. Clark (2011) suggests that bullying is a threatening situation, reflective of a form of abuse that requires further consideration independent of incivility. Bullying among children is not a new concept, but its transition into adult life and professional life is an increasing concern in the workplace, the health care environment, and the nursing profession. The findings have noted that bullying can cause significant psychological and physical distress, including feelings of alienation, lack of control over working conditions, and feelings of low self-esteem and powerlessness. If these conditions are left unchecked, the victims of bullying may develop problems sleeping, exhibit signs of depression, posttraumatic stress syndrome, and low morale. They may use sick time excessively and wind up leaving school or the profession (Meierdierks-Bowllan, 2015).

The vulnerable role of nursing students and graduate nurses as they socialize to the profession of nursing can be filled with fears of incompetence and powerlessness. In addition, these new nurses experience multiple stressors such as juggling personal and work demands, financial pressures, time management difficulties, perceived lack of faculty and peer support, and potential mental health problems or personal issues—all of which can further impact students' capacity to effectively cope on a daily basis.

EVIDENCE-BASED TEACHING PRACTICE

Leong and Crossman (2016) conducted a qualitative study of 26 new nurses and five preceptors in five hospitals in Singapore and Japan. The data analysis gave rise to a movement of "tough love" from senior nurses to new nurses not described in the literature. The "tough love" was rationalized as well intentioned, but nevertheless it was an abusive strategy used to condition new nurses to conform to expected professional and organizational behaviors. The authors concluded that this "tough love" behavior damages the transitional experience of new nurses and has the potential to determine whether the new nurses will remain in the health care organization and nursing profession.

PREVENTION IS KEY

So, what can be done to help with this situation? Prevention is the key. Some suggested solutions are the use of an organization's resources and conduct policies, to educate staff to be accountable for their own behavior, to have staff model appropriate behavior, and to not allow disruptive behavior to go unchecked (McNamara, 2012). TJC further outlined preventive strategies, including skill-based training and coaching, ongoing nonconfrontation surveillance, embedded systems to assess staff perceptions of seriousness and extent of nonprofessional behavior, and integration of policies to ensure early reporting without fear of intimidation. To prevent, one must first identify at-risk behaviors. This would incorporate a zero-tolerance policy and a nonpunitive reporting mechanism. Education and awareness are also key components (Meierdierks-Bowllan, 2015).

Within the classroom similar situations need to occur. Faculty and administration must provide programs to identify and educate against uncivil behavior. This must include policies to hold the faculty and students accountable for their actions. Role modeling, coaching, open forums for discussion, stress-reduction activities like yoga and meditation, opportunities for counseling, and communication-building activities need to be used within and outside of the classroom to change this trend.

EVIDENCE-BASED TEACHING PRACTICE

Clark, Barbosa-Liker, Larecia-Money, and Nguyen (2015) obtained a convenience sample of nursing faculty and students from 20 schools of nursing in the United States who participated in a mixed-methods study to test the psychometric properties of the Incivility in Nursing Education-Revised (INE-R) Survey. They found the INE-R is a psychometrically sound instrument to measure faculty and student perceptions of incivility; to examine differences regarding levels of nursing education, program type, gender, age, and ethnicity; to compare perceptions of incivility between and among adjunct, clinical, teaching, and research faculty; and to conduct pre- and postassessments of the perceived levels of faculty and student incivility in nursing programs to inform evidence-based interventions.

CASE STUDIES

CASE STUDY 9.1

The nurse educator is working in a 12-month accelerated nursing program. As a result of the time constraints of only having the learners for 12 months, the nurse educator realizes it is essential to incorporate only the most important facts in the course. The program has successfully graduated four groups of accelerated learners. The university sends out a follow-up survey to see how these learners are doing in the clinical environment. The survey reals comments like, "I didn't realize nursing was going to be this hard," "I wasn't really ready for the demands of working in this fast-paced environment," "I didn't think it would be this hard fitting in on the floor where I work," "No one really helps me," "I am not sure I am going to remain in nursing," "I wish I knew it was going to be like this." The nurse educator realizes that, perhaps by focusing so much on getting in all the content needed for learners to pass their licensure examinations, the university missed out on providing an important lesson. The program did not take time to "socialize" these learners to the role of nursing. List some ideas of how you might better address the socialization of nursing learners in the future, in both your course and at the university level.

CASE STUDY 9.2

The nurse educator has been teaching in a university setting for the past 3 years. The nurse educator's class typically has 50 learners and meets in a large auditorium. The nurse educator tries to keep the learners engaged and actively involved in the learning process, but frequently notices that learners are talking among themselves while teaching is going on. Is this an example of learners being uncivil? If so, what might the nurse educator do to curtail this in the classroom?

CASE STUDY 9.3

The nurse educator is teaching a course that has a clinical component. The nurse educator notices that a particular learner does exceptionally well in the clinical area. The learner is professional, completes excellent assessments, and interacts beautifully with patients. However, in the classroom, this learner seems to be the last one done when taking a test and is barely passing the course. What might the nurse educator think is going on with this learner? What should the nurse educator do to help the learner? Should the nurse educator assume this learner may have a learning disability? Answer "yes" or "no," and support your answer.

PRACTICE QUESTIONS

1. The nurse educator needs additional understanding when she states that the following is incivil behavior:

A. The student falls asleep in class

B. The student is texting on her cell phone while in class

C. The student rolls his eyes at the professor

D. The student is taking notes on the computer

2. Which of the following methods is a positive way to socialize a newly licensed nurse into the nursing profession?

A. Invite the new nurse to go out drinking with "the gang"

B. Say to the new nurse "I got your back"

C. Invite the new nurse to attend a professional nursing conference with you

D. Be nice to the nurse, but when you are with senior nurses say what you really think of her abilities

3. The nurse educator is working in an institution and notices a new nurse and her preceptor interacting on a weekend shift. The nurse educator notices that the preceptor is in fact bullying the new nurse who quietly stands by and does not react when her preceptor embarrasses her in front of their patient. What would be the best strategy to employ to correct this behavior?

A. Ask the patient whether he or she likes the care he or she is receiving?

B. Tell your nurse manager on Monday that you don't think the preceptor should have new orientees anymore

C. Do nothing as this is not your preceptee

D. Ask to speak with the preceptor in private and share with her your perceptions and offer solutions as to how she might better interact with the student

4. Which of the following is an acceptable teaching strategy when teaching low-literacy patients?

A. Create a professional authoritative relationship with them because you are the educator

B. Use repetition to reinforce information

C. Use the direct question-and-answer method

D. Give them large amounts of information at a time as availability of a translator is limited

5. Which of the following statements is true about learning styles?

A. When a teacher uses a variety of teaching methods, it confuses the learner and the student learns less

B. Learners feel less stressed when using just one style of learning

C. Using learning methods that are consistent with the learner is considered the best way to effect the best learning achievement

D. The educator applying learning styles theory to each learner allows the educator to recognize whether learners will process information correctly

6. The nurse educator has a learner in the class who has an accommodation for increased time for testing. The educator needs to:

A. Understand the nature of the disability

B. Meet privately with the learner

C. Accommodate the learner

D. Keep a copy of the letter from the physician

7. The nurse educator is teaching a large class that is very diverse. Which population of learners is at an increased risk for failure? Learners who:

A. Decided to pursue a second career

B. Just graduated from high school

C. Speak English as a second language

D. Transferred from another nursing program

8. The nurse educator is discussing graduation with learners. One of the learners says that being responsible for patients without the instructor is very frightening. Which statement by the nurse educator would be most appropriate?

A. "The nurse manager will be available to guide you in decision making that is related to patient care"

B. "Most hospitals have an orientation program that will make sure you are prepared"

C. "The procedure manual is always available to assist you in making patient care decisions"

D. "Your mentor will provide a structured process to guide your decisions and behaviors"

9. The nurse educator assesses the written work of a millennial learner and is surprised that among the references the learner uses is a(n):

A. Textbook

B. Internet source

C. Encyclopedia

D. Article

10. Learners are encouraged to become members of the National Student Nurses Association (NSNA). The framework of this organization indicates that the learner will gain experience:

A. Making decisions and being accountable for those decisions

B. Following regulations determined by elected officers

C. Learning how to engage in social activities while in school

D. Discussing health information and presenting projects

REFERENCES

Amaro, D., Abriam-Yago, K., & Yoder, M. (2006). Perceived barriers for ethnically diverse students in nursing programs. *Journal of Nursing Education, 45*(7), 247–254.

American Association of Colleges of Nurses. (2016). Cultural competency in nursing education. Retrieved from http://www.aacn.nche.edu/education-resources/cultural-competency, http://www.aacn.nche.edu/publications/position/diversity-and-equality

Amos, K. (2013). *Nursing faculty members' perspectives of faculty-to-faculty workplace incivility among nursing faculty members* (Unpublished doctoral dissertation). Capella University, Minneapolis, MN.

Andersson, L. M., & Pearson, C. M. (1999). Tit for tat? The spiraling effect of incivility in the workplace. *The Academy of Management Review, 24*, 452–471. Retrieved from http://journals.aomonline.org/amr

Bandura, A. (1977). *Social learning theory.* Englewood Cliffs, NJ: Prentice Hall.

Barretti, M. (2004). What do we know about the professional socialization of our students? *Journal of Social Work Education, 40*(2), 255–283.

Bastable, S. B. (2013). *Nurse as educator: Principles of teaching and learning from nursing practice* (4th ed.). Boston, MA: Jones & Bartlett.

Benner, P. (1984). *From novice to expert: Excellence and power in clinical nursing practice.* Boston, MA: Addison-Wesley.

Blevins, S. (2014). Nurses as educators: Understanding learning styles. *MEDSURG Nursing, 23*(1), 59–60.

Boyle, D. K., Popkess-Vawter, S., & Taunton, R. L. (1996). Socialization of new graduate nurses in critical care. *Heart & Lung, 25*(2), 141–154.

Burruss, N., & Popkess, A. (2012). The diverse learning needs of students. In D. M. Billings & J. A. Halstead (Eds.), *Teaching in nursing: A guide for faculty* (4th ed., pp. 15–33). St. Louis, MO: Elsevier Saunders.

Cassidy, S. (2004). Learning styles: An overview of theories, models, and measures. *Educational Psychology, 24*(4), 419–444.

Cherry, B., & Jacob, S. R. (2005). *Contemporary nursing: Issues, trends, and management.* St. Louis, MO: Elsevier.

Clark, C. M. (2009). Faculty field guide for promoting civility in the classroom. *Nurse Educator, 34*(5), 194–197.

Clark, C. M. (2006). *Incivility in nursing education: Student perceptions of uncivil faculty behavior in the academic environment* (Unpublished doctoral dissertation). University of Idaho, Moscow, ID.

Clark, C. M., & Kenaley, B. (2011). Faculty empowerment of students to foster civility in nursing education: A merging of two conceptual models. *Nursing Outlook, 59*, 158–165.

Clark, C. M., Barbosa-Liker, C., Larecia-Money, G., & Nguyen, D. (2015). Revision and psychometric testing of the Incivility in Nursing Education (INE) survey: Introducing the INE-R. *Journal of Nursing Education, 54*(6), 306–315.

Clark, C. M., & Springer, P. J. (2007). Incivility in nursing education: A descriptive study of definitions and prevalence. *Journal of Nursing Education, 46*(1), 7–14.

Clements, P. T. (2012). Defusing incivility. *Nurse Faculty Matters Newsletter.*

Czepula, A. I., Bottacin, W. E., Hipolito, E., Baptista, D. R., Pontarolo, R., & Correr, C. J. (2016). Predominant learning styles among pharmacy students at the Federal University of Paraná, Brazil. *Pharmacy Practice, 14*(1), 650.

Educational Testing Services. (2016). The TOEFL® test. Retrieved from http://www.toeflgoanywhere.org

Felder, R. M., & Solomon, B. A. (1998). Learning styles and strategies. Retrieved from http://www4.ncsu.edu/unity/lockers/users/f/felder/public/ILSdir/styles.htm

Fleming, N. (2001). VARK: A guide to learning styles. Retrieved from http://www.vark-learn.com/english/page.asp?p=categories

Fleming, N., & Mills, C. (1992). Not another inventory, rather a catalyst for change. In D. Wulff & J. Nygist (Eds.), *To improve the academy: Resources for faculty, instructional, and organizational development* (Vol. 11, pp. 137–155). Stillwater, OK: New Forums.

Frank, B. (2012). Teaching students with disabilities. In D. M. Billings & J. A. Halstead (Eds.), *Teaching in nursing: A guide for faculty* (4th ed., pp. 55–75). St. Louis, MO: Elsevier Saunders.

Hansen, E., & Beaver, S. (2012). Faculty support for ESL nursing students: Action plan for success. *Nursing Education Perspectives, 33*(4), 246–250.

Johnston, A., Hamill, J., Barton, M. J., Baldwin, S., Percival, G., Williams-Pritchard, J., . . . Todorovic, M. (2015). Student learning styles in anatomy and physiology courses: Meeting the needs of nursing students. *Nursing Education in Practice, 15*, 415–420.

Incivility. (n.d.) In *Merriam-Webster's online dictionary.* Retrieved from http://www.merriam-webster.com/dictionary/incivility

Knowles, M. S., Houlton, E. F., & Swanson, R. A. (2015). *The adult learner* (8th ed.). Boston, MA: Taylor & Francis.

Kolanko, K. M., Clark, C. M., Heinrich, K. T., Olive, D., Serembus, J. F., & Sifford, K. S. (2006). Academic dishonesty, bullying, incivility, and violence: Difficult challenges facing nurse educators. *Nursing Education Perspectives, 27*(1), 34–43.

Kramer, M. (1974). *Reality shock: Why nurses leave nursing.* St. Louis, MO: Mosby.

Leong, Y. M. J., & Crossman, J. (2016). Tough love or bullying: New nurses transitional experience. *Journal of Clinical Nursing, 25*(9), 1356–1366.

Letourneau, R., & Fater, K. H. (2015). Nurse residency programs: An integrative review of the literature. *Nursing Education Perspectives, 36*(2), 96–101. doi:10.5480/13-1229

Li, Y., Wen-Pin, L., Chinb-Fang, S., Shieh, S., & Yang, B. (2014). An exploratory study of the relationship between learning styles and academic performance among students in different nursing programs. *Contemporary Nurse: A Journal for the Australian Nursing Profession, 48*(2), 229–239. doi:10.5172/conu.2014.48.2.229

Lichtenthal, C. (1990). A self-study module of readiness to learn. Unpublished manuscript re-printed in Bastable, S. (2013). *Nurse as educator: Principles of teaching and learning for nursing practice* (4th ed.). Boston, MA: Jones & Bartlett.

Mahoney, P. (2007). *Certified nurse educator preparation course.* Philadelphia, PA: Villanova University.

McNamara, S. (2012). Incivility in nursing: Unsafe nurse, unsafe patients. *Association of Perioperative Registered Nurses, 95*(4), 535–540.

Meierdierks-Bowllan, N. (2015). Nursing student's experience of bullying, prevalence, impact, and interventions. *Nurse Educator, 40*(4), 194–198.

Mooney, M. (2007). Professional socialization: The key to survival as a newly qualified nurse. *International Journal of Nursing Practice, 13*, 75–80.

National League for Nursing. (2016). Certified nurse educator (CNE) 2016 candidate handbook. Retrieved from http://www.nln.org/docs/default-source/professional development-programs/certified-nurse-educator-%28cne%29-examination-candidate -handbook.pdf?sfvrsn=2

Nesler, M. S., Hanner, M. B., Melburg, V., & McGowan, S. (2001). Professional socialization of baccalaureate nursing students: Can students in distance nursing programs become socialized? *Journal of Nursing Education, 40*(7), 293–302.

Orkiszewski, P., Pollitt, P., Leonard, P., & Hayes-Lane, S. (2016). Reaching millennials with nursing history. *Creative Nursing, 22*(1), 60–64.

Overton, T., Fielding, C., & Simonsson, M. (2004). Decision making in determining eligibility of culturally and linguistically diverse learners. *Journal of Learning Disabilities, 37*(4), 319–330.

Pellico, L. H., Duffy, T. C., Fennie, K. P., & Swan, K. A. (2012). Looking is not seeing and listening is not hearing: Effect of an intervention to enhance auditory skills of graduate-entry nursing students. *Nursing Education Perspectives, 33*(4), 234–239.

Philipin, S. M. (1999). The impact of project 2000 educational reforms on the occupational socialization of nurses: An exploratory study. *Journal of Advanced Nursing, 29*(6), 1326–1331.

Smith, P., Ooms, A., & Marks-Maran, D. (2016). Active involvement of learning disabilities service users in the development and delivery of a teaching session to pre-registration nurses: Students' perspectives. *Nurse Education in Practice, 16*(1), 111–118.

Suplee, P., Lachman, V., Siebert, B., & Anselmi, K. (2008). Managing nursing student incivility in the classroom, clinical setting and on-line. *Journal of Nursing Law, 12*(2), 68–77.

Thomson, S. (2011). A comparison of outcomes between associate- and baccalaureate-prepared nurses participating in a nurse residency program. *Journal for Nurses in Staff Development, 27*(6), 266–271.

Tiberius, R. G., & Flak, E. (1999). Incivility in dyadic teaching and learning. *New Directions for Teaching and Learning, 77*, 3–12.

Tomey, A. M. (2008). *Nursing management and leadership* (8th ed.). St. Louis, MO: Mosby/ Elsevier.

U.S. Department of Education. (2016). No child left behind. Retrieved from http://www2 .ed.gov/nclb/landing.jhtml

Vinales, J. (2015). The learning environment and learning styles: A guide for mentors. *British Journal of Nursing, 24*(8), 454–457.

Facilitating Learner Development Through Service Learning Experiences

FRANCES H. CORNELIUS, MARYANN GODSHALL, AND RUTH A. WITTMANN-PRICE

The only person who is educated is the one who has learned how to learn and change.

—Carl Rogers

This chapter addresses the Certified Nurse Educator Exam Content Area 2: Facilitate Learner Development and Socialization (National League for Nursing [NLN], 2016, p. 5).

- Content Area 2 is 14% of the examination
- It is estimated that there will be approximately 21 questions from Content Area 2

LEARNING OUTCOMES

- Describe the characteristics of service learning (SL)
- Understand the types of SL
- Examine the benefits of SL
- Discuss methods used to operationalize SL experiences
- Analyze safety issues associated with SL
  * Discuss studying abroad
  * Understand student exchange opportunities
  * Understand building cultural competence
  * Explore the use of the global classroom

Integrating values with learning experiences can be done in a multitude of ways, including use of global classrooms, exchange programs, and SL. One of the most popular methods is the participation of faculty and students in SL. SL is community based, and the community can be defined as local, national, or global. SL is a way for students to give back to the community through a partnership that delivers a needed service (Wittmann-Price, 2007). SL became an educational concept in the late 1960s and has gained in popularity as a learning activity (Griffith & Clark, 2016). SL is "a teaching and learning strategy that integrates meaningful community service with instruction and reflection to enrich the learning experience, teach civic responsibility, and strengthen communities" (National Service-Learning Clearinghouse, 2016, p. 1). The benefits of using SL as a learning activity are:

- It can be used to enhance cultural competence for learners in a variety of settings (Wittmann-Price, 2007)
- It can change attitudes toward homeless people
- SL can build competencies for working with diverse populations
- SL can increase nursing intervention skills
- SL fosters therapeutic communication
- It can engage learners with hands-on experiences
- SL can encourage skills and knowledge needed for real-life experiences
- SL can explore preconceived ideas and assumptions (Long, 2016)

EVIDENCE-BASED TEACHING PRACTICE

Krishnan, Richards, and Simpson (2016) studied audiology, the effect of students' (N = 12) cultural competence of participating, in a study abroad program. Data were collected qualitatively by using the Public Affairs Scale (Levesque-Bristol & Cornelius-White, 2012) and qualitative data were collected in the form of journals. The Public Affairs Scale pre- and postscores demonstrated an increase in cultural competence and journals demonstrated that students' cultural awareness increased.

CHARACTERISTICS OF SERVICE LEARNING

SL allows students to experience the community and forms partnerships. The students learn from the experience as they provide a needed service to humanity. SL encourages interaction, caring, cultural competence, and dialogue; an SL project can be integrated into a curriculum as an assignment.

- SL is guided by learning outcomes that include relevant content of a course.
- Learner reflection is usually incorporated as a learning and/or evaluative tool.
- SL may take place in local, community-based settings or even internationally.
- It entails recognizing the needs of the community or of a given patient population.
- SL develops cultural competency among students through reflection and through the discussion of real-life experiences.
- SL develops collaboration skills among students. A cooperative purpose is always a powerful tool in education (Wittmann-Price, Anselmi, & Espinal, 2010).

Bringle and Clayton (2012) maintain that the most effective SL design is a

[C]ourse or competency-based, credit-bearing educational experience in which students (a) participate in mutually identified service activities that benefit the community, and (b) reflect on the service activity in such a way as to gain further understanding of course content, a broader appreciation of the discipline, and an enhanced sense of personal values and civic responsibility. (pp. 114–115)

The overall educational goal is not to practice skills but to fundamentally influence the long-term actions of students. Students stated that participating in SL made them more anxious to finish nursing school and start their careers as a nurse and will influence their future careers in that they plan to seek further mission trips and find ways to serve the underprivileged as a health care provider. It enriched their personal appreciation for cultural understanding and diversity (Hawkins & Vialet, 2012).

EVIDENCE-BASED TEACHING PRACTICE

Tapley and Patel (2016) examined the use of SL along with a precede–proceed model in physical therapy students ($N = 45$) and found that the combination increased students' interest, confidence, and willingness to participate in SL health–promotion programs in the community after graduation.

STUDYING ABROAD

Study-abroad opportunities can be developed to enable students to study in another country for one course, a semester, or a year or more. This is often marketed as an opportunity for students to develop global awareness and cultural competence. *Cultural competence* is defined by the nursing profession as being an essential element of nursing practice in which the nurse is enabled to recognize the impact of globalization of individual health and nursing practice (Carlton, Ryan, Ali, & Kelsey, 2007). The evidence suggests that students who participate in study-abroad courses improve their knowledge of culture and global health and enjoy enhanced personal and professional development (Ruddock & Turner, 2007). Saenz and Holcomb (2009) report that research results indicate that study-abroad programs have positive learning outcomes. They identify basic educational components and learning activities that can be used to maximize students' learning in a study-abroad program in a low-resource country. Four elements of global health are prerequisite content for the pretrip educational preparation portion of the course. They are:

1. Epidemiology—causality, risk, and rates of occurrence of health and illness
2. Environmental health—environmental factors affecting health, like food and water
3. Community resources—availability and access to health care
4. Social welfare and the role of nursing in health care availability of nurses and nursing schools and the health care system

The final module of a study-abroad program consists of posttrip debriefing and discussion of the emotional and personal effects of the field experience. Many times, global health content is included in community health courses, exploring at greater depth the international population's health concerns and cultural factors that influence health access and disparity are needed.

These study-abroad opportunities expand on SL trips in that they enable students to gain deeper insight into culture, global health systems, and policy. They have proven to be valuable for students in developing their global health awareness and cultural competence.

To be successful, study-abroad experiences need a lot of preplanning—a minimum of 6 months to a year is needed. It is important to review course objectives, expectations of the student, planned clinical experiences while abroad, and to prepare the students for hardships of the trip, all of which may help to remove the "vacation" expectation some students may have of a study-abroad opportunity (Foronda & Belknap, 2012). Making expectations of the students clear prior to departure will help to promote positive outcomes and learning experiences for the students. If going to a poverty-stricken country, it is highly recommended that faculty accompany the students. Time spent abroad can be negotiated with the administration.

Palmer, Wing, Miles, Heaston, and de la Cruz (2013) suggest using graduate students and alumni as affiliate faculty members or adjuncts in study-abroad programs. In fact, this may be a resource for hiring adjunct faculty and those who are interested in nursing education. This eliminates one of the barriers to continued nursing faculty participation, which has been the personal financial cost and time investment by full-time faculty. Hiring adjunct faculty gives university backing to function as a teacher with all the inherent roles and responsibilities as well as encourages continual interest and support of the program.

There are study-abroad opportunities that may be set up with other colleges and universities for nonclinical courses, which involve classroom activity only. For these experiences students can go alone or in groups. Housing, tuition exchange, flights, and overall costs can be negotiated with the sending and receiving universities.

Studying abroad differs from SL in that the time commitment is usually longer in duration. It may or may not involve faculty members as the time commitment part of the experience, depending on whether a clinical component is involved. It also focuses on a more in-depth examination of culture, roles, policy, and experiences than providing a service of care to an underprivileged population. This experience can be as broad or narrow in scope as the faculty imagines it to be. SL differs from volunteering in that SL is a blend of learning and volunteering at the same time during the same experience.

SL and study-abroad also differ primarily in four ways. For example, much study-abroad research focuses on how international experience affects an individual's personal growth. SL, on the other hand, tends to emphasize reciprocal learning and growth for faculty and community members as well as for students. SL has longer term outcomes, with research showing that civic participation or social responsibility—the action component of connective learning—is an important SL outcome. The longer term objective for study-abroad programs focuses on more personalized outcomes such as improved job skills or enhanced opportunities for graduate education, careers, or international travels. Cultural learning acquired through study-abroad and SL programs is also different. Study-abroad frequently emphasizes content learning about one's own and other cultures, whereas SL concentrates less on cultures per se and more on results of cultural interactions such as reduced racism or greater tolerance for diversity. Lastly, study-abroad management programs typically feature visits to for-profit organizations; SL usually involves a nonprofit organization. Study-abroad opportunities frequently include student free time that may involve interactions with international students, community, or interviews with host nationals and independent travel, whereas SL does not (Parker & Altman, 2007).

STUDENT EXCHANGE PROGRAMS

Student exchange programs involve "exchanging" a student at one university for a student at another. This can be done nationally or internationally. This is ideal in that it gives the students a chance to experience studying various topics in another learning environment or country. This can be done for credit or non-credit coursework. When done for credit, both faculty must agree on courses and content that meet both institutions' curriculum needs. Forming partnerships with nursing colleges and universities can be started with an e-mail and then followed up with site visits. Many universities have departments that assist with these processes. In fact, in some universities the student exchange can be interdepartmental. For example, University A can send an engineering major to University B in exchange for a nursing major. The exchange can also be cross-departmental. Exchange tuition rates will need to be negotiated by the university. This is usually a very beneficial situation not only for both universities but also the relevant departments and enables more students the ability to participate in gaining intercultural competence.

BUILDING INTERCULTURAL COMPETENCE

SL experiences—whether composed of on-campus diverse interactions and integrative learning or international study-abroad experiences—provide opportunities to build intercultural competence among students (Salisbury, An, & Pascarella, 2013; Stebleton, Soria, & Cherney, 2013). SL experiences build both hard (cognitive) and soft (social/relational) skills. Kohlbry (2016) reports that immersive international SL experiences strengthens the process of becoming culturally competent and that nurses "graduating with enhanced cultural understanding will contribute to decreased health disparities and improved patient care quality and safety" (p. 304).

Rawthorn and Olsen (2014) point out that the level of interest in global health among undergraduate and graduate students has grown dramatically over the past decade. This growth has heightened the need for interdisciplinary education and collaboration to address the complex factors impacting the health of individuals and communities worldwide. Interprofessional global health education builds global health competency and comprises both substantive content but also "noncognitive individual and interpersonal skills, such as perseverance, openness, and ability to work as part of a team" (Rowthorn & Olsen, 2014, p. 550). International SL experiences will provide students with the opportunity to not only build intercultural competency but also *teamwork competency*. Teamwork competency is critical and requires "the ability to work on a team" and "a broad range of skills, attitudes, and knowledge including team values, understanding relevant roles and responsibilities, and communication skills" (Rowthorn & Olsen, 2014, p. 550).

THE GLOBAL CLASSROOM

The traditional methods of teaching "lecture style" are beginning to decrease in popularity, shifting toward more integrated global-learning experiences. With the increasing growth of technology and social networking, there is an increased demand for nurses to have a more developmental learning curriculum that instructs as well as brings the students other experiences as well.

Videoconferencing has played a significant role in enhancing nursing education experiences through clinical case discussions, educational learning, and exploration of research. These conferences can be from other countries, providing a different cultural learning experience as well as enhancing the educational experience. Videoconferencing provides an innovative, active learning methodology that challenges and engages students (Amendola, Fisher, Schaffer, & Howarth, 2016).

Global learning can be done through learning collaborative classroom delivery formats or through new technologies like "FaceTime" or "Zoom." There are many new evolving classroom delivery systems that allow online courses that can be delivered in a synchronous (at the same time) or asynchronous (to be viewed later at the students' available time) teaching method. These have grown with online classroom instruction.

Thinking out of the box with courses like research and health policy enables faculty to not only conduct a conference, but deliver online courses across the world. This enhances cultural diversity, student experience, and opens one's mind to new ideas and collaboration with nurses worldwide. This is a new modality and challenges faculty to explore.

FACULTY AND INSTITUTIONAL ROLES IN INTERNATIONAL SL

Faculty involvement in SL is critical because, in its most common form, SL is a course-driven feature of the curriculum. Therefore, it is important that the faculty become involved at an advisory-committee level in any SL initiative.

The academic organization must be committed to the SL initiative. A mechanism of support for the faculty must be in place to:

- Generate interest among the faculty in SL
- Provide the faculty with support to make the curricular changes necessary to add an SL component to a course

EVIDENCE-BASED TEACHING PRACTICE

Wilson and colleagues (2012) used an online survey of English- and Spanish-speaking respondents ($N = 542$) to test their perceptions of global health competencies. Although the respondents thought that the competencies were important for nursing education, they also voiced concerns about the additive curriculum.

An overview of the faculty and institutional activities that support SL is presented in Table 10.1.

TABLE 10.1 Institutional SL Support		
	INSTITUTION	**FACULTY**
Planning	• Form a planning group of key persons • Survey institutional resources and climate • Attend the Campus Compact Regional Institute • Develop a campus action plan for SL • Form an advisory committee	• Survey faculty interests and SL courses that are currently offered • Identify faculty for an SL planning group and advisory committee
Awareness	• Inform key administrators and faculty groups about SL and program development • Join national organizations (e.g., Campus Compact, National Society for Experiential Education, Partnership for SL) • Attend SL conferences	• Distribute information on SL (e.g., brochures, newsletters, and articles) • Identify a faculty liaison in each academic unit
Prototype	• Identify and consult with exemplary programs in higher education	• Identify or develop prototype course(s)
Resources	• Obtain administrative commitments for an SL office (e.g., budget, office space, personnel) • Develop a means for coordinating SL with other programs on campus (e.g., student support services, faculty development) • Apply for grants	• Identify interested faculty and faculty mentors • Maintain a syllabus file by discipline • Compile a library collection on SL • Secure faculty development funds for expansion • Identify existing resources that can support faculty development in SL • Establish a faculty award that recognizes service

(continued)

TABLE 10.1
Institutional SL Support (*continued*)

	INSTITUTION	FACULTY
Expansion	• Discuss SL with a broader audience of administrators and staff (e.g., deans, counselors, student affairs) • Support attendance at SL conferences • Collaborate with others in programming and applying for grants • Arrange campus speakers and forums on SL	• Offer faculty development workshops • Arrange one-on-one consultations • Discuss SL with departments and schools • Provide course development stipends and grants to support SL • Focus efforts on underrepresented schools • Develop faculty mentoring program • Promote the development of general education and sequential and interdisciplinary SL courses
Recognition	• Publicize the university's SL activities to other institutions • Participate in conferences and workshops • Publish research • Publicize SL activities in local media	• Publicize faculty accomplishments • Include SL activities on faculty annual report forms • Involve faculty in professional activities (e.g., publications, workshops, conferences, forums) • Publicize recipients of the faculty service award
Monitoring	• Collect data within the institution (e.g., number of courses, number of faculty teaching SL courses, number of students enrolled, number of agency partnerships)	• Collect data on faculty involvement (e.g., number of faculty involved in faculty development activities, number of faculty offering SL courses)
Evaluation	• Compile an annual report for the SL office • Include SL in institutional assessments	• Provide assessment methods and designs to faculty (e.g., peer review, portfolios) • Evaluate course outcomes (e.g., student satisfaction, student learning)
Research	• Conduct research on SL within the institution and across institutions	• Facilitate faculty research on SL • Conduct research on faculty involvement in SL

(continued)

TABLE 10.1
Institutional SL Support (*continued*)

	INSTITUTION	FACULTY
Institutionalization	• Service is part of the university mission statement and SL is recognized in university publications • SL is an identifiable feature of general education • SL courses are listed in bulletins, schedules of classes, and course descriptions • University sponsors regional or national conferences on SL • Hard-line budget commitments sustain SL programs	• SL is part of personnel decisions (e.g., hiring, annual reviews, promotion, and tenure) • SL is a permanent feature of course descriptions and the curriculum • SL is an integral part of the faculty's professional development program

SL, service learning.

FACULTY AND LEARNER SAFETY IN SL INTERNATIONAL SITUATIONS

A prime consideration for international SL is safety. Careful preparation prior to the trip will help to ensure safety. Some considerations include the following:

> **Teaching Gem:** All learners who take regular medications should carry enough with them for the entire trip, including a surplus in case the return trip is detained.

- Review best practice and current literature related to SL
  - Understand the political conditions of the destination country
- Register at the U.S. Embassy in the destination country
- Understand the health care system and the role of the nurse in the destination country
- Align with an educational health care organization in the destination country
- Ensure faculty and learners have the proper immunizations, medications, and identifications
- Hold preparatory sessions prior to leaving to review learning outcomes and evaluation expectations as well as predeparture cultural preparation
- Understand the food preparation and water safety of the destination country
- Include learner medications that may be needed
- Have emergency contacts on standby while away (Wittmann-Price et al., 2010)
- Have opportunities for formal debriefing and reflections after the trip

> ### CRITICAL THINKING QUESTION
>
> What precautions should the nurse educator take when traveling to countries and places that have significantly different altitudes than the learners' place of origin?

CASE STUDY

> ### CASE STUDY 10.1
>
> Two faculty members are arranging an international SL trip for six prelicensure learners to an underdeveloped country. The hostel in which their group is being housed is 90 miles from the airport in a small town. What are some of the safety issues that must be addressed before the learners and faculty depart? What are the appropriate evaluation mechanisms to assess learning that took place while the learners were on the trip?

PRACTICE QUESTIONS

1. According to Bringle and Clayton (2012), the optimal service learning (SL) design includes:

    A. A formal buddy assignment

    B. Separation from a formal academic course

    C. Benefits to the community

    D. Mandatory core competencies

2. A student is going to travel to Cuba for a student learning (SL) experience. To build intercultural competence predeparture, which of the following will help the most?

    A. Dining weekly in restaurants in a Hispanic neighborhood

    B. Binge watching HBO's *Havana* series

    C. Attend the predeparture training session offered by the Study Abroad office

    D. Take a conversational Spanish course

3. An example of implementing a global classroom would be to:

    A. Collaborate with students and faculty using video-teleconferencing

    B. Assign research articles to students to review nursing around the globe

    C. Have students find a research article about nursing in another country

    D. Have a class utilizing Internet videos about other countries

4. Which of the following exemplifies study-abroad opportunities?

    A. A student going to take blood pressures in a well clinic in another country

    B. A student taking a course in research at the University of Sydney, Australia

    C. Participating in an online virtual class from his or her apartment

    D. Going to South America to help rebuild homes after a hurricane

5. Which of the following programs enables students to spend a year in a different country learning at an institution of higher learning?

    A. Studying abroad

    B. Faculty enhancement program

    C. Service learning

    D. Global classroom

6. Which of the following is an important element for students to utilize when returning from an international learning experience to enable them to share and verbalize feelings and experiences?

    A. Write a paper summarizing the experience

    B. Conduct a debriefing experience

    C. Do a role-play to reenact the experience

    D. Write a case study of an individual they met and present it

7. Which of the following statements best reflects what *cultural competence* means?

    A. Understanding people react differently depending on their religion

    B. Being aware that language plays a key role in one's ability to access health care

    C. Allowing the nurse to recognize the impact of globalization of individual health and nursing practice

    D. Having a cognitive understanding of what each member of the health care team's role is in different areas of the world

8. A university has an exchange program with a university in Europe. The best description of a well-managed exchange program is:

    A. The foreign university will accommodate English-speaking students

    B. The foreign university is gaining tuition funds by participating

    C. The foreign university will grant course credit

    D. The foreign university cannot grant transferable courses

9. A nurse educator is taking a group of interprofessional students on a service learning (SL) trip. A safety feature that is encouraged it to:

    A. Take cash for exchange purposes

    B. Carry school texts for reference

    C. Be generous with people who beg for cash or goods

    D. Develop a social media site

10. During a debriefing from an service learning (SL) experience, which student comment best indicates cultural awareness:

    A. "This experience allowed me to see how others live"

    B. "I think we should go back, the people need more resources from us"

    C. "I think we made a difference today"

    D. "This experience was different than what I expected"

11. The culture of service learning (SL) is currently developed in learners by:

A. Nurse educators, in order to emphasize the caring aspects of nursing

B. Parents, to better prepare their children for the world

C. Primary and secondary schools, to develop global citizens

D. Organizations, to increase fund-raising

12. The best format to publicize service learning (SL) done by learners and faculty would be to:

A. Produce flyers about the trip

B. Hold an SL conference with poster presentations

C. Post an advertisement in the local newspaper

D. Comment on the experiences on Facebook

REFERENCES

Amendola, B., Fisher, K., Schaffer, D., & Howarth, K. (2016). Creating and evaluating a global classroom to teach nursing research. *Journal of Nursing Education and Practice, 6*(4), 117–121.

Bringle, R. G., & Clayton, P. H. (2012). Civic education through service learning: What, how, and why? In L. McIlraith, A. Lyons, & R. Munck (Eds.), *Higher education and civic engagement: Comparative perspectives* (pp. 101–124). New York, NY: Palgrave Macmillan. Retrieved from https://tulane.edu/cps/faculty/upload/Research-on-Service-Learning -An-Introduction.pdf

Carlton, K. H., Ryan, M., Ali, N. S., & Kelsey, B. (2007). Global health concepts. *Nursing Education Perspectives, 28*(3), 124–129.

Foronda, C., & Belknap, R. A. (2012). Short of transformation: American ADN students' thoughts, feelings, and experiences of studying abroad in a low-income country. *International Journal of Nursing Education Scholarship, 9*(1), 1–16.

Generator School Network. (2016). National service-learning clearing house. Retrieved from https://gsn.nylc.org/clearinghouse

Griffith, T., & Clark, K. R. (2016). Teaching techniques: Service learning. *Radiologic Technology, 87*(5), 586–588.

Hawkins, J., & Vialet, C. (2012). Service learning abroad: A life-changing experience for students. *Journal of Christian Nursing, 29*(3), 173–177.

Kohlbry, P. W. (2016). The impact of international service-learning on nursing students' cultural competency. *Journal of Nursing Scholarship, 48*, 303–311. doi:10.1111/jnu.12209

Krishnan, L. A., Richards, K. A. R., & Simpson, J. M. (2016). Outcomes of an international audiology service-learning study-abroad program. *American Journal of Audiology, 25*(1), 1–13. doi:10.1044/2015_AJA-15-0054

Levesque-Bristol, C., & Cornelius-White, J. (2012). The Public Affairs Scale: Measuring the public goods mission of higher education. *Journal of Public Affairs Education, 18*, 695–716.

Long, T. (2016). Influence of international service learning on nursing students' self efficacy towards cultural competence. *Journal of Cultural Diversity, 23*(1), 28–33.

National League for Nursing. (2016). Certified nurse educator (CNE) 2016 candidate handbook. Retrieved from http://www.nln.org/docs/default-source/professional -development-programs/certified-nurse-educator-(cne)-examination-candidate- handbook.pdf?sfvrsn=2

Palmer, S., Wing, D., Miles, L., Heaston, S., & de la Cruz, K. (2013). Study abroad programs: Using alumni and graduate students as affiliate faculty. *Nurse Educator, 38*(5), 198–201.

Parker, B., & Alman-Dautoff, D. (2007). Service learning and study abroad: Synergistic learning opportunities. *Michigan Journal of Service Learning, 13*(2), 40–53.

Rowthorn, V., & Olsen, J. (2014). All together now: Developing a team skills competency domain for global health education. *Journal of Law Medicine & Ethics, 42*(4), 550–563. doi:10.1111/jlme.12175

Ruddock, H. C., & Turner, D. S. (2007). Developing cultural sensitivity: Nursing students experiences of a study abroad programme. *Journal of Advanced Nursing, 59*(4), 361–369.

Saenz, K., & Holcomb, L. (2009). Essential tools for studying abroad in nursing courses. *Nurse Educator, 34*(4), 172–175.

Salisbury, M. H., An, B. P., & Pascarella, E. T. (2013) The effect of study abroad on intercultural competence among undergraduate college students. *Journal of Student Affairs Research and Practice, 50*(1), 1–20. Retrieved from http://www.tandfonline.com/doi/pdf/10.1515/jsarp-2013-0001

Stebleton, M. J., Soria, K. M., & Cherney, B. (2013). The high impact of education abroad: College students' engagement in international experiences and the development of intercultural competencies. *Frontiers: Interdisciplinary Journal of Study Abroad, 22.* Retrieved from http://works.bepress.com/michael_stebleton/22

Tapley, H., & Patel, R. (2016). Using the precede-proceed model and service-learning to teach health promotion and wellness: An innovative approach for physical therapist professional education. *Journal of Physical Therapy Education, 30*(1), 47–59.

Wilson, L., Harper, D. C., Tami-Maury, I., Zarate, R., Salas, S., Farley, J., . . . Ventura, C. (2012). Global health competencies for nurses in America. *Journal of Professional Nursing, 28*(4), 213–222. doi:10.1016/j.profnurs.2011.11.021

Wittmann-Price, R. A. (2007). Promoting reflection in groups of diverse nursing students. In B. Moyer & R. A. Wittmann-Price (Eds.), *Nursing education: Foundations for practice excellence*. Philadelphia, PA: F. A. Davis.

Wittmann-Price, R. A., Anselmi, K. K., & Espinal, F. (2010, March/April). Creating opportunities for successful international student service-learning experiences. *Holistic Nursing Practice, 24*(2), 89–98. doi:10.1097/HNP.0b013e3181d3994a

11

Using Assessment and Evaluation Strategies

ROSEMARY FLISZAR

Learning without thought is labor lost.
—Confucius

This chapter addresses the Certified Nurse Educator Exam Content Area 3: Use Assessment and Evaluation Strategies (National League for Nursing [NLN], 2016, p. 5).

- Content Area 3 is 17% of the examination
- It is estimated that there will be approximately 25 or 26 questions from Content Area 3

LEARNING OUTCOMES

- Identify internal and external factors that influence admission, progression, and graduation in a nursing program
- Utilize nursing program standards related to admission and progression
- Describe the process of program evaluation to assess outcomes in a nursing curriculum
- Use a variety of strategies to assess learning in the cognitive, affective, and psychomotor domains within the context of fair testing guidelines
- Understand various frameworks and models upon which evaluation and assessment are based
- Analyze assessment and evaluation data in determining learner achievement and program outcomes
- Use assessment and evaluation data to enhance the teaching–learning process and influence program outcomes

This chapter focuses on the factors that influence nursing education program outcomes. The relationship of standards related to admission and progression within the parent institution in general, and in the nursing program in particular, is discussed. Methods of assessing learning and outcomes are presented to provide a mechanism for the nurse educator to determine program effectiveness and identify strategies to improve the quality of the nursing program.

DEFINITIONS

To understand the assessment and evaluation process involved in a nursing education program, it is important to understand the terminology related to this process.

- "[A] nursing education program refers to any academic program offered in a postsecondary education institution, which results in initial licensure or advanced preparation in nursing" (Sauter, Gillespie, & Knepp, 2012, p. 467).
- Nursing programs that offer initial licensure are of three types:
  1. Baccalaureate degree—A 4-year program offered by a college or university
  2. Associate degree—A 2-year program typically offered by a community college
  3. Diploma—A 2- or 3-year program that is hospital based and offered in a school of nursing
- Nursing programs offering advanced preparation in nursing occur at the college or university level and include:
  * RN–BSN programs
  * RN–MSN programs
  * MSN degree
  * Doctorate (doctor of philosophy [PhD] or doctor of nursing practice [DNP])
- Second-degree programs or accelerated BSN degree programs deliver a baccalaureate in an accelerated format in which a student with a previous bachelor's degree in any field attends a condensed baccalaureate degree program. This can range from as little as 11 months to longer time frames, but is usually less than 2 years.
- *Assessment* is a process in which information is gathered to determine whether learning has occurred. Multiple methods may be used to gather this information, analyze the information, and interpret the findings. This may result in making changes to improve learner outcomes, which is similar to formative evaluation (Billings & Halstead, 2012; Fardows, 2011; Keating, 2011).
- *Evaluation* is a systematic and continuous process in which information is gathered to determine the worth and value of the program, outcomes, and achievement of the learner. It is equated to summative evaluation, in which a judgment is made about the outcome (Billings & Halstead, 2012; Fardows, 2011; Keating, 2011).
- *Program evaluation* refers to "the assessment of all components of the program" (Sauter et al., 2012, p. 467).
- *Standards* and *guidelines* are "Statements of expectations and aspirations providing a foundation for professional nursing behaviors of graduates of baccalaureate, master's, professional doctoral, and postgraduate APRN

certificate program. Standards are developed by a consensus of professional nursing communities who have a vested interest in the education and practice of nurses" (CCNE [Commission on Collegiate Nursing Education] Accreditation Manual, 2013, p. 23). Accreditation Commission for Education in Nursing (ACEN [2015]) defines *standards* as "Agreed-upon rules to measure quantity, extent, value, and quality" (*ACEN Manual,* December, 2013, p. 7).

- "Key elements as defined by CCNE are designed to enable a broad interpretation of each standard in order to support institutional autonomy and encourage innovation while maintaining the quality of nursing programs and the integrity of the accreditation" (CCNE Accreditation Manual, 2013, p. 23).
- *Criteria* are "Statements that identify the variables that need to be examined in evaluation of a standard" (*ACEN Manual*, December, 2013, p. 8).

The *admission* policies of an institution are the first standards with which a learner is evaluated for admission into a nursing program. The policies must be clearly defined and published by the institution. The nursing program in an academic setting may further refine these standards and criteria to ensure the academic quality of the learners entering the program. Criteria for admission into a nursing program may include:

- Standardized testing, such as the Scholastic Aptitude Test (SAT) for undergraduate education and Graduate Record Examination (GRE) for graduate applications
- Courses taken in high school or college with a strong science and math base
  - Nursing program entry examinations such as Health Education Systems Incorporated Admission Examination (HESI A2 Exam), Educational Resources Inc. Nurse Entrance Test (NET), or the Assessment Technology Incorporated Test of Academic Skills (ATI TEAS)
- Minimum grade point average (GPA)
- Personal letter of intent
- Letters of reference
- Background checks (Farnsworth & Springer, 2006; Serembus, 2016)

Learner success on the National Council of Licensure Examination (NCLEX®) is the benchmark for all nursing programs for achieving minimum standards of competency and quality. Predictive criteria have been studied to determine the attributes of a nursing learner that are necessary for passing the NCLEX. Yin and Burger (2003) found that the following criteria were excellent predictors of which learners enrolled in an associate degree nursing program would successfully pass the NCLEX:

- College GPA before admission into the nursing program was found to be the most important predictor of success
- High GPAs in natural science courses—biology, chemistry, and anatomy and physiology
- Course grade in an introductory psychology course
- High school rank

Sayles, Shelton, and Powell (2003) found that other predictors, in addition to the aforementioned, also improved success rates of learners on the NCLEX:

* Scores on the NET Comprehensive Achievement Profiles, administered by Educational Resources, Inc.
* Pre-RN assessment scores

Carrick (2011) suggests that other factors related to learning outcomes assessment are essential to predicting NCLEX success and include the following:

* Assessment of learning outcomes on examinations using higher level questions at the analysis and application level should be initiated after nurse educators help learners change their approach to learning.
* Nurse educators should address the underlying needs of the learner.

Personal and situational factors, such as learner anxiety and frustration, may need to be examined (p. 82). High GPAs in the natural sciences and other college courses taken prior to admission into baccalaureate nursing programs have also been predictive of learner success when taking the NCLEX. Based on this success rate, many nursing programs of all three types now require learners to complete all college requirements before admission into a nursing program. Admission into the nursing major has become very selective, based on specific criteria, as identified by the individual nursing program. In a baccalaureate program with this admission requirement, learners enter the nursing major at the junior level if they have met the strict criteria for admission into the program.

EVIDENCE-BASED TEACHING PRACTICE

Carrick (2011) used systems theory and student's approach to learning (SAL) to analyze the interdependency of the nursing education system and the nursing student learning system to help understand why certain learners are at risk for failure of the NCLEX. Learner outcomes were used to determine effectiveness of the nursing education system. Personal and situational factors were examined to determine how learners approach learning. Suggestions are made for nursing education interventions to improve the success rate on the NCLEX. Academic policies, curriculum and teaching approaches, assessment of learning outcomes, and remediation and learner support are the targeted areas for interventions.

Admission criteria for graduate nursing education must be clearly developed for applicants to this program. The policies must be congruent with the institution's overall policy but, as is seen in undergraduate education, criteria may be more selective for admission into the nursing program. Predictors of success in a graduate programs have been based on the undergraduate GPA and scores on the GRE. However, Newton and Moore (2007) found that the undergraduate GPA was not always predictive of success when taking GREs and, as such, should be used with caution when making decisions related to admission into a graduate nursing program. Many nursing programs waive the standardized testing requirement if applicants have a GPA of 3.3 or 3.5 or higher.

EVIDENCE-BASED TEACHING PRACTICE

Serembus (2016) outlined a plan to improve NCLEX-RN® pass rates and comprehensive standardized examination scores based on Deming's four phases of the continuous-improvement model (CIP): Plan, Do, Study, Act. This is a comprehensive systems approach to program evaluation. In the *Plan phase* of the CIP, strategies for improving NCLEX pass rates are established. Strategies are enacted in the *Do phase*. During the *Study phase*, the results of the plan are evaluated. The educator accepts or rejects the plan in the *Act phase* based on the outcomes. If the outcomes are successful, then the strategies are implemented and continuously assessed. If outcomes are negative, then the Plan phase is reassessed and new approaches are identified as part of the cycle.

Progression Policies

Progression policies within the nursing major must be congruent with the program goals and institutional standards and must be clearly identified and published. Criteria that are often included in progression policies are:

- Minimum course grades for nursing and science courses
- Minimum cumulative GPA for progression in the program
- Number of times a learner may repeat selective courses at both the undergraduate and graduate levels
- Standards in place if a learner takes a leave of absence during the program of study
- Achievement of a minimum grade on standardized achievement tests based on established benchmarks for prelicensure learners

THE EVALUATION/ASSESSMENT PROCESS

The terms *assessment* and *evaluation* are often used interchangeably but in reality they have different meanings.

Evaluation is the process of systematically collecting and analyzing data that has been gathered through various measurements to determine the merit, worth, and value of something and to render a judgment about the subject of the evaluation (Billings & Halstead, 2012; Fardows, 2011; Keating, 2011). Evaluation in the educational setting is conducted to determine (a) learner progress toward achieving program outcomes, (b) effectiveness of the educational process to foster learning, and (c) accomplishment of the mission of the institution to prepare nurses for entry into practice (Billings & Halstead, 2012; O'Connor, 2006).

Assessment is the process of obtaining information about learners, educators, programs, and institutions and is often used interchangeably with the term *evaluation*. More specific, assessment involves setting standards and criteria for learning, gathering, analyzing, and interpreting data to determine how performance matches the standards and criteria and using that information to improve learning, teaching, courses, and programs (Angelo, 1993; Billings & Halstead, 2012; Bourke & Ihrke, 2012; Fardows, 2011; Keating, 2011).

Philosophies of Evaluation

The evaluation process is influenced by the evaluator's beliefs about evaluation and his or her philosophical perspective. Some examples of evaluation philosophies include:

- Practice orientation
  - Practice goals are reflected in course outcomes
  - Performance achieved at the end of the course, clinical experience, or program is the most important consideration
- Service orientation
  - This perspective is based on a values approach to evaluation
  - This view takes a more global or holistic view of the goals of the educational process beyond course outcomes
  - This perspective includes goals that are integrated into a model of performance that represents the typical or ideal learner at a particular level of development
  - With this approach, instructors view the evaluation process as a means to identify learner strengths and weaknesses in various components of performance
  - This view facilitates learner progress toward model performance
- Judgment orientation
  - This perspective reflects a focus on the determination of acceptability of learner performance and the value or grade that should be assigned based on the performance
  - Instructors assign a pass/fail grade or letter or numerical grade—pass/fail is used most often in clinical grading
- Constructivist orientation
  - Assigns heaviest consideration to stakeholders who will be affected by the success or failure of the program. In nursing, the stakeholders are the employers of graduates and the recipients of the graduates' nursing care
  - The evaluation process involves input from patients and staff who contribute to the assignment of the grade in the clinical setting (O'Connor, 2006)

Teaching Gem: The best test combines aspects of both norm-referenced and criterion-referenced tests.

Purposes of Evaluation

The purpose of the evaluation process must be clearly delineated for nurse educators and learners. Purposes of evaluation include:

- Identification of learning
- Diagnosis of problems such as learning needs or deficits in teaching practices, courses, or the curriculum
- Decision making related to assignment of grades, tenure, and promotion

- Improvement of products such as textbooks or course content
- Judgment of effectiveness of learner goal achievement and the meeting of standards and program outcomes (Bourke & Ihrke, 2012; O'Connor, 2006)

Formative Evaluation

- Refers to the evaluation of learning while it is occurring.
- Identifies a learner's readiness to learn and his or her learning needs.
- May be used to improve learner performance before the end of the course or program.
- Assigns no final grade.
- Shares the evaluation with the learner informally throughout the learning process, but formally presents it in clinical courses at midsemester (Oermann & Gaberson, 2014).

Summative Evaluation

- Refers to the level of performance of the learner at the end of the course, program, or activity.
- Makes a judgment as to whether or not the standards and criteria have been met for the event (course, clinical, and program).
- Uses data collected throughout the learning experience as the basis for evaluation.
- Assigns a final grade (letter, number, pass/fail, and satisfactory/unsatisfactory).
- Evaluator determines evaluation and shares with the learner being evaluated while the summative period is in effect, particularly in clinical courses or activities (Oermann & Gaberson, 2014).

Evaluation Models

An evaluation model is useful for explaining the process on which variables, items, or events are evaluated and provides a systematic plan or framework for evaluation. Several models are used in nursing education and should be selected based on the context, needs of the stakeholders, and the question to be evaluated. Some of the evaluation models are included here (Bourke & Ihrke, 2012):

> **Teaching Gem:** The learner should never be surprised to be told that he or she has not met course requirements in either the classroom or clinical setting. The nurse educator must keep the learner informed of his or her progress throughout the entire learning experience.

- *Logic Model*
  - Useful in designing program evaluations
  - Helps conceptualize, plan, and communicate with others about the program

* Uses flowcharts to help clarify key elements of a program
* Inputs are resources that are needed to run the program
* Educational strategies
* Outputs are learner demographics, contact hours, assignments, and tests
* Initial outcomes—changes noted in learners in response to the learning activities
* Intermediate outcomes—longer term learner outcomes
* Ultimate outcomes—vision of what should be accomplished when learners have completed the program

- *Decision-Oriented Models: CIPP (Context, Input, Process, and Product)*
  * Provides information on which decisions can be made, measures strengths and weaknesses of a program, identifies target populations, and identifies options
  * Uses context evaluation to identify the target population and assess needs
  * Uses input evaluation to assess the capabilities of the system, uses alternative program strategies and procedural designs to implement the strategy
  * Process evaluation detects defects in the design or implementation of the strategy, as well as satisfaction with the experience
  * Product evaluation reflects the outcomes and results of the program

- *Fourth-Generation Models*
  * Incorporates evaluator observations, interviews, and participant evaluations to elicit views, meaning, and understanding of the stakeholders (Bourke & Ihrke, 2012, p. 396)
  * Provides meaning, consensus, and understanding of all involved

- *Accreditation Model: Evidence-Based Evaluation*
  * Process used in institutions of higher learning and professional programs to determine the extent to which a program achieves its mission, goals, and outcomes
  * Focus is on ongoing self-evaluation and the achievement of outcomes to support quality improvement of the program
  * Two main organizations accredit nursing programs
    – ACEN (http://www.acenursing.org)
    – CCNE (www.aacn.nche.edu)

Evaluation Methods

After an evaluation model has been determined, the method(s) of evaluation must be selected to assess the effectiveness of learning and the achievement of course and program outcomes in both their theoretical and clinical components. Multiple methods are often used as learning is evaluated in the three domains: cognitive, affective, and psychomotor. Using a single evaluation method does not adequately measure all three domains (see Table 11.1).

TABLE 11.1 Evaluation Strategies		
ASSESSMENT STRATEGY	**DOMAIN OF LEARNING ASSESSED**	**USES OF ASSESSMENT STRATEGY**
Papers/essays	Affective Higher cognitive levels	Demonstrates organizational skills Encourages creativity Improves critical thinking skills
Portfolios	Affective Higher cognitive levels	Measures program outcomes Shows evidence of learner progress in a specific class Advanced placement of learners within courses
Critiques	Higher cognitive levels Affective	Active learner involvement Builds critical thinking skills Reinforces expected standards
Journals	Higher cognitive levels Affective	Allows for learner reflection on experiences Promotes active learning Assesses learning Enhances critical thinking skills Helps improve writing skills
Concept maps	Cognitive (all levels) Affective	Visual representation of concepts and connections Improves critical thinking Promotes understanding of complex relationships among concepts Integrates theoretical knowledge into practice
Audiotape	Cognitive (all levels) Affective	Demonstrates communication skills Demonstrates interview skills
Videotape	Higher cognitive levels Affective Psychomotor	Reviews learner performance of skills Allows learner to observe his or her performances Reflects on the experience
Role-playing	Cognitive Affective Psychomotor	Explores feelings about an experience or issue Develops problem-solving skills Reflects on the experience Effects changes in attitude, beliefs, or values

(continued)

TABLE 11.1
Evaluation Strategies (*continued*)

ASSESSMENT STRATEGY	DOMAIN OF LEARNING ASSESSED	USES OF ASSESSMENT STRATEGY
Oral presentations	Cognitive Affective	Improves communication skills Enhances critical thinking Improves organizational skills
Simulations	Cognitive Affective Psychomotor	Practice skills in a nonthreatening environment Improves critical thinking skills Improves prioritization of activities Active learning Assesses learner learning

In any case, the learner must be informed of the evaluation methods to be used to assess his or her learning. Grading rubrics are one method of evaluation that includes rating scales used to evaluate written work and assign a grade. Grading rubrics are usually shared with the learner before the evaluation process so the learner is aware of the criteria. Grading rubrics are useful when evaluating:

- Tests/examinations (paper/pencil, computer)
- Written work
- Papers and essays
- Portfolios
- Critiques
- Journals
- Nursing care plans
- Concept maps
- Audiotape and videotape
- Role-playing
- Oral presentations
- Simulations
- Observations by the instructor
- Rating scales
- Skills checklists

Many nurse educators use grading rubrics to assess participation in electronic discussion boards. Rubrics range from being extremely detailed to rating scales that are more general and therefore contain some subjectivity. Table 11.2 offers an example of a grading rubric used for a journal assignment.

Achievement Tests and Assessments

To ensure effective evaluation, achievement tests should be related to the instruction given. The test questions should measure the achievement of

TABLE 11.2
Grading Rubric Example

TASK	1 POINT	2 POINTS	3 POINTS	4 POINTS
Identify goals and attainment	Goals not clearly identified No description of attainment of goals	Goals not clearly identified Minimal description of attainment of goals	Goals clearly identified Attainment of goals mentioned, but not described completely	Goals clearly identified Attainment of goals thoroughly discussed
Score: (/4)				
Summary of interactions	Briefly summarized interactions with preceptor No identification of situations encountered	Briefly summarized interactions with preceptor Minimal identification of situations encountered	Summarized interactions with preceptor Identified situations encountered	Thoroughly summarized interactions with preceptor Identified situations encountered
Score: (/4)				
Analysis of significant events	No critical reflection evident in the analysis of the experience Minimal to no description of feelings, reactions, or responses Last journal includes little or no discussion of attainment of objectives and lessons learned	Analysis shows minimal reflection of the experience Minimal description of feelings, reactions, or responses Last journal includes minimal discussion of attainment of objectives and lessons learned	Analysis shows some critical reflection of the experience Feelings, reactions, and responses described Last journal includes discussion of attainment of objectives and lessons learned	Analysis shows critical reflection of the experience Feelings, reactions, and responses described in depth Last journal includes discussion of attainment of objectives and lessons learned
Score: (/4)				
Submission of journals		Journals submitted late		Journals submitted by due date
Score: (/4)				
Total Score: (/16) = %				

the learning outcomes and should fit the learner population's learning characteristics. The results of achievement tests should be reliable and valid, and learners should benefit from the test's feedback. The results should also provide the nurse educator with feedback about content areas for which more emphasis is needed or areas that were interpreted differently than expected (Gronlund, 1993). Achievement testing can be an effective evaluative mechanism for both learner and faculty if tests are developed based on sound, evaluative principles.

Guidelines for Developing Classroom Tests

According to Gronlund (1993), there are three types of evaluative mechanisms used in nursing education. *Achievement tests* usually denote tests that have sound psychometric reliability; many times, these are standardized tests created by an outside vendor. *Norm-referenced tests* are those that rank a group of learners. Someone gets the highest score, someone else receives the lowest, and the scores in between are compared to the shape of a "bell curve" for that evaluation. A *criterion-referenced test* is one that is closely aligned to an achievement test. The criteria are set, and the score is compared to a criterion, not to other scores. The specific characteristics of each type of test are listed here.

Achievement Tests
- Achievement tests should measure clearly defined learning outcomes.
  * These tests are measured in terms of learner performance.
- Achievement tests should be concerned with all intended learning outcomes.
  * These tests must include outcomes based on knowledge, skill, understanding, application, and complex learning.
- Achievement tests should measure a representative sample of instructionally relevant learning skills.
  * These tests are based on sampling.
  * Instructors need to use a systematic procedure to obtain a representative sample of the test items relevant to the instruction.
  * Instructors need to prepare learners for test specifications.
- Achievement tests should include the types of test items that are most appropriate for measuring the intended outcomes.
  * The tests need a means of determining whether the specified performance and learning have occurred.
  * Key: Select the most appropriate item type and construct it to elicit the desired response.
- Achievement tests should be based on plans for using the results.
- Achievement tests should provide scores that are relatively free from measurement errors.
  * The test should provide consistent results (it should be reliable).

* The following factors increase the amount of error in test scores:
  – Ambiguous test items
  – Testing a specific skill with too few test items yields scores that are influenced by chance rather than by learner performance
  – Essay tests are subjective
  – Learners' attention, effort, fatigue, and guessing on tests

Norm-Referenced Tests

- Interpreted in relation to the ranking of learners in the class
- Tell how a learner's scores compare with those of his or her peers
- Provide a wide range of scores to discriminate among levels of achievement
- Focus on a broad range of learning tasks
- Feature relatively few test items per task
- Focus on learner ranking
- Provide a percentile rank of learners from high to low achievers
  * These are commonly used in national standardized tests, such as SATs and ATIs (Billings & Halstead, 2012; Gronlund, 1993; McDonald, 2007)

Criterion-Referenced Tests

- These tests are expressed in terms of the specific knowledge and skills a learner can demonstrate
- Include test items that are directly relevant to the learning outcomes regardless of the degree of difficulty
- Focus on a detailed learning domain
- Should be designed to measure the ability of a learner in a particular area
- Feature a relatively large number of test items per task
- Most are teacher made and are based on course objectives
- Items provide a detailed description of learner performance
- Scores are reported as the percentage correct based on preset standards
- Example: 100% of the learners will correctly calculate medication dosages on the calculation examination (Billings & Halstead, 2012; Gronlund, 1993; McDonald, 2007)

PLANNING THE TEST

The first step in planning a test is to determine what type of test should be given. This decision is based on the purpose of the test. The type of test given should effectively measure the learning or capability to be measured and the desired outcome of the test. Some examples of reasons why a test may be given include:

- To determine eligibility before entry into a nursing program as part of the admission criteria
- To determine appropriate academic placement

- To monitor learning progress
- To determine levels of mastery of content at the end of an instruction period

Identifying and Defining Learning Outcomes

The next step in planning a test is to identify and define intended learning outcomes. The use of Bloom's taxonomy of learning is one method to accomplish this step. (Refer to Chapter 2 to review Bloom's taxonomy.)

- The cognitive domain addresses areas related to intellectual abilities.
- The affective domain is concerned with values and attitudes.
- The psychomotor domain addresses motor skills (Table 11.3)

TABLE 11.3
Bloom's Taxonomy for Affective Domains

LEVEL	CONCEPTS	VERBS USED IN WRITING OBJECTIVES AND LEARNING OUTCOMES, WITH EXAMPLES
Receiving	Awareness Willingness to receive Control of selected attention	**Verbs:** Ask, listen, focus, attend, take part, discuss, acknowledge, hear, be open to, retain, follow, concentrate, read, do, feel **Examples:** Listens to teacher or trainer, takes interest in session or learning experience, takes notes, attends; makes time for learning experience, participates passively
Responding	Acquiescence in responding Willingness to respond Satisfaction with response	**Verbs:** React, respond, seek, interpret, clarify, provide, contribute **Examples:** Participate actively in group discussion, active participation in activity, show interest in outcomes, enthusiasm for action, question, and probe ideas, suggest interpretations
Valuing	Acceptance of a value Preference for a value Commitment	**Verbs:** Argue, challenge, debate, refute, confront, justify, persuade, criticize **Examples:** Decide worth and relevance of ideas or experiences; accept or commit to particular stance or action

(continued)

TABLE 11.3
Bloom's Taxonomy for Affective Domains (continued)

LEVEL	CONCEPTS	VERBS USED IN WRITING OBJECTIVES AND LEARNING OUTCOMES, WITH EXAMPLES
Organization	Conceptualization of a value Organization of a value system	**Verbs:** Build, develop, formulate, defend, modify, relate, prioritize, reconcile, contrast, arrange, compare **Examples:** Qualify and quantify personal views, state personal position and reasons, state beliefs
Characterization by a value or a value complex	General set of behaviors that characterize a person Characterization of the whole person—an internal consistency	**Verbs:** Act, display, influence, solve, practice **Examples:** Self-reliant; behaves consistently with personal value set

Achievement testing is focused primarily on the cognitive domain, with the following six main areas to consider (Gronlund, 1993):

1. *Knowledge (remembering previously learned material)*
   * Intellectual abilities and skills
   * Comprehension (grasping the meaning of material)
2. *Translation (converting from one form to another)*
   * Interpretation (explaining material)
   * Extrapolation (extending the meaning beyond data)
3. *Application (using information in a concrete situation)*
4. *Analysis (breaking down material into its parts)*
   * Identify the parts
   * Identify the relationships
   * Identify the organization
5. *Synthesis (putting parts together to create a whole)*
   * Uniqueness
   * Abstract relations
6. *Evaluation (judging the value for a given purpose using specific criteria)*
   * Judgment in terms of internal evidence
   * Judgment in terms of external criteria

Another method used to plan a test is to use the NCLEX Test Plan (2016). Patient needs are the basis of the test plan and include four major areas:

1. Safe, effective care environment
2. Health promotion and maintenance
3. Psychosocial integrity
4. Physiological integrity

TABLE 11.4 **NCLEX Test Plan**
CLIENT NEEDS TESTED
Safe and effective care environment - Management of care—20% - Safety and infection control—12% Health promotion and maintenance—9% Psychosocial integrity—9% Physiological integrity - Basic care/comfort—9% - Pharmacological and parenteral therapies—15% - Reduction of risk potential—12% - Physiological adaptation—14%

Source: National Council of State Boards of Nursing (2016).

Each area is assigned a percentage of the number of questions on the NCLEX (Table 11.4). Most items are concerned with the application or higher levels of cognitive ability, but the examination also includes knowledge and comprehension questions.

Determining the Types of Test Questions to Use

Once the nurse educator has determined the purpose of the test and the plan to be used in its construction, the next step is to decide on the types of test questions to be included. This decision is based on the objectives and outcomes for the test and should include a variety of types of questions that are consistent with formats used on the NCLEX-RN exam (NCLEX 2016), such as:

- Multiple choice
- Multiple response
- True/false
- Matching
- Fill in the blank
- Essay
- Ordered response
- Hot spots
- Multimedia, including charts, graphs, audio, sound, and tables

A table of specifications (test plan, test blueprint) should be used as the basis for developing achievement tests (see Table 11.5 for a test blueprint for the nursing process).

The following factors should be taken into consideration when developing a table of specifications:

- Matches the purpose of the test—be sure that the test is measuring a representative sample of the content and learning outcomes
- Relates learning outcomes to content
- Indicates the relative weight for each area based on several factors (see Table 11.5)
- How much time was spent on each area during instruction? This should be the most important consideration
- Which outcomes are most important in regard to retention and transfer value?

Another consideration that should be part of the table of specifications would be to determine the number of questions for each part of the content being tested based on the criteria listed earlier (see Table 11.6 for an example of the distribution of test questions by content).

TABLE 11.5
Test Blueprint

CONTENT AREA	ASSESSMENT	ANALYSIS	PLANNING	IMPLEMENTATION	EVALUATION	TOTAL NUMBER OF ITEMS
Cardiac %						
Renal %						
Endocrine %						
Total number of items						

TABLE 11.6
Distribution of Test Questions

OUTCOMES/ CONTENT	KNOWLEDGE		COMPREHENDS PRINCIPLES	APPLIES PRINCIPLES	TOTAL NUMBER OF ITEMS
	TERMS	FACTS			
Role of nurse in decision making	4	4	3	5	16
Osteoarthritis	3	2	4	5	14
Total number of items	7	6	7	10	30

Validity and Reliability of Tests

Validity refers to the appropriateness, meaningfulness, and usefulness of the *inferences* from the test scores (Billings & Halstead, 2012; Gronlund, 1993). A test's validity is the judgment one makes to determine whether the test measured what was intended.

Approaches for testing validity include the following (Billings & Halstead, 2012; Gronlund, 1993):

- Content-related evidence
  * How well does the test measure the intended learning outcomes?
  * Did the test feature an adequate sampling of material?
  * Was the test properly constructed, administered, and scored?
- Criterion-related evidence
  * How accurately does test performance predict future performance?
  * Can one use test performance to estimate current performance on a criterion?
  * What is the degree of relationship between the test scores and the criterion—the key element?
  * What was the correlation coefficient (r)?
    - Positive relationship—high or low scores on one measure are accompanied by high or low scores on another
    - Negative relationship—high scores on one measure are accompanied by low scores on another measure
- Construct-related evidence
  * How well can test performance be explained in terms of psychological characteristics?

Reliability refers to the degree of consistency of test scores. Factors that may affect reliability include insufficient test length and group variability (Twigg, 2012). Reliability is measured by a correlation coefficient. The simplest method of estimating the reliability of test scores from a single administration of a test is using the Kuder–Richardson formulas (KR-20 or KR-21). The KR-20 reflects the accuracy or power of discrimination of the test (Kehoe, 1995). Three types of information are required to determine the KR: (a) the number of items in the test, (b) the mean, and (c) the standard deviation (Gronlund, 1993). The formula for the KR-21 is shown in Exhibit 11.1.

EXHIBIT 11.1

KR-21 Formula

Reliability estimate (KR21) $= 1 - \dfrac{M(k-M)}{K(s^2)}$

K = number of items in the test
M = mean of test scores
s = standard deviation of test scores

Reported reliabilities for standardized achievement tests are .90 or better for KR formulas. Reliability coefficients for classroom tests should be between .50 and .80 (1.0 is the maximum; Kehoe, 1995).

Factors That Lower Reliability of Test Scores

- Too few items on the test
- Excessive numbers of very easy or very hard questions
- Inadequate testing conditions
- Items are poorly written and do not discriminate
- Scoring is subjective (remedy: prepare scoring keys and follow them carefully when scoring essay answers and performance tasks; in other words, prepare a rubric; Gronlund, 1993; Kehoe, 1995)

Exhibit 11.2 provides an example of test statistics. Try to interpret the meaning of the statistics.

Item Analysis

Item analysis is done to determine whether tests have separated the learners from the nonlearners (discrimination). Software packages can provide statistical data about the overall analysis of a test and provide a detailed analysis of each item. The following key concepts are necessary to consider when reviewing the item analysis on a classroom test.

EXHIBIT 11.2	
Example of Test Statistics	
Total possible points	50
Students in this group	17
Standard deviation	3.53
Reliability coefficient (KR-20)	0.56
Point biserial	0.18
Total group	64.71%
Upper 27% of group	80.00%
Median score	40.33
Mean score	40.35

- Item difficulty (p-value; Gronlund, 1993)
- Percentage of the group that answered the item correctly
- $p = .5$ (50% correct) is a good discrimination index
- Upper limit = 1.00 (100% of learners answered the question correctly)
- Lower limit depends on the number of possible responses and probability of guessing correctly
- If there are four options, then $p = .25$ is the lower limit or probability of guessing

See Exhibit 11.3 for a formula for calculating item difficulty.

Item Discrimination

- Differentiates between learners who knew the content from those who did not
- Measured by point-biserial correlation (measures each learner's item performance with each learner's overall test performance)
  - Questions that discriminate well have point-biserial correlations that are highly positive for the correct answer and negative for the distractors
  - Learners who knew the content answered correctly; those who did not chose the distractors
  - Indices greater than .3 are good; greater than .4 are very good
  - Item difficulty of $p = .5$ shows a discrimination index that is maximized. If the index is too high or too low, the index is attenuated and the item is a poor discriminator
- Distractor evaluation
  - Need to evaluate each distractor individually
  - Distractors should appeal to the nonlearner

EXHIBIT 11.3				
Calculating Item Difficulty				
EXAMPLE				
ITEM 1. ALTERNATIVES	A	B[a]	C	D
Upper 10	0	6	3	1
Lower 10	3	2	2	3
$P = \dfrac{R}{T} \times 100$				
$P = \dfrac{8}{20} \times 100 = 40\% \ (.40)$				

P = the percentage who answered the item correctly, R = the number who answered the item correctly, T = total number who attempted the item.

[a]B is correct answer.

⁂ Distractors that have a point biserial of zero means learners did not select them and they need to be revised or replaced—learners probably got the question correct by guessing.

⁂ Negative discriminating power occurs when more learners in the lower group than in the upper group choose the correct answer. These items need to be revised or replaced.

- Compute item analysis
  1. Mean score—the average of all the learners
  2. Median—the point at which 50% are higher and 50% are lower
  3. Standard deviation—measures the variability of test scores; the degree test scores deviate from the mean
  4. D-value = $\dfrac{R_u - R_L}{1/2T}$

- D = index of discriminating power; R_u = number in the upper group who answered the item correctly; R_L = number in the lower group who answered the item correctly; $1/2\,T$ = one half of the total number of learners included in the item analysis

In other words, for a multiple-choice question to be discriminating, it should be answered correctly by the upper one third of the class and answered incorrectly by the lower one third of the class. See Exhibit 11.4 for a formula for calculating point biserials.

EXHIBIT 11.4

Formula for Calculating Point–Biserial Correlation

ITEM 1. ALTERNATIVES	A	B[a]	C	D
Upper 10	0	6	3	1
Lower 10	3	2	2	3
D-value = $\dfrac{R_u - R_L}{1/2T}$				
$D = \dfrac{0-3}{10} = -0.3$ (for answer A)				
$D = \dfrac{6-2}{10} = 0.40$ (for answer B)				
$D = \dfrac{3-2}{10} = 0.1$ (for answer C)				
$D = \dfrac{1-3}{10} = -0.2$ (for answer D)				

[a]B is the correct answer.

Some evaluators like to purposely include one or two easy questions at the beginning of an examination to decrease learners' anxiety (Exhibit 11.5; a Gronlund, 1993).

Item Revision

- Completed after item analysis
- Revise items with the following characteristics:
  - p-values that are too high or too low.
  - Correct answers with low positive or negative point biserials.
  - Distractors with highly positive point-biserial correlations.
  - Items that correlate less than .15 with total test scores should be restructured. They are probably confusing or misleading to those taking the examination (Kehoe, 1995).
  - The distractor was not chosen by any learner. This prevents discriminating the good learners from the poor learners (Kehoe, 1995).
  - Items that all test takers get right. These questions do not discriminate among learners and should be replaced by more difficult ones.

EXHIBIT 11.5

Nondiscriminating Questions

(1) What do you do if you have a question that 100% of the class gets right?

D-value $= \dfrac{0-0}{0} = 0$ for the D-value or split-biserial value

Is this a discriminating question?

(2) Five learners out of the top third of the class chose the correct answer on an examination question; six out of the middle third, and eight out of the lower third. Calculate the point biserial for this question as indicated in the following.

D-value $= \dfrac{5-8}{10} = \dfrac{-3}{10} = -0.3$ for the D-value or split-biserial value

Is this a discriminating question? YES _____ NO __✓__
Rationale for answer: The question is too difficult or unclear.

(3) All learners ($n = 10$) in the upper group answered an item correctly on an examination, but none of the learners in the lower group got it correct.

$D = \dfrac{10-0}{10} = 1.00$

Is this a discriminating question? YES _____ NO __✓__
Rationale for answer: Question is too difficult and does not discriminate.

COLLABORATIVE TESTING/EVALUATION

Nurses work collaboratively with other health care team members in all aspects of care for the patient. To develop cooperation and collaboration in the learning process and to foster accountability in the learner, educators often assign learners to work in groups or teams on specific assignments. Group projects can also be used in the clinical component to evaluate whether learning has occurred.

There are some important considerations that the nurse educator must take into account when developing collaborative learning assignments and evaluation of learning (Billings & Halstead, 2012):

- The assignments must be meaningful and should be designed for small groups whenever possible.
- The educator must ensure that members of the group understand the role of each person in the group.

Teaching Gem:
Eliminate the following from test items:
- Ethnocentrism such as "death practices in the Western culture"
- Elitism such as using words like "estate"
- Tone of language such as comments like "soul food, regatta"
- Inflammatory material as when using the issue of abortion
- Making judgments such as using "unfortunately"
- Avoid words such as never, always, and all

Also:
- Avoid "none of the above" and "all of the above"
- Randomize the correct options (Su, Osisek, Montgomery, & Pellar, 2009)

- The groups should be structured heterogeneously with regard to gender, ethnicity, ability, experience, and so on, to increase learning.
- Enough time must be given for the group to complete and process its work.

The nurse educator must also decide how the group will be evaluated or graded on the project. Some considerations for evaluation include (Gaberson & Oermann, 2010):

- All members of the group receive the same grade.
- Learners might be asked to indicate which part of the assignment they completed and receive an individual grade based on the quality of that section.
- Peer assessment of the project may be used to contribute to the grade (e.g., peer evaluation counts for 40% of the grade, educator evaluation for 60% of the grade).
- Learners can prepare a group and an individual project.
- Educators must use grading rubrics to assess group projects and assign a grade.

EVIDENCE-BASED TEACHING PRACTICE

Sandahl (2010) examined the effect of collaborative testing on learning and retention of course content, and group process skills and learner retention. Collaborative testing in which learners worked together on a test was used to determine examination scores, retention of course content, and learner perceptions of learning. Even though test scores did not significantly increase in collaborative testing, learners reported a perception of increased learning.

ROLE OF STANDARDIZED TESTING IN THE CURRICULUM

To assess learning in the nursing curriculum, many programs require learners to pass standardized tests to progress through the curriculum and also as a measure to predict success of a student's passing the NCLEX-RN on the first attempt (Mee & Hallenbeck, 2015; Molsbee & Benton, 2016; Spurlock, 2013). The NLN defines using a test to predict individual student performance on the NCLEX-RN or to make decisions about progression and graduation in a program based on learner scores on standardized tests as *high-stakes testing* (NLN, 2012b).

The NLN created a task force to develop guidelines for the use of standardized tests as a prerequisite for learner progression in the nursing program (NLN, 2010). Outcomes of this task force included the development of a position statement on fair testing that was approved by the NLN Board of Governors (NLN, 2012b), and the development of Fair Testing Guidelines for Nursing Education (NLN, 2012a). The guidelines include the following:

- Faculty have an ethical obligation to ensure that test and decisions made based on tests are valid, supported by solid evidence, consistent across courses, and fair to all test takers.
- Faculty have the responsibility to assess students' abilities to practice nursing competently, but recognize that current approaches to assessment of learning are limited.
- Multiple sources of evidence and approaches to assessment are critical to evaluating competency in knowledge and clinical abilities, especially if high-stakes decisions are based on the assessment.
- A variety of measures, including tests, are used to evaluate students' competencies, to support student learning, improve teaching, and guide program improvements.
- Standardized tests must have information available to faculty and show evidence of reliability, content, and predictive validity before faculty administer, grade, and distribute results from, or write policies related to, the use of standardized tests (NLN, 2012a, 2012b).

Standardized tests are useful in predicting success of high-performing learners in passing the NCLEX, but they are less accurate in identifying learners who will fail the NCLEX. Companies that sell standardized tests are less clear in their ability to report who will fail the NCLEX-RN (Spurlock, 2013).

When selecting standardized tests for use in a nursing curriculum or specific course(s), nurse educators need to consider the following:

- Does research support the validity and reliablity of the test?
- Who are the test-item writers and what are their qualifications as content experts?
- Does the test blueprint adhere to the NCLEX-RN blueprint?
- Does the test include key concepts and content areas that faculty want to assess?
- Are the scoring reports easy for faculty to interpret with regard to data for groups and individual learners?
- Does the item content include categories based on the requirements of accrediting agencies such as the CCNE, ACEN, Quality and Safety in Nursing Education

(QSEN), Essentials documents of the American Association of Colleges of Nursing (AACN), and the nursing process, to name a few (Mee & Hallenbeck, 2015)?

CRITICAL THINKING QUESTION

Should passing a standardized test be part of the course grade and, if so, what percentage should it be counted as?

OUTCOME EVALUATION

"Educational evaluation occurs while assessing the program for its quality, currency, relevance, projections into the future, and the need for possible revisions in light of these factors" (Keating, 2006, p. 260). Program evaluation encompasses all aspects of the program, including the curriculum, learner satisfaction, congruence of the mission of the nursing program with that of the institution, faculty and staff qualifications, learner policies and development, and resources to promote achievement of the outcomes. Accreditation of nursing programs is voluntary but encouraged, as it is a public statement attesting to the quality of the program. Several accrediting bodies oversee this process:

- State Commissions of Higher Education—the entire academic institution and programs of study are evaluated by this body
- ACEN—evaluates diploma, baccalaureate, master's, and clinical doctorate nursing programs; also licensed practical nurse programs
- CCNE—evaluates baccalaureate, graduate, and residency programs in nursing

Evaluation of the nursing program is an ongoing process. Table 11.7 gives an example of a program evaluation plan.

An essential component of program evaluation is the assessment of learner outcomes. This can be achieved in several ways:

- Satisfaction surveys
  - Exit interviews—which are conducted at the conclusion of the program, before graduation.
  - Employer and graduate surveys—conducted at a designated period of time, such as 9 months, 1 year, and so on. The purpose of the survey is to determine the satisfaction of the employer with the graduate nurse's ability to function effectively within the work environment. Graduates of the program are also surveyed to determine their satisfaction with the nursing program in preparing them for the responsibilities of a graduate nurse.
- Graduation and retention rates of the program
- Standardized examination pass rates—NCLEX, certification examinations
- Employment opportunities

A summation of program outcomes is discussed in Exhibit 11.6.

TABLE 11.7
Program Evaluation Example

Standard curriculum: The curriculum prepares learners to achieve the outcomes of the nursing education unit, including safe practice in contemporary health care environments

	PROCESS				IMPLEMENTATION	
Component	Where documentation is found	Person responsible	Frequency of assessment	Assessment method(s).	Results and analysis of data collection and levels of achievement	Actions needed/ not needed
Curriculum flows in a logical progression	Curriculum committee minutes, class, and clinical evaluation tools	Curriculum committee chair person	Every 8 years or when revisions occur	Comparison of curriculum elements for internal consistency	Due date	Criterion met, no action required

EXHIBIT 11.6

Summation of Program Outcomes

Evaluation of learning demonstrates that graduates have achieved identified competencies consistent with the institutional mission and professional standards and that the outcomes of the nursing education unit have been achieved.

EVIDENCE-BASED TEACHING PRACTICE

Molsbee and Benton (2016) initiated a process in an associate degree nursing program to move away from high-stakes testing to a model of comprehensive competency but still utilized standardized testing in a senior capstone course. A new course was developed consisting of theory and preceptor components. The theory component consists of review sessions in content taught by faculty experts in the content area. Faculty-made exams are given on the content. The HESI exam is required when students enter the course for diagnostic purposes to identify strengths and weakness. The results have shown that NCLEX-RN pass rates have remained stable, retention rates increased, and student complaints and grade appeals have decreased. These changes were implemented to ensure alignment with the NLN fair testing guidelines.

CASE STUDIES

CASE STUDY 11.1

The NCLEX pass rate for first-time test takers graduating from a nursing program has been 80% for the past 2 years. The program evaluation committee is charged with assessing all aspects of the nursing curriculum, including admission and progression criteria, course evaluations, and scores on standardized and classroom tests. The current admission policy into the nursing program is congruent with the university's admission policies. They include the following criteria: SAT scores of 980 or better, upper half of graduating class, minimum GPA of 2.0. Once enrolled in the nursing major, learners must maintain a minimum cumulative GPA of 2.5, and grades of C or better (75%) in the nursing and science courses. At this university, learners must meet admission and progression requirements established by the university, but individual programs may require more stringent policies for the major. As a member of the admission and progression committee in the nursing department, what recommendations would you make regarding admission into the nursing major? What recommendations would you make regarding progression in the nursing major through each level? What, if any, changes would you make relative to grading criteria, teacher-made tests, and the use of standardized achievement tests? Develop a program evaluation plan based on your recommendations.

CASE STUDY 11.2

The nurse educator is a member of the admission, progression, and graduation committees. There is a concern regarding declining pass rates on the NCLEX. The committee has been charged with reviewing and revising the admission and progression standards. What areas should the nurse educator consider priorities to address as part of the revision of the standards to improve NCLEX pass rates?

PRACTICE QUESTIONS

1. The program evaluation committee is reviewing the nursing program evaluation data. The nursing program has established an 86% pass rate as the benchmark for graduates taking the National Council of Licensure Examination (NCLEX) for the first time. This goal has not been met for the past 3 years. Which of the following recommendations would be a *priority* for the committee to make?

   A. Increase the passing-grade benchmark for each nursing course to 93%

   B. Require a minimum GPA of 3.0 in the natural science and nursing courses

   C. Lower the NCLEX pass-rate benchmark for first-time takers to 78%

   D. Institute a pre-RN assessment test with a minimum benchmark for admission into the nursing program

2. The clinical educator is preparing to write the summative evaluation for the learners in her clinical group. The educator believes in the constructivist philosophy of evaluation. Therefore when completing the evaluation, she will do which of the following?

   A. Determine whether the objectives of the course have been met

   B. Compare the learner to others to determine level of development

   C. Seek input from clinical staff regarding the learner's clinical performance

   D. Assign a grade of pass/fail for the clinical performance

3. The nursing curriculum committee is revising the curriculum to be more congruent with changes in health care delivery. The most important consideration of the committee should be which of the following?

   A. Be sure the new curriculum is aligned with the mission and philosophy of the governing institution

   B. Develop curriculum objectives and program outcomes

   C. Establish benchmarks for first-time pass rates on the National Council of Licensure Examination (NCLEX)

   D. Require a standardized exit exam with a benchmark pass rate of 85%

4. The nurse educator is reviewing the item analysis on a course test for a multiple-choice question. The following statistics were calculated for one item:

Point Biserial = −0.27	Correct Answer = B		Total Group = 88.24%	
Distractor Analysis	A	B	C	D
Point biserial	0.27	−0.27	0.00	0.00
Frequency	12%	88%	0%	0%

The educator realizes the cause for this frequency distribution is that:

   A. The distractors were not clear

   B. The distractors were too hard for learners to choose

   C. Learners who scored lower on the examination got the item correct

   D. Learners who knew the content answered the item correctly

5. The following statistics were calculated on a multiple-choice question on an examination:

Point Biserial = 0.61	Correct Answer = C		Total Group = 76.47%	
Distractor Analysis	A	B	C	D
Point biserial	−0.59	0.00	0.61	−0.24
Frequency	6%	0%	88%	6%

The reason for this frequency distribution is that:

   A. Learners who scored lower on the exam got the item correct

   B. The distractors were not clear

   C. This item has been used on previous exams

   D. Learners who scored higher on the exam got the item correct

6. The item analysis revealed the following data for a multiple-choice question:

Point Biserial = 0.19	Correct Answer = D		Total Group = 5.88%	
Distractor Analysis	A	B	C	D
Point biserial	−0.25	0.39	−0.35	0.19
Frequency	41%	41%	12%	6%

Based on these statistics, the professor should do which of the following when using this item on future exams?

A. Nothing, as the upper third of the class answered the item correctly

B. Revise distractor A

C. Revise distractor B

D. Revise distractor C

7. An item-analysis report for a multiple-choice examination revealed that the KR-20 was 0.56. Based on this statistic, which of the following interpretations can be made regarding this exam?

A. The exam is reliable in measuring learner knowledge of the material

B. There are too few items on the exam

C. The items are poorly written and do not discriminate

D. There is an excess of very easy questions

8. A professor administered a multiple-choice exam and performed an item analysis, which revealed the following data:

Point Biserial = 0.56	Correct Answer = A		Total Group = 52%	
Distractor Analysis	A	B	C	D
Point biserial	0.56	−0.31	−0.44	0.02
Frequency	52%	18%	18%	12%

The likely cause for this frequency distribution is:

A. The distractors are too hard

B. Learners who scored highest on the exam got the item correct

C. The distractors are too easy

D. Learners guessed the answer to this question

9. The following statistics were obtained in an item analysis for a multiple-choice exam:

Point Biserial = 0.00	Correct Answer = C		Total Group = 100%	
Distractor Analysis	A	B	C	D
Point biserial	0.00	0.00	0.00	0.00
Frequency	0%	0%	100%	0%

What action should be taken based on this data?

A. No action is needed as all learners answered the question correctly

B. Revise distractor C

C. Add another distractor to the choices

D. Rewrite all of the distractors

10. Which of the following activities would be the *best* strategy to engage the visual learner at the cognitive and affective levels?

A. Audiotaping a lecture

B. Writing a case study

C. Developing a concept map

D. Writing an essay

REFERENCES

Accreditation Commission for Education in Nursing. (2013). Accreditation manual. Retrieved from http://www.acenursing.org

Angelo, T. A. (1993). Teacher's dozen: Fourteen general, research-based principles for improving higher learning in our classrooms. Retrieved from http://ir.atu.edu/Retention_Info/retentionother/Thomas_Angelo's_14_Principles.pdf

Billings, D., & Halstead, J. A. (2012). *Teaching in nursing: A guide for faculty* (4th ed.). St. Louis, MO: Elsevier Saunders.

Bourke, M. P., & Ihrke, B. A. (2012). The evaluation process: An overview. In D. M. Billings & J. A. Halstead (Eds.), *Teaching in nursing: A guide for faculty* (4th ed., pp. 422–436). St. Louis, MO: Elsevier Saunders.

Carrick, J. A. (2011). Student achievement and NCLEX-RN success: Problems that persist. *Nursing Education Perspectives, 32*(2), 78–83. doi:10.5480/1536-5026-32.2.78

Commission on Collegiate Nursing Education. (2013). *Procedures for accreditation of baccalaureate and graduate degree nursing programs*. Washington, DC: Author. Retrieved from http://www.aacn.nche.edu

Fardows, N. (2011). Investigating effects of evaluation and assessment on students learning outcomes at undergraduate level. *European Journal of Social Sciences, 23*(1), 34–40.

Farnsworth, J., & Springer, P. (2006). Background checks for nursing students: What are schools doing? *Nursing Education Perspectives, 27*(3), 48–53.

Gaberson, K. B., & Oermann, M. H. (2010). *Clinical teaching strategies in nursing* (3rd ed.). New York, NY: Springer Publishing.

Gronlund, N. E. (1993). *How to make achievement tests and assessments* (5th ed.). Boston, MA: Allyn & Bacon.

Keating, S. B. (2006). *Curriculum development and evaluation in nursing*. Philadelphia, PA: Lippincott Williams & Wilkins.

Keating, S. B. (2011). *Curriculum development and evaluation in nursing* (2nd ed.). New York, NY: Springer Publishing.

Kehoe, J. (1995). Basic item analysis for multiple-choice tests. *Practical Assessment, Research & Evaluation, 4*(10). Retrieved from http://PAREonline.net/getvn.asp?v = 4 & n = 10

McDonald, M. E. (2007). *The nurse educator's guide to assessing learning outcomes* (2nd ed.). Boston, MA: Jones & Bartlett.

Mee, C. L., & Hallenbeck, V. J. (2015). Selecting standardized tests in nursing education. *Journal of Professional Nursing, 31*(6) 493–497.

Molsbee, C. P., & Benton, B. (2016). A move away from high-stakes testing toward comprehensive competency. *Teaching and Learning in Nursing, 11*, 4–7.

National Council of State Boards of Nursing. (2016, April). *NCLEX-RN examination detailed test plan*. Chicago, IL: Author. Retrieved from http://www.ncsbn.org

National League for Nursing. (2010). *High-stakes testing*. New York, NY: Author. Retrieved from www.nln.org/aboutnln/reflection_diaglogue/refl_dial_7.htm

National League for Nursing. (2012a). NLN fair testing guidelines for nursing education. Retrieved from www.nln.org/facultyprograms/facultyresources/fairtestingguidelines.pdf

National League for Nursing. (2012b). The fair testing imperative in nursing education. Retrieved from www.nln.org/aboutnln/livingdocuments/pdf/nlnvision_4.pdf

National League for Nursing. (2016). Certified nurse educator (CNE) candidate handbook. Retrieved from http://www.nln.org/docs/default-source/professionaldevelopment -programs/certified-nurse-educator-%28cne%29-examination-candidate-handbook .pdf?sfvrsn=2

Newton, S. E., & Moore, G. (2007). Undergraduate grade point average and graduate record examination scores: The experience of one graduate nursing program. *Nursing Education Perspectives, 28*(6), 327–331.

O'Connor, A. B. (2006). *Clinical instruction and evaluation: A teaching resource* (2nd ed.). Boston, MA: Jones & Bartlett.

Oermann, M. H., & Gaberson, K. (2014). *Evaluation and testing in nursing education* (4th ed.). New York, NY: Springer Publishing.

Sandahl, S. S. (2010). Collaborative testing as a learning strategy in nursing education. *Nursing Education Perspectives, 31*(3), 142–147.

Sauter, M. K., Gillespie, N. N., & Knepp, A. (2012). Educational program evaluation. In D. M. Billings & J. A. Halstead (Eds.), *Teaching in nursing* (4th ed., pp. 503–547). St. Louis, MO: Elsevier Saunders.

Sayles, S., Shelton, D., & Powell, H. (2003, November/December). Predictors of success in nursing education. *ABNF Journal, 14*(6), 116–120.

Serembus, J. F. (2016). Improving NCLEX first-time pass rates: A comprehensive program approach. *Journal of Nursing Regulation, 6*(4), 38–44.

Spurlock, D. (2013). The promise and peril of high-stakes tests in nursing education. *Journal of Nursing Regulation, 4*(1), 4–8.

Su, W. M., Osisek, P. J., Montgomery, C., & Pellar, S. (2009). Designing multiple-choice test items at higher cognitive levels. *Nurse Educator, 34*(5), 223–231.

Twigg, P. (2012). Developing and using classroom tests. In D. M. Billings & J. A. Halstead (Eds.), *Teaching in nursing: A guide for faculty* (4th ed., pp. 464–483). St. Louis, MO: Elsevier Saunders.

Yin, T., & Burger, C. (2003). Predictors of NCLEX-RN success of associate degree nursing graduates. *Nurse Educator, 28*, 232–236.

Curriculum Design and Evaluation of Program Outcomes

MARYLOU K. McHUGH

*The materials of instruction should be selected and organized
with a view to giving the learner that development most
helpful in meeting and controlling life experiences.*
—D. E. Walker and J. Soltis

**This chapter addresses the Certified Nurse Educator Exam Content Area 4: Participate
in Curriculum Design and Evaluation of Program Outcomes (National League for Nursing
[NLN], 2016b, p. 5).**

- Content Area 4 is 17% of the examination
- It is estimated that there will be approximately 25 to 26 questions from Content Area 4

LEARNING OUTCOMES

- Discuss leadership and change behaviors that assist in curriculum development
- Analyze the process of curriculum development
- Discuss current trends in curriculum development
- Analyze evaluation methods appropriate to measuring program outcomes
- Evaluate teaching methods/strategies for classroom and clinical teaching

Curriculum development can be the most creative and satisfying part of the
educational process. It is not only dynamic and vibrant, but also demands the
nurse educator's time. In today's educational environment, with so much content needed for thoughtful practice with an emphasis on higher level thinking, the
educator is challenged even more than ever.

Curriculum is a living entity and must be reviewed regularly for its relevance
to the environment in which it exists. Faculty need to consider the environmental

and human factors that influence the curriculum. These factors are called "the frame" and are classified as either internal or external factors (Keating, 2006). External frame factors consist of the elements of the environment that are outside of the parent institution that influence the curriculum. All of these elements must be considered when developing a curriculum. External frame factors include the following issues and prompt the questions that follow.

Financial Support

- How will the program be financed? Are there resources available for the latest technology?
- Does the institution have available room for the program's needs?

Regulations and Accreditation

- What state regulations need to be considered?
- Will the program apply for national accreditation?
- Are there resources available to assist in these efforts?
- How will the program meet professional standards?

Nursing Profession

- Are there nursing leaders and staff nurses who will support the program and act as mentors?
- Are the professionals active in and interested in the education of future nurses?

Need for the Program

- Does the community really need the program?
- Is there adequate interest in the program?
- What are the employment possibilities for the graduates?

Demographics

- What are the age ranges and age groups, predicted population changes, ethnic and cultural groups, and typical socioeconomic status of people in the community?
- What is the effect of globalization on the curriculum?

Political Climate and the Body Politic

- Who are the individuals who exert influence within the community?
- Who are the players and are they supportive of the program?

Health Care System and Health Needs of the Populace

- What are the major health care systems in the area?
- Can they be utilized for clinical experiences?
- What are the major health care problems?
- What effect has the Patient Protection and Affordable Care Act had on the health care system and nursing education?

Characteristics of the Academic Setting

- What are the characteristics of the setting?
- Is it a private liberal arts college or a major research university?
- How will these characteristics inform the program?

Internal frame factors refer to those elements that are internal to the institution and inform the program. All of these elements must be considered when developing the curriculum. Internal frame factors and clarifying questions include (Keating, 2006) the items that follow.

Potential Faculty and Learner Characteristics

- Are there enough available, experienced nurse educators who have expertise in the various curriculum areas?
- What is the quantity and quality of the potential student body?

Description and Organization of Structure of the Parent Institution

- What is the quality of the physical campus and its buildings?
- What is the role of the nursing program in the institution?

Resources Within the Institution and the Nursing Program

- Who will develop the business plan that focuses resources for program support?
- Are there endowments, financial aid programs, and/or governmental and private grants available to the program?
- Are there appropriate support services for learners and faculty, such as advising, academic help, library services, technology, and research support?

Internal Economic Situation and Its Influence on the Curriculum

- Is the economic status of the parent institution sound?
- Does the administration support the goals of the nursing program?

Mission or Purpose, Philosophy, and Goals of the Parent Institution

- How will the three areas of institutional focus—research, service, and teaching—inform the nursing program and which will be prominent?
- Will there be some attempt at balance?

CRITICAL THINKING QUESTION

Have you carefully assessed your program in light of the preceding requirements that will impinge on curriculum development and the success of the program? Can you identify those external and internal factors that will be most influential in your curriculum development?

LEADING THE PROGRAM

In any major academic endeavor, such as curriculum development, deciding on leadership is an important part of the process. What defines leadership? Where does the leader come from? Who should lead? What are the qualities that the leader will need? Leadership is the process of showing the way by going in advance, by directing the performance or activities of a group (Morris, 1970). The leader may be the dean, chair, or director in a small school or department of nursing. In a bigger institution, the leader may be a seasoned faculty member with some prior experience in curriculum development. Leaders may emerge from the group or may be appointed by the dean.

A leader should possess knowledge of both the content and process of curriculum development as well as a caring and compassionate attitude (Yoder-Wise, 2013). Leaders emerge in the following ways:

- *Emergent leadership*—The members of the group view the leader as someone who is knowledgeable and trustworthy; they recognize and accept the leader's influence to lead.
- *Imposed or organizational leadership*—The leader is appointed by someone outside the group. If the group members do not have confidence in the appointed leader's abilities, they may not perform to their highest potential (Figure 12.1).

EVIDENCE-BASED TEACHING PRACTICE

Hofmeyer, Sheingold, Klopper, and Warland (2015) found that successful leaders invest time in getting to know the people they lead and help everyone to focus. Developing relationships is the first step in developing and inspiring others: A good leader promotes others at the same time, so it's not just all about them.

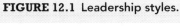

FIGURE 12.1 Leadership styles.

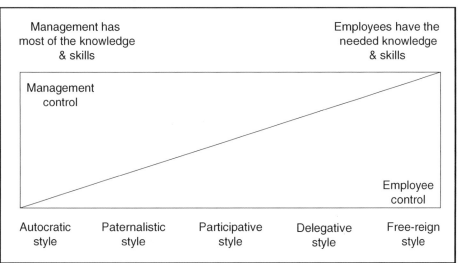

Wiles and Bondi (1998) have identified the following 19 roles that a curriculum leader needs to fulfill:

Expert	Linker
Confronter	Analyzer
Instructor	Demonstrator
Counselor	Diagnostician
Trainer	Modeler
Advisor	Designer
Retriever	Advocate
Observer	Manager
Referrer	Evaluator
Data collector	

Five practices associated with exceptional leadership are (Huber, 2000) as follows:

1. Challenging the process by searching for opportunities, experimenting, and taking risks
2. Inspiring a shared vision by envisioning the future and enlisting the support of others
3. Enabling others to act by fostering collaboration and strengthening others
4. Modeling the way by setting an example and planning small successes
5. Encouraging the heart by recognizing contributions and celebrating accomplishments

Refer to Chapter 13 for a complete discussion of leadership attributes.

RESPONSIBILITIES OF FACULTY IN CURRICULUM DEVELOPMENT

Although the leader is responsible for guiding the faculty through the curriculum process, individual faculty members have their own sets of responsibilities. Many nursing leaders believe that the faculty "own" the curriculum because of their expertise in content, along with a good sense of the practice world. Because of the concept of academic freedom, faculty members may investigate new theories and ideas and express opinions in the classroom that are relevant to the course being taught (Finke, 2012). This does not mean that faculty members may develop course content in isolation; rather, they must work together to develop the plan and then follow the plan they have developed. Curriculum must build in a structured way that enables the learner to incorporate the art, science, and practice of nursing in a coherent manner. Faculty must strive to ensure that the program outcomes are achieved. The curriculum must also meet the requirements of both the state board of nursing and external accrediting bodies.

Faculty responsibilities include the following:

- Develop policies and procedures that affect learner and faculty conduct and the curriculum
- Advise administration and learners on educational issues
- Participate in administrative actions that affect the institution and community
- Ensure that content and learning experiences are sequenced toward educational outcomes
- Collect and analyze relevant information pertaining to the need for curriculum development and revision
- Prepare graduates to function in the changing and complex health care environment
- Develop strategies to facilitate the exchange of ideas and decision making relevant to curriculum development and revisions (Johnson, as cited in Keating, 2006, p. 37)

There are certain attributes related to academic freedom, including the following three aspects, as set forth by the American Association of University Professors (1940/1970). These are:

1. Teachers are entitled to full freedom in research and in the publication of the results, subject to the adequate performance of their other academic duties, but research for pecuniary return should be based on an understanding with the authorities of the institution.
2. Teachers are entitled to freedom in the classroom in discussing their subject, but they should be careful not to introduce into their teaching controversial matter that has no relation to their subject. Limitations of academic freedom because of religious or other aims of the institution should be clearly stated in writing at the time of the appointment.
3. College and university teachers are citizens, members of a learned profession, and officers of an educational institution. When they speak or write as citizens,

they should be free from institutional censorship or discipline, but their special position in the community imposes special obligations. As scholars and educational officers, they should remember that the public may judge their profession and their institution by their utterances. Therefore, they should at all times be accurate, should exercise appropriate restraint, should show respect for the opinions of others, and should make every effort to indicate that they are not speaking for the institution.

There are many factors that nurse educators have to consider in curriculum design; some of these are similar to the considerations of the total program design as mentioned previously. These factors include:

- Institutional philosophy and mission, which provide a belief and value base for the curricular structure and content (Leddy, 2007). This operationalizes the following:
  1. Institution's reason for being, with outcome goals
  2. Program's philosophy and mission, which reflect those of the parent institutions
- Organizing framework
  1. The curriculum framework provides a way for faculty to conceptualize and organize knowledge, skills, values, and beliefs that are critical to the delivery of a coherent curriculum
  2. It facilitates the sequencing and prioritizing of knowledge in a way that is logical and internally consistent (Boland & Finke, 2012)
- Current nursing and health care trends
  1. Faculty should consider the economic and political issues that influence health care issues
  2. Issues such as bioterrorism; genetics; interdisciplinary education; an aging population; cultural illiteracy; violence; lesbian, gay, bisexual, transgender, and queer issues; quality and safety; and the use of technology such as electronic medical records, Simulation (SIM) people, and standardized patients (SPs) are important
- Community and societal needs
  1. Changes in social perceptions about ageism, sexism, gender discrimination, and racism, are pertinent topics for inclusion
  2. There is a need for primary care practitioners and health educators in community settings
- Educational principles
  1. Active teaching strategies for both traditional and nontraditional learners should be considered
  2. Discussion about various educational theories should precede the actual curriculum plan
- Theory and research
  1. Evidence-based practice (EBP) is a current mandate
  2. The theory and research supporting all procedures is a priority

- Use of technology
  1. Smartphones, electronic medical records, SIM people, and SPs are a part of health care education
  2. Faculty needs to discuss its integration into the curriculum (Keating, 2006; Leddy, 2007)

There are also standards from accrediting bodies that need to be incorporated into curriculum design. The three specialty accrediting bodies in nursing are the National League of Nursing's Commission for Nursing Education Accreditation (CNEA), American Association of Colleges of Nursing's Commission on Collegiate Nursing Education (CCNE), and the Accreditation Commission for Education in Nursing (ACEN). The standards for curriculum development are clearly stated and nurse educators systematically review curriculum to ensure that the criteria in the standard is being met. Examples from ACEN (2016) regarding curriculum include:

Standard 4—Curriculum*

The curriculum supports the achievement of the identified student learning outcomes and program outcomes of the nursing education unit consistent with safe practice in contemporary health care environments.

4.1. The curriculum incorporates established professional standards, guidelines, and competencies, and has clearly articulated student learning outcomes and program outcomes consistent with contemporary practice.

4.2. The student learning outcomes are used to organize the curriculum, guide the delivery of instruction, direct learning activities, and evaluate student progress.

4.3. The curriculum is developed by the faculty and regularly reviewed to ensure integrity, rigor, and currency.

4.4. The curriculum includes general education courses that enhance professional nursing knowledge and practice.

4.5. The curriculum includes cultural, ethnic, and socially diverse concepts and may also include experiences from regional, national, or global perspectives.

4.6. The curriculum and instructional processes reflect educational theory, interprofessional collaboration, research, and current standards of practice.

4.7. Evaluation methodologies are varied, reflect established professional and practice competencies, and measure the achievement of the student learning outcomes.

4.8. The length of time and the credit hours required for program completion are congruent with the attainment of identified student learning outcomes and program outcomes and consistent with the policies of the governing organization, state and national standards, and best practices.

4.9. Practice learning environments support the achievement of student learning outcomes and program outcomes.

4.10. Students participate in clinical experiences that are evidence based and reflect contemporary practice and nationally established patient health and safety goals.

---

* Reprinted from the 2013 Standards and Criteria, Standard 4 Curriculum, by the Accreditation Commission for Education in Nursing (ACEN) by permission of the ACEN. The ACEN 2013 Standards and Criteria will be replaced by the ACEN 2017 Standards and Criteria available at www.acenursing.org, effective January 1, 2017, mandatory, January 1, 2018.

4.11. Written agreements for clinical practice agencies are current, specify expectations for all parties, and ensure the protection of students.

4.12. Learning activities, instructional materials, and evaluation methods are appropriate for all delivery formats and consistent with the student learning outcomes.

THEORETICAL AND CONCEPTUAL FRAMEWORKS

After completing the first step toward curriculum development, the careful review of the mission statement of both the parent institution and the nursing unit, the next step is for faculty to begin to identify the organizing framework to be used as the model for building the curriculum. All nursing programs are based on some sort of model, whether the faculty recognizes it or not (Barnum, 1998). There are many models to choose from. Remember, the framework selected for use will eventually provide learners with the basis for the conceptualization of their profession. It should be clear and practical, and faculty must be consistent in the way they use it. The nurse educator must realize that the amount of knowledge, both scientific and nursing, is increasing at a frightening rate. This necessitates nurse educators quickly add and/or eliminate content in order to provide learners with the best and most current practice modalities. What to add and what to delete can be a real challenge. The basic goal may be to teach learners to become lifelong learners. The basic curriculum models, as well as newer models, and their characteristics include the items that follow.

Curriculum Model

- Students learn the disciplines inherent to the profession
- The model may take varied forms, such as medical models
- Courses include Medical Surgical Nursing, Pediatric Nursing, Psychiatric Mental Health Nursing, and so on

Courses developed under the curriculum model will be very traditional. They would treat each area separately with courses such as fundamentals of nursing, Care of the Adult I, II, and III, Pediatric Nursing, and so on. The nursing process steps—assessment, diagnosis, planning, implementation, and evaluation—would be integrated into each traditional course. This model is often called the *additive curriculum*.

Integrated Model

- This model addresses problems such as circulatory, respiratory, and orthopedic care.
- It addresses the nursing care of patients at all developmental levels (infancy, childhood, adolescence, adulthood, and elderly).

In contrast, courses in the integrated model would be more integrated throughout the curriculum. Examples of course titles include Circulatory Problems Across the Life Cycle or Care of the Infant, which would then include all of the health–illness issues associated with that topic. Many educators feel that content is often lost in this kind of model, yet for some programs, this model works extremely well.

TABLE 12.1 Dorothea Orem Theoretical Model			
SECONDARY STEPS OF THE NURSING PROCESS	WHOLLY COMPENSATORY SYSTEM	PARTLY COMPENSATORY SYSTEM	SUPPORTIVE EDUCATIVE SYSTEM
Assessment	–	–	–
Diagnosis	–	–	–
Planning	–	–	–
Intervention	–	–	–
Evaluation	–	–	–

Discipline Model or Nursing Theorist Model

- Curriculum is informed by a conceptual model of nursing (e.g., Levine, Orem, Neuman, or Roy)
  - It may also be designed by the faculty from an intuited image of nursing (Barnum, 1998).
  - The courses are specifically designed to the model (e.g., if using Levine, courses would include Problems of Conservation of Energy, Problems of Conservation of Structural Integrity).

Courses in the Discipline Model are integrated into the concepts of the theory used. Table 12.1 illustrates how a nursing process may be integrated into the Dorothea Orem Theoretical Model for patients who need wholly compensatory care.

DECONSTRUCTED, CONCEPTUAL, OR EMANCIPATOR CURRICULUM MODELS

Courses in these curricular models focus on concepts rather than on specific disease entities. Instead of teaching the same material for many populations, the concept curriculum focuses on concepts that are more useful in practice. These models promote the "development of cognitive skills necessary for knowledge transfer across contexts and the ability to transform learners into lifelong learners" (Hardin & Richardson, 2012, p. 155). They reflect the complex nature of nursing care better than some of the other models.

Authors (Diekelmann, 2002; Forbes & Hickey, 2009; Giddens & Brady, 2007; Giddens, et al., 2008; Hickey, Forbes, & Greenfield, 2010; Ironsides, 2004) have responded by supporting the concept and offering suggestions for curricular revisions. Diekelmann (2002) suggested increasing attention to the pedagogies with less attention to the content. She stressed that reading, writing, thinking, and dialogue replace the push to include more content. Ironsides (2004) conducted a qualitative study and concluded that "challenging additive curricula and the relationship between covering content and teaching thinking by enacting new pedagogies provides teachers with ways to pursue substantive reform" (p. 11). Candela, Dalley, and Benzel-Lindley (2006) agreed that there is too much content and advocated learning-centered curricula. They offered practical suggestions for any faculty moving to a learning-centered curriculum. One of the keys to this kind of learning is conceptual learning. Giddens and Brady (2007) summarized their work by stating, "A concept based curriculum coupled with a conceptual learning approach can prepare nursing graduates who are skilled at conceptual thinking and learning; such skills are necessary to respond to a rapidly changing profession and health care environment" (p. 68). Giddens and colleagues (2008) addressed developing and implementing a new "deconstructed" curriculum along with the problems they encountered.

Some of the unique features of the curriculum included:

- A conceptual approach
- New approach to clinical education
- An innovative, web-based teaching platform has been created that is known as the *Neighborhood* (Giddens, 2007)

In 2009, Forbes and Hickey summarized the literature addressing curricular reform and identified the following four themes:

- Incorporating safety and quality competencies in nursing education
- Redesigning conceptual frameworks
- Strategies to reduce content-laden curricula
- Teaching using alternative pedagogies. They called for educational research in nursing to study newer, nontraditional pedagogies, such as narrative pedagogy, integrative teaching, and active learning strategies, along with their effects on student learning.

Concepts can be defined as a collection of social, cultural, and historical constructions and ideas that, over time, maintain similar form, structure, and patterns (Hardin & Richardson, 2012, p. 155).

Components of the Conceptual Curriculum

- Addressing misconceptions—all learners bring their own history and experiences to the educational setting, which must be addressed and corrected prior to learning new content.
- Building enduring understanding—when learners understand concepts, they will endure and transfer across educational and clinical contexts.
- Developing metacognition—this is the ability to understand and monitor one's own thinking (refer to Chapter 2 for a further description of metacognition).
- Teaching methods include:
  * Misconception and preconception check—may take the form of a short and simple questionnaire.

* Discrepant event—an event that is a situation contrary to what is expected that provokes learners to search for the discrepancy.
* Concept map—this is a diagram that links concepts to one another.
* Approximate analogies—the nurse educator provides the first half of the analogy; the learners provide the second. For example, perfusion is to oxygenation as X is to Y. This increases creativity and is an important part of developing metacognition.
* Check-your-knowledge quiz—a short and ungraded quiz to determine the learners' understanding of the material at one point in time (Hardin & Richardson, 2012).

Models that demonstrate the deconstructed curriculum include those that originate from the Institute of Medicine (IOM) or The Joint Commission. These curricular models may be based on Quality and Safety Education for Nurses (QSEN), the IOM priority areas, or Healthy People 2020 (Office of Disease Prevention and Health Promotion, 2016). In addition, concepts, such as infection, preparedness, environmental health, and community-based health, can thread through many courses. The learner focuses on thinking about connections among many health care problems and solves prototypes. Coaching as a teaching strategy is helpful in broadening the competency base of students (Shostrom & Schofe, 2016).

A model using the IOM's priority areas would include courses such as:

- Preventive Care
- Behavioral Health
- Chronic Conditions
- End of Life
- Children and Adolescents
- Inpatient/Surgical Care

Nurse educators would select prototypes from Healthy People 2020 to determine specific content for each course.

A model based on QSEN would focus on the following areas. Again, nurse educators can select specific content areas from Healthy People 2020.

- Patient-centered care
- Teamwork and collaboration
- EBP
- Quality improvement
- Safety
- Informatics

EVIDENCE-BASED TEACHING PRACTICE

In 2002, The Joint Commission established its National Patient Safety Goals (NPSGs) program. The NPSGs were established to help accredited organizations address specific areas of concern in regard to patient safety (The Joint Commission, 2016).

A model based on the recommendations of The Joint Commission National Patient Safety Goals (2003) would focus on safety issues. Concepts that organize the curriculum would include:

- Improving the accuracy of patient identification
- Improving staff communication
- Improving the timely reporting of critical test results and values
- Improving the safety of using high-alert medications
- Preventing health care-associated infections
- Reducing the risk of patient harm resulting from falls
- Preventing health care-associated pressure ulcers
- Using the Universal Protocol for Preventing Wrong Site, Wrong Procedure, and Wrong Person Surgery™

Nurse educators would structure courses around prototypical health problems taken from Healthy People 2020 (Office of Disease Prevention and Health Promotion, 2016).

EVIDENCE-BASED TEACHING PRACTICE

Lewis, Stephens, and Ciak (2016) threaded the concepts of QSEN throughout the curriculum using classroom, clinical, and simulation strategies. A qualitative analysis of preceptors perceptions after a year demonstrated an increase in student's and faculty's ability to meet QSEN competencies.

The Carnegie Foundation for the Advancement of Teaching

In the spring of 2009, the Carnegie Foundation for the Advancement of Teaching (2013) released its study of nursing education. The purpose of this study was to understand the demands of learning to be a nurse and the most effective strategies for teaching nursing. The Preparation for the Professions Program (PPP) took a comparative perspective to the issues of teaching, learning, assessment, and curriculum in nursing education. The PPP has identified three dimensions of apprenticeships for professional education. In nursing education, these are high-end apprenticeships and include:

- Intellectual training to learn the academic knowledge base and have the capacity to think in ways important to the profession
- A skill-based apprenticeship of practice, including clinical judgment
- An apprenticeship to the ethical standards, ethical comportment, social roles, and responsibilities of the profession through which the novice is introduced to the meaning of an integrated practice of all dimensions of the profession, grounded in the profession's fundamental purposes

Benner, Sutphen, Leonard, and Day (2009) have authored a book explaining the findings of the PPP and offer suggestions for nursing education. Highlights follow; you can also go to the Carnegie Foundation website for more information. The key PPP findings are:

- Major gap in practice versus education
- Radical separation of classroom and clinical teaching
- Faculty development needed for classroom teaching

There are three cross-professional frames for the five Carnegie Foundation studies of professional education (they are in the process of releasing their findings on medical education).

First Framework

- Civic professionalism rather than technical professionalism: Focus is on civic responsibilities to the client and society rather than solely on technology. It emphasizes autonomy and control over professional knowledge development and professional participation.

Second Framework

Cognitive apprenticeship: Knowledge of science, theory, and principles required for practice

- Practice apprenticeship: Clinical reasoning and decision-making
- Formation and ethical comportment apprenticeship: Learning to embody and enact upstanding professional practice

Third Framework

Experiential teaching and learning

- Situated cognition or learning how to think in action
- Situated teaching and learning or readiness to respond to a situation
- Reflection on particular cases and situations in relation to patient outcomes
- Development of ethical comportment or doing the right thing

---

CRITICAL THINKING QUESTION

How would you include the Carnegie Foundation's suggestions into your curriculum? What other institutional departments would you include as you implement these suggestions?

Table 12.2 illustrates a curriculum grid for incorporating the nursing health–illness concerns into the integrated model approach.

Whatever curricular model is chosen, time for including the process of debriefing should be included as faculty develop the curriculum. The NLN (2015), in collaboration with the International Nursing Association for Clinical Simulation

TABLE 12.2
Integrated Model Approach

SECONDARY DEVELOPMENTAL LEVELS	DOMINANT NURSING PROBLEM COMPONENTS					
	CIRCULATORY HEALTH TO ILLNESS	RESPIRATORY HEALTH TO ILLNESS	NEUROLOGIC HEALTH TO ILLNESS	ENDOCRINE HEALTH TO ILLNESS	GASTRO-INTESTINAL HEALTH TO ILLNESS	RENAL HEALTH TO ILLNESS
Infancy	–	–	–	–	–	–
Childhood	–	–	–	–	–	–
Young adult	–	–	–	–	–	–
Middle-aged adult	–	–	–	–	–	–
Elderly	–	–	–	–	–	–

CRITICAL THINKING QUESTION

What kind of curriculum model do you feel is most appropriate for your unit, faculty, and learners, and why? How will you choose which concepts to teach?

---

and Learning (INACSL), concluded that it is critical for nurse educators to have a chosen theory-based method, formal training, and ongoing assessment of competencies. They also believe that "integrating debriefing across the curriculum not just in simulation has the potential to transform nursing education" (p. 2).

EVIDENCE-BASED TEACHING PRACTICE

Bulman, Llathlean, and Gobbi (2012) found that reflection helped students and teachers make sense out of experiences. It helped teachers and students to move on after becoming self-aware about experiences.

MULTICULTURALISM IN NURSING EDUCATION

Significant changes are taking place in the population demographics of the United States, with shifts occurring in both ethnic and minority groups. A *diverse population* can refer to a population that differs in ethnicity, age, gender, sexual orientation, ability, or life experiences. Because of these changes, nurse educators must adapt and adjust both curricula and teaching methods to assist these diverse populations. The five dimensions of multicultural education are (Banks & Banks, 2010):

1. Content integration
2. Knowledge construction
3. Equity pedagogy
4. Prejudice reduction
5. Empowering school and social culture

Lou (1994) identified three prerequisites for equity in teaching a diverse population:

1. Attitude—the nurse educator is open to make changes in classroom teaching, using active rather than passive methods
2. Personal perception—the nurse educator gains an insight into his or her own cultural perspective that might be brought into the classroom
3. Knowledge—the nurse educator must be knowledgeable about the learning styles of students

Multicultural teaching and teaching for cultural competency includes:

• Understanding one's own cultural values
• Assisting learners to understand their cultural values
• Taking cultural considerations into all stages of course development
• Delivering instruction that is free from bias
• Encouraging group activity and involvement
• Assessing knowledge of cultural competency (Rowles, 2012)

CRITICAL THINKING QUESTION

What are your biases? Do they affect your behavior when dealing with students? Do they affect your behavior when dealing with peers?

VIOLENCE IN THE NURSING CURRICULUM

The statistics on domestic violence indicate the magnitude of this problem, as a result of this significant issue, many nursing organizations have addressed the role of nursing in this public health problem. The American Association of Colleges of Nursing (AACN) has developed a position statement and suggested content that nurse educators should consider for inclusion in the curriculum.

"Because of the prevalence of physical and psychological violence in our society, nurses frequently care for the victims, the perpetrators, and the witnesses of physical and psychological violence. In addition, nurses also may be at risk for experiencing violence in the workplace. As members of the largest group of health care providers, nurses should be aware of assessment methods and nursing interventions that will interrupt and prevent the cycle of violence.

In particular, the AACN recognizes domestic violence as a special form of violence with a high incidence and prevalence that requires health care interventions. AACN recommends that faculty in educational institutions preparing nurses in baccalaureate and higher degree programs ensure that the curricula contain opportunities for all learners to gain factual information and clinical experience regarding domestic violence (Table 12.3). The content should include:

- Acknowledgment of the scope of the problem
- Assessment skills to identify and document abuse and its health effects
- Interventions to reduce vulnerability and increase safety, especially of women, children, and elders
- Competence in recognizing how cultural factors influence the patterns of and responses to domestic violence to individuals, families, and communities
- Legal and ethical issues in treating and reporting domestic violence
- Activities to prevent domestic violence (American Association of Colleges of Nursing, 2016a, 2016b)

Many nurse educators today are sensitized to the importance of including content on violence and victim/survivor care in various nursing education programs. Although a survey of Ontario's schools of nursing in Canada revealed a considerable number of hours devoted to this topic, the approach is largely incidental, depending heavily on individual faculty interests. To achieve this goal and avoid pitfalls such as an "add-on" approach to curriculum revision, nurse educators' needs in Ontario were addressed in a series of workshops involving collaboration among faculty, clinical preceptors, and community-based experts in victim/survivor care (Hoff, 1995).

TABLE 12.3
Content and Activities for Inclusion

CONTENT	ACTIVITIES
Screening and assessment	Didactic content Physical assessment course work Screening with valid and reliable tools All clinical settings are appropriate for these activities
Intervention and documentation	Clinical experiences in all settings using skills obtained in course and college laboratory Early case finding Appropriate referrals
Ethical, legal, and cultural issues	Didactic content in sociology, ethics, and nursing courses Know state and local regulations
Prevention activities	Participate in health fairs, public awareness activities

The majority of university schools of nursing provided experiential instruction in the area of violence, but the other types of schools of nursing provided very little such instruction. Findings revealed sensitivity to the importance of including content on violence in nursing curricula; however, the approach to this content is largely incidental and heavily dependent on individual faculty interests. Implications of this study point to the need for the systematic inclusion of violence-related content and the sharing of resources among schools of nursing (Connor, Nouer, Speck, Mackey, & Tipton, 2013; Ross, Hoff, & Coutu-Wakulczyk, 1998).

In addition to issues such as domestic violence and bullying, faculty need to include content addressing natural disasters and terrorist attacks.

EVIDENCE-BASED TEACHING PRACTICE

Connor et al. (2014) examined graduate nursing curriculum for the topic of intimate partner violence (IPV) to study knowledge, attitudes, beliefs, and self-reported behaviors. Results indicated that previous IPV training promoted significantly higher perceived preparation and knowledge. In addition, 40% of nursing students surveyed had personally experienced some type of domestic violence, including IPV.

INTERPROFESSIONAL CURRICULUM

In 2011, the AACN was part of group that developed competencies for interprofessional learning. The goal of interprofessional learning is to prepare all health professions students for deliberatively working together with the common goal of building a safer and better patient-centered and community/population-oriented U.S. health care system. Interprofessional education (IPE) occurs when two or more professions learn about, from, and with each other to enable effective collaboration and improve health outcomes. Collaborative practice in health care occurs when multiple health workers from different professional backgrounds provide comprehensive services by working with patients, their families, careers, and communities to deliver the highest quality of care across settings. Practice includes both clinical and nonclinical health-related work, such as diagnosis, treatment, surveillance; health communications; management; and sanitation engineering. Health and education systems consist of all the organizations, people, and actions whose primary intent is to promote, restore, or maintain health and facilitate learning, respectively (Inter Professional Education Collaboration Expert Panel, 2011). While in its infancy, this panel began to develop core competencies to guide curriculum development. The core competencies developed include:

- Create a coordinated effort across the health professions to embed essential content in all health professions education curricula
- Guide professional and institutional curricular development of learning approaches and assessment strategies to achieve productive outcomes

---

EXHIBIT 12.1

The Core Competencies of IPE

Interprofessional Education (IPE) is necessary for all health professional education programs. The Association of American Colleges of Nursing (2011) describes IPE in terms of:

- Values and ethics
- Roles and responsibilities
- Interprofessional communication
- Teams and teamwork

Each component of IPE concentrates on the fundamental principles of teamwork, which include building respect; understanding each other's roles and communicating with patients, families, and each other clearly; and building team relationships that enhance the concept of working together for a common patient care goal.

- Provide the foundation for a learning continuum in interprofessional competency development across the professions and the lifelong learning trajectory
- Acknowledge that evaluation and research work will strengthen the scholarship in this area
- Prompt dialogue to evaluate the "fit" between educationally identified core competencies for interprofessional collaborative practice and practice needs/demands
- Find opportunities to integrate essential IPE content consistent with current accreditation expectations for each health professions education program
- Offer information to accreditors of educational programs across the health professions that they can use to set common accreditation standards for IPE, and so they know where to look in institutional settings for examples of implementation of those standards
- Inform professional licensing and credentialing bodies in how to define potential testing content for interprofessional collaborative practice (Exhibit 12.1)

CRITICAL THINKING QUESTION

What teaching and learning strategies would you include in an IPE course and clinical experience?

PROGRAM GOALS, OBJECTIVES, AND OUTCOMES

The next stage of curriculum development is to identify the program goals, outcomes, and terminal objectives of the program and to identify how one will measure these outcomes to determine whether they were achieved. The science of writing objectives was discussed in Chapter 2. This section discusses how to articulate a program's outcomes and develop the objectives for each level of learning. These are called *level objectives* and are used to guide the shaping of course selection and content throughout the years (or levels) through which the learners progress. These statements must be specific and must reflect the institution's and the program's mission statements. Faculty should discuss the following questions:

1. What exactly should the graduating students look like?
2. What characteristics and competencies does the student need to possess upon completion of the program?
3. How do these objectives address the mission and terminal objectives of the program?

> **Teaching Gem:** The curriculum has moved from being politically correct to being theoretically pluralistic; it now incorporates caring and humanitarianism as core values rather than being dominated by technology; and the centrality of the student–teacher relationship is now prized over esoteric scholarship (NLN, 1993).

The development of specific program outcomes and goal objectives will flow from the answers derived from the discussion of these three pertinent and important questions. Leveling a program is an important concept in curriculum development; it orchestrates where to place course materials and what can be expected from learners in the clinical area.

LEVEL OBJECTIVES

The next task pertaining to leveling and course placement is to develop level objectives that delineate what skills the learner will need to develop if he or she is to achieve the program outcomes. Level objectives are meant to guide course design while feeding into the program outcomes.

> **Teaching Gem:** Program objectives and level objectives for the program reflect program outcomes and plan for the sequential development of the knowledge and competencies necessary to achieve those outcomes. The objectives address the same core competencies, but at different levels of sophistication and with different populations. The related course objectives mirror the program and level objectives, but express how the objective is achieved within the content and related clinical experiences learners cover in the course (O'Connor, 2006).

Level objectives can be teased out to reflect specific program objectives, course objectives, and clinical objectives. Table 12.4 illustrates how program, course, and clinical objectives for each level lead to the final outcomes of a program.

- Level One: Learners begin to identify the ethical issues that may affect the care of their patients.
- Level Two: Building on level one, the learners apply these concepts.
- Level Three: Learners are required to analyze the effects of the legal–ethical system on the care of patients, families, and communities.
- By the end of the program, learners are expected to be able to integrate these concepts into their patient care.

On the basis of the program outcomes and the level objectives, faculty will develop courses that will lead to the learners' achievement of the goals. Competencies at the course level are much more specific and lead the faculty to prepare content, learning activities, and clinical experiences.

TABLE 12.4
Level Objectives

LEVEL ONE	LEVEL TWO	LEVEL THREE	LEVEL FOUR
Identify legal and ethical issues that affect the professional nurse's delivery of care to patients and their families.	Apply ethical and legal concepts to the care of patients and their families.	Analyze the effect of legal and ethical issues to the care of patients, families, and communities.	Integrate ethical/legal concepts and principles, the Code of Ethics for Nurses, and professional standards into practice within professional, academic, and community settings.
COURSE OBJECTIVES			
LEVEL ONE	LEVEL TWO	LEVEL THREE	LEVEL FOUR
Discuss the content inherent in the ANA's Code of Ethics for Nurses.	Apply legal/ ethical content to case studies involving patients and families.	Develop care plans based on criteria found in the Standards of Practice of the American Nurses Association and the Code for Nurses.	Compare and contrast the appropriate Standards of Practice and Code of Ethics to various practice situations.
CLINICAL OBJECTIVES			
LEVEL ONE	LEVEL TWO	LEVEL THREE	LEVEL FOUR
Using the Code of Ethics for Nurses, identify one issue that has impinged on your nursing care of a patient and/or the family.	Apply legal/ ethical principles in caring for your patient and family.	Analyze the effects of the Health Insurance Portability and Accountability Act (HIPAA) on the care of your patient and family.	Consciously practice using the Code of Ethics for Nurses and the appropriate Standards of Practice when caring for patients, families, or communities.

BACCALAUREATE OUTCOMES OF THE AACN AND NLN

In October 2008, the AACN identified outcomes for the baccalaureate-prepared nurse that faculty should consider when planning their curricula. The AACN (2008) nursing outcomes include:

1. Conduct comprehensive and focused physical, behavioral, psychological, spiritual, socioeconomic, and environmental assessments of health and illness parameters in patients, using developmentally and culturally appropriate approaches.

2. Recognize the relationship of genetics and genomics to health, prevention, screening, diagnostics, prognostics, selection of treatment, and the monitoring of treatment effectiveness using a constructed pedigree from collected family history information as well as standardized symbols and terminology.

3. Implement holistic, patient-centered care that reflects an understanding of human growth and development, pathophysiology, pharmacology, medical

management, and nursing management across the health/illness continuum, across the life span, and in all health care settings.

4. Communicate effectively with all members of the health care team, including the patient and the patient's support network.

5. Deliver compassionate, patient-centered, evidence-based care that respects patient and family preferences.

6. Implement patient and family care around the resolution of end-of-life and palliative care issues, such as symptom management, support of rituals, and respect for patient and family preferences.

7. Provide appropriate patient teaching that reflects developmental stage, age, culture, spirituality, patient preferences, and health literacy considerations to foster patient engagement in their care.

8. Implement evidence-based nursing interventions as appropriate for managing the acute and chronic care of patients and promoting health across the life span.

9. Monitor client outcomes to evaluate the effectiveness of psychobiological interventions.

10. Facilitate patient-centered transitions of care, including discharge planning and ensuring the caregiver's knowledge of care requirements to promote safe care.

11. Provide nursing care based on evidence that contributes to safe and high-quality patient outcomes within health care microsystems.

12. Create a safe care environment that results in high-quality patient outcomes.

13. Revise the plan of care based on an ongoing evaluation of patient outcomes.

14. Demonstrate clinical judgment and accountability for patient outcomes when delegating to and supervising other members of the health care team.

15. Manage care to maximize health, independence, and quality of life for a group of individuals that approximates a beginning practitioner's workload.

16. Demonstrate the application of psychomotor skills for the efficient, safe, and compassionate delivery of patient care.

17. Develop a beginning understanding of complementary and alternative modalities and their roles in health care.

18. Develop an awareness of patients' and health care professionals' spiritual beliefs and values and how those beliefs and values impact health care.

19. Manage the interaction of multiple functional problems affecting patients across the life span, including common geriatric syndromes.

20. Understand one's role and participation in emergency preparedness and disaster response with an awareness of environmental factors and the risks they pose to oneself and patients.

21. Engage in caring and healing techniques that promote a therapeutic nurse–patient relationship.

22. Demonstrate tolerance for the ambiguity and unpredictability of the world and its effect on the health care system as related to nursing practice.

In 2010, the NLN developed outcomes and competencies for graduates of practical/vocational, diploma, associate degree, baccalaureate, master's, practice doctorate, and research doctorate programs in nursing. The NLN stated that nursing educators must prepare individuals who

- Are grounded in values and ethics
- Understand that knowledge is continually evolving
- Are able to evaluate that knowledge
- Apply it in situations where nurses touch the lives of others

Graduates of any program should have several things in common. All nurses should be able to:

- Provide safe care that is culturally and developmentally appropriate and that is centered on building and sustaining positive, healthful relations with individuals, families, groups, and communities
- Practice within a legal, ethical, and professional scope that is guided by accepted standards of practice
- Continually learn and grow as professionals whose practice is supported by evidence
- Advocate for access to and quality of health care (NLN, 2016a, p. 9)

In addition, the NLN has defined program outcomes as

> [T]he expected culmination of all learning experiences occurring during the program, including the mastery of essential core nursing practice competencies, built upon the seven core values and the six integrating concepts. Course outcomes are the expected culmination of all learning experiences for a particular course within the nursing program, including the mastery of essential core competencies relevant to that course. Courses should be designed to promote synergy and consistency across the curriculum and lead to the attainment of program outcomes. (NLN, 2016a, p. 32)

The NLN's competencies model consists of the following elements:

1. Core values
   * Caring
   * Diversity
   * Excellence
   * Holism
   * Integrity
   * Patient centeredness
2. Integrating concepts
   * Context and environment
   * Knowledge and science
   * Personal and professional development
   * Quality and safety
   * Relationship-centered care
   * Teamwork

TABLE 12.5
Competencies for Graduates of Baccalaureate Programs

OUTCOME	COMPETENCY
Human flourishing	Incorporate the knowledge and skills learned in didactic and clinical courses to help patients, families, and communities continually progress toward fulfillment of human capacities.
Nursing judgment	Make judgments in practice, substantiated with evidence, that synthesize nursing science and knowledge from other disciplines in the provision of safe, quality care, and promote the health of patients, families, and communities.
Professional identity	Express one's identity as a nurse through actions that reflect integrity, a commitment to EBP; caring; advocacy; and safe, quality care for diverse patients, families, and communities; and a willingness to provide leadership in improving care.
Spirit of inquiry	Act as an evolving scholar who contributes to the development of the science of nursing practice by identifying questions in need of study, critiquing published research, and using available evidence as a foundation to propose creative, innovative, or evidence-based solutions to clinical practice problems.

EBP, evidence-based practice.

Source: NLN (2010, p. 39).

3. Program outcomes
   * Enhance human flourishing
   * Show sound nursing judgment
   * Develop professional identity
   * Approach all issues and problems in a spirit of inquiry
4. Nursing practice
   * Unbounded by any closed structures, the four program outcomes converge into nursing practice depending on the program type

Competencies for graduates of baccalaureate programs are provided as an example in Table 12.5.

CRITICAL THINKING QUESTION

How do you measure the outcomes of your curriculum to determine if goals and objectives are truly being met?

Answer: There are many ways to determine if goals and objectives are being met, including through objective measures like testing, simulation, and observed clinical performance.

When building curricular models, nurse educators must realize that there are many ways to conceptualize the curricula. The goal is to develop curricula so that the entire faculty are in agreement and are willing to keep the model clear and simple enough so that the learners develop an understanding of the practice of nursing as a whole, not just of discrete parts of a medical model.

CHANGING OR REVISING THE CURRICULUM

Changing an existing curriculum is sometimes more difficult than developing a curriculum from scratch because faculty members have a history with the outgoing curriculum. A contemplated change process must be used to change an existing curriculum effectively. When leaders or managers are planning to manage change, there are six key principles that need to be kept in mind:

1. Different people react differently to change
2. Everyone has fundamental needs that must be met
3. Change often involves a loss, and people go through the "loss curve"
4. Expectations need to be managed realistically
5. Fears have to be dealt with
6. There should be a good reason for the change

Here are some tips for applying the above principles when managing change.

- Give people information—be open and honest about the facts, but don't give into overly optimistic speculation. Meet people's openness needs, but in a way that does not set unrealistic expectations.
- For large groups, produce a communication strategy that ensures that information is disseminated efficiently and comprehensively to everyone (don't let the grapevine take over). Tell everyone at the same time. However, follow this up with individual interviews to produce a personal strategy for dealing with the change. This helps to recognize and deal appropriately with the individual reactions to change.
- Give people choices and be honest about the possible consequences of those choices. Meet their control and inclusion needs.
- Give people time to express their views and support their decision making. Provide coaching, counseling, or information as appropriate to help them through the loss curve.
- Where the changes involve a loss, identify what will or might replace that loss—loss is easier to cope with if there is something to replace it. This will help assuage potential fears.
- When it is possible to do so, give individuals the opportunity to express their concerns and provide reassurances—this also helps to assuage potential fears.
- Maintain good management practices, such as making time for informal discussions and feedback. Even though the pressure might make it seem that it is reasonable to let such things slip, during difficult change such practices are even more important (Team Technology, 2008).

Treat change as a project. Do this by applying all the rigors of project management to the change process: produce plans, allocate resources, appoint a steering board and/or project sponsor, and so on. The six principles listed earlier should form part of the project objectives (Team Technology, 2008).

CHANGE THEORIES

First-Order and Second-Order Changes

- First-order change does not challenge or contradict the established context of an organization. This type of change does not usually threaten people, either personally or collectively.
- The deeper changes that frustrate leaders and threaten followers are planned second-order changes. These changes intentionally challenge widely shared assumptions, disintegrate the context of "organization," and, in general, reframe the social system. This, in turn, generates widespread ambiguity, discontinuity, anxiety, frustration, confusion, paranoia, cynicism, and anger as well as temporary dysfunction.

The varieties of change theories often used in nursing are reviewed in Chapter 14. To provide a theoretical example that could be used in changing a curriculum, Lewin's force-field analysis model is used to illustrate elements of change and resistance to change. A force field relates to all the behaviors of a group in its environment during a given period of time.

According to this model, pressing for change tends to threaten stability and thus increases the power of those forces maintaining the system. Therefore, the most effective way to bring about change is to *reduce the forces of resistance*. The major concepts of the model are outlined in the following list (Goad & Hough, 1993):

- Driving forces—The past, present, and future elements, along with hopes, aspirations, and emotional investments that tend to affect a social event in a positive direction
- Restraining forces—The past, present, and future elements, along with hopes, aspirations, and emotional investments that tend to affect a social event in a negative direction
- Status quo—A dynamic equilibrium composed of a balance between the driving and restraining forces
- Motivators—The initial stimuli that convince the concerned parties there is a need for change
- Confirmation of nonaccomplishment—Information that confirms the fact that the desired job is not being accomplished
- Confirmation of lack of obtainment—Information that confirms the fact that what is wanted, needed, or expected is not being obtained
- Confirmation of lack of growth or maturation—Information that confirms the fact that growth or maturation is not being achieved

Stages

- Unfreezing—The stage in the change process during which the change agents create dissatisfaction, followed by inspiring the motivation to accept some type of change

- Moving—A cognitive redefinition by the participants of attitude and behavior toward the planned change
- Refreezing—The new behaviors are practiced and reinforced
- Change agent—The responsible person who moves those to be affected by change through the stages of change in a logical manner

Curriculum development and curriculum change are complex endeavors that require nursing education expertise, leadership, and vision. These processes should be done often and systematically to meet the goals of today's health care systems.

PLANNING LEARNING WITHIN THE CURRICULUM

Planning learning activities requires considerable faculty preparation time. Activities should be planned to enhance critical thinking and can be very important for enhancing students' learning. Planning learning activities involves the following six steps:

1. Developing the learning outcomes for the specific learning session
2. Creating an anticipatory set
3. Selecting a teaching strategy (refer to Chapter 3 for classroom teaching strategies)
4. Considering implementation issues
5. Designing closure for the session
6. Designing formative and summative evaluation strategies (Scheckel, 2012, p. 205)

CASE STUDIES

CASE STUDY 12.1

Marjorie is a seasoned nursing faculty member at a major university. She has been asked by the dean to serve as the curriculum coordinator and as mentor to a new faculty member, Stephanie. Stephanie is also on the curriculum committee and comes to the university with 8 years of teaching experience at a midsized university. Discuss the mentor–mentee relationship in this situation. What are some of the assets they can both bring to the curriculum committee? How should Marjorie approach this responsibility? What are the key elements of mentorship that she should be certain to address? What is Stephanie's responsibility in this relationship?

CASE STUDY 12.2

You are chosen to lead the curriculum committee in its efforts to update your school's curriculum from one that follows a medical model to a conceptually based curriculum. What is the process you would initiate to accomplish this task? Consider change theory, conceptual base, concepts to include, and teaching strategies.

PRACTICE QUESTIONS

1. When developing an interprofessional curriculum, the planning committee should:
   A. Communicate with and include community members to decide on areas that need improvement
   B. Try to align the entire curriculum with the various programs
   C. Allow each discipline to plan its own clinical activities
   D. Invite students at the same level in the same programs to participate

2. A teaching strategy appropriate for an interprofessional education course would include all EXCEPT a(n):
   A. Interdisciplinary case study
   B. Low-risk simulation experience
   C. Panel presentation by an interprofessional team of experts
   D. Concept map from each discipline

3. Which technique may have the potential for "transforming" nursing education?
   A. Simulation
   B. Journaling
   C. Debriefing
   D. Questioning

4. Which is an example of first-order change?
   A. The faculty moves the pediatric content to a different semester
   B. The new curriculum stresses concepts, not diseases
   C. The library becomes completely electronic
   D. Testing is done completely via simulation

5. The Preparation for the Professions Program (PPP) has identified three dimensions of apprenticeships for professional education. They include the following: (Select all that apply.)
   A. Acquired skill-based learning that includes clinical judgment
   B. Dependence on authority
   C. Intellectual training
   D. Ethical standards

6. Which course would be appropriate for a conceptual curriculum?
   A. Respiratory care in the intensive care unit
   B. Respiratory care over the life cycle
   C. Pediatric respiratory problems
   D. Issues in respiratory care

7. An objective that is appropriate for the first nursing course in a baccalaureate nursing program is:
   A. List the nutritional needs of clients of all ages.
   B. Choose foods appropriate for a low-sodium diet
   C. Analyze the nutrients in a diabetic diet
   D. Develop a nutritional plan for a client with kidney disease

8. Graduates of any program should be able to:

   A. Develop research questions related to patient safety

   B. Practice according to ethical standards

   C. Feel confident that they have mastered the practice of nursing

   D. Provide care that is appropriate to individuals

9. Competencies for graduates of baccalaureate programs include all EXCEPT:

   A. Human flourishing

   B. Professional identify

   C. Research expertise

   D. Nursing judgment

10. Which is the most appropriate topic for a simulation used in an interprofessional education (IPE) course with several disciplines?

    A. Disaster training

    B. Difficult childbirth

    C. Cardiac failure

    D. Infectious disease training

REFERENCES

Accreditation Commission for Education in Nursing. (2016). ACEN 2013 standards and criteria baccalaureate. Retrieved from http://www.acenursing.net/manuals/SC2013 _BACCALAUREATE.pdf

American Association of Colleges of Nursing. (2008). *The essentials of baccalaureate education for professional nursing practice*. Washington, DC: Author.

American Association of Colleges of Nursing. (2011). Core competencies for intercollaborative practice. Retrieved from http://www.aacn.nche.edu/education-resources/ ipecreport.pdf

American Association of Colleges of Nursing. (2016a). Position statement on violence as a public health problem. Report of the AACN Task Force on Violence as a public health problem. Retrieved from http://www.aacn.nche.edu/publications/position/ violence-problem

American Association of Colleges of Nursing. (2016b). Commission on collegiate nursing education (CCNE). Retrieved from http://www.aacn.nche.edu/ccne-accreditation

American Association of University Professors. (1970). Statement of principles on academic freedom and tenure with interpretive comments. Retrieved from http://www.aaup .org/statement/Redbook/1940 stat.htm (Original work published 1914)

Banks, J. A., & Banks, C. A. M. (2010). *Multicultural education: Issues and perspectives* (7th ed.). Hoboken, NJ: Wiley.

Barnum, B. J. (1998). The advanced nurse practitioner: Struggling toward a conceptual framework. *Nursing Leadership Forum, 3*(1), 14–17.

Benner, P., Sutphen, M., Leonard, V., & Day, L. (2009). *Educating nurses: A call for radical reform*. Hoboken, NJ: Jossey-Bass/Carnegie Foundation for the Advancement of Teaching.

Boland, L., & Finke, L. (2012). Curriculum designs. In D. M. Billings & J. A. Halstead (Eds.), *Teaching in nursing: A guide for faculty* (4th ed., pp. 119–137). St. Louis, MO: Elsevier Saunders.

Bulman, C., Lathlean, J., & Gobbi, M. (2012). The concept of reflection in nursing. Qualitative findings on student and teacher perspectives. *Nurse Education Today, 32*, e8–e13.

Candela, L., Dalley, K., & Benzel-Lindley, J. (2006). A case for learning-centered curricula. *Journal of Nursing Education, 43*(2), 59–65.

Carnegie Foundation for the Advancement of Teaching. (2013). Retrieved from https://www.carnegiefoundation.org/resources/publications

Connor, P. D., Nouer, S. S., Speck, P. M., Mackey, S. N., Tipton, N. G. (2013). Nursing students and intimate partner violence education: Improving and integrating knowledge into health care curricula. *Journal of Professional Nursing, 29*(4), 233–239.

Diekelmann, N. (2002). "Too much content" . . . . epistemologies' grasp and nursing education. *Journal of Nursing Education, 41*(11), 469–470.

Finke, L. M. (2012). Teaching in nursing: The faculty role. In D. M. Billings & J. A. Halstead (Eds.), *Teaching in nursing: A guide for faculty* (4th ed., pp. 1–14). St. Louis, MO: Elsevier Saunders.

Forbes, M., & Hickey, M. (2009). Curricular reform in baccalaureate nursing education: Review of the literature. *International Journal of Nursing Education Scholarship, 6*, 27.

Giddens, J. (2007). The neighborhood: A web-based platform to support conceptual teaching and learning. *Nursing Education Perspectives, 28*(5), 251–256.

Giddens, J., & Brady, D. (2007). Rescuing nursing education from content saturation: The case for a concept-based curriculum. *Journal of Nursing Education, 46*(26), 5–12.

Giddens, J., Brady, D., Brow, P., Wright, M., Smith, D., & Harris, J. (2008). A new curriculum for a new era of nursing education. *Nursing Education Perspectives, 29*(4), 2000–2004.

Goad, S., & Hough, L. (1993). Lewin's field theory with emphasis on change. In S. Zeigler (Ed.), *Theory-directed nursing practice* (pp. 183–192). New York, NY: Springer Publishing.

Hardin, P., & Richardson, S. (2012). Teaching the concept curricula: Theory and method. *Journal of Nursing Education, 51*(3), 155–159. doi:10.3928/014834-20120127-01

Hickey, M., Forbes, M., & Greenfield, S. (2010). Integrating the institute of medicine competencies in a baccalaureate curricular revision: Process and strategies. *Journal of Professional Nursing, 26*(4), 214–222.

Hoff, L. A. (1995). Violence content in nursing curricula: Strategic issues and implementation. *Journal of Advanced Nursing, 21*(1), 137–142.

Hofmeyer, A., Sheingold, B., Klopper, H. C., & Warland, J. (2015). Leadership in learning and teaching in higher education: Perspectives of academics in non-formal leadership roles. *Contemporary Issues in Education Research, 8*, 181–192.

Huber, D. (2000). *Leadership and nursing care management* (2nd ed.). Philadelphia, PA: W. B. Saunders.

Interprofessional Education Collaboration Expert Panel. (2011). *Core competencies for expert practice in collaboration: Report of an expert panel*. Washington, DC: Interprofessional Collaborative.

Ironsides, P. (2004). "Covering content" and teaching thinking: Deconstructing the additive curriculum. *Journal of Nursing Education, 43*(4), 5–12.

Keating, S. (2006). *Curriculum development and evaluation in nursing*. Philadelphia, PA: Lippincott Williams & Wilkins.

Leddy, S. (2007). Curriculum development in nursing education. In B. Moyer & R. A. Wittmann-Price (Eds.), *Foundations of practice excellence* (pp. 66–81). Philadelphia, PA: F. A. Davis.

Lewis, D. Y., Stephens, K. P., & Ciak, A. D. (2016). QSEN: Curriculum integration and bridging the gap to practice. *Nursing Education Perspectives, 37*(2), 97–100. doi:10.5480/14-1323

Lou, R. (1994). Teaching all students equally. In H. Roberts, J. C. Gonzales, & O. Scott (Eds.), *Teaching from a cultural perspective* (pp. 28–44). Thousand Oaks, CA: Sage.

Morris, W. (Ed.). (1970). *American Heritage dictionary of the English language* (3rd ed.). Boston, MA: American Heritage Publishing Company.

National League for Nursing. (1993). *A vision for nursing education*. New York, NY: Author.

National League for Nursing. (2010). *Outcomes and competencies for graduates of practical/ vocational, diploma, associate degree, baccalaureate, master's, practice doctorate, and research doctorate programs in nursing*. New York, NY: Author.

National League for Nursing. (2016a). Certified nurse educator (CNE) 2016 candidate handbook. Retrieved from http://www.nln.org/docs/default-source/professional

development-programs/certified-nurse-educator-%28cne%29-examination-candidate-handbook.pdf?sfvrsn=2

National League of Nursing. (2016b). Commission for Nursing Education Accreditation (CNEA). Retrieved from http://www.nln.org/accreditation-services/the-nln-commission-for-nursing-education-accreditation-%28cnea%29

National League of Nursing. Board of Governors. (2015). *Debriefing across the curriculum: A living document from the National League for Nursing in collaboration with the International Nursing Association for Clinical Simulation and Learning.* New York, NY: Author.

O'Connor, A. (2006). *Clinical instruction and evaluation: A resource guide* (2nd ed.). Sudbury, MA: Jones & Bartlett.

Office of Disease Prevention and Health Promotion. (2016). Healthy people 2020: Improving the health of America. Retrieved from http://www.healthypeople.gov

Ross, M. M., Hoff, L. A., & Coutu-Wakulczyk, G. (1998). Nursing curricula and violence issues. *Journal of Nursing Education, 2,* 53–60.

Rowles, C. J. (2012). Strategies to promote critical thinking and active learning. In D. M. Billings & J. A. Halstead (Eds.), *Teaching in nursing: A guide for faculty* (4th ed., pp. 258–284). St. Louis, MO: Elsevier Saunders.

Scheckel, M. (2012). Selecting learning activities to achieve curriculum outcomes. In D. M. Billings & J. A. Halstead (Eds.), *Teaching in nursing: A guide for faculty* (4th ed., pp. 170–187). St. Louis, MO: Elsevier Saunders.

Shostrom, B., & Schofer, K. (2016). A case-based curriculum with nurse as coach. *Journal of Nursing Education, 55*(5), 292–296.

Team Technology. (2008). MMDI™ personality test. Retrieved from http://www.team technology.co.uk

The Joint Commission. (2016). Performance measurement. Retrieved from https://www .joint commission.org/performance_measurement.aspx

The Joint Commission National Patient Safety Goals. (2003). *TIPS, 10*(1), 4–6.

Walker, D. E., & Soltis, J. (2009). *Curriculum and aims* (5th ed.). New York, NY: Teachers College Press.

Wiles, J., & Bondi, J. (1998). *Curriculum development: A guide to practice* (5th ed.). Upper Saddle River, NJ: W. B. Saunders.

Yoder-Wise, P. S. (2013). *Leading and managing in nursing* (5th ed.). St. Louis, MO: Elsevier.

Pursuing Continuous Quality Improvement in the Academic Nurse Educator Role

LINDA WILSON AND FRANCES H. CORNELIUS

If you don't know where you are going,
any road will take you there.
—Lewis Carroll, *Alice in Wonderland*

This chapter addresses the Certified Nurse Educator Exam Content Area 5: Pursue Continuous Quality Improvement in the Academic Nurse Educator Role (National League for Nursing [NLN], 2016a, pp. 5 & 8).

- Content Area 5 is 9% of the examination
- It is estimated that there will be approximately 13 to 14 questions from Content Area 5

LEARNING OUTCOMES

- Identify activities that promote one's socialization to the nurse educator role
- Discuss the importance of a mentor across the career trajectory
- Discuss the importance of a commitment to lifelong learning
- Discuss the importance of membership and active participation in professional organizations
- Identify professional development opportunities that increase one's effectiveness in the nursing role
- Identify sources of feedback to improve role effectiveness

The National League for Nursing (NLN) states that "academic nurse educators engage in a number of roles and functions, each of which reflects the core competencies of nursing faculty. The extent to which a specific nurse educator implements these competencies varies according to many factors, including the mission of the nurse educator's institution, the nurse educator's rank, the nurse educator's academic preparation, and the type of program in which the nurse educator teaches" (NLN, 2016a, p. 2).

To pursue systematic self-evaluation and improvement in the nurse educator role, it is necessary that he or she:

- "Engages in activities that promote one's socialization to the role
- Maintains membership in professional organizations
- Participates actively in professional organizations
- Demonstrates a commitment to lifelong learning
- Participates in professional development opportunities that increase one's effectiveness in the role
- Manage[s] the teaching, scholarship, and service demands as influenced by the requirements of the institution
- Uses feedback gained from self, peer, student, and administrative evaluation to improve role effectiveness
- Practice[s] according to legal and ethical standards relevant to higher education and nursing education
- Mentor[s] and support[s] faculty colleagues in the role of an academic nurse educator
- Engage[s] in self-reflection to improve teaching practices" (NLN, 2016a, p. 8)

This chapter focuses on the essential elements required in the pursuit of continuous quality improvement. These include:

1. Socialization to the faculty role
2. Role of mentorship across the career continuum
3. Active membership in professional organizations
4. Commitment to lifelong learning
5. Balancing teaching, scholarship, and service
6. Self-reflection to promote professional development

SOCIALIZATION TO THE EDUCATOR ROLE

The role of a new academic nurse educator can be both exciting and challenging. One of the most important support systems for a new educator is appropriate mentoring (NLN, 2006). An orientation program should include:

1. Introduction to key personnel
2. Introduction to other faculty members
3. A review of available resources within the department and organization
4. A review of courses and their related content (curriculum matrix)
5. A review of job benefits (done by the human resource department)
6. A review of administrative and governance structures (chain of command)

7. An introduction to the culture and political environment (full university faculty meetings and voting procedures for university committees)

8. Presentations on key aspects of the curriculum (what is emphasized in the curriculum has to do with the educational unit's core values)

9. A review of expectations for teaching, research, and service (for promotion and tenure—see Chapters 15 and 16 for further explanation)

10. Assignment of a faculty mentor

Many nurse educator orientation programs are completed one on one with a mentor. Some larger schools of nursing have developed extensive faculty orientation programs.

MENTOR AND SUPPORT FACULTY COLLEAGUES

Academic nurse educators have many roles and responsibilities, including the responsibility of mentoring. Nursing faculty have a responsibility to mentor colleagues, assisting them in their development as both educators and scholars (Billings & Halstead, 2012). Faculty mentorship includes guiding, coaching, and supporting faculty as they advance in their careers. Mentoring is extremely important, particularly for novices, because graduate school often provides little preparation for the academic nurse educator role. Mentoring is also important throughout all career stages.

Bruner, Dunbar, Higgins, and Martyn (2016) identify top five priorities for mentorship. These include:

1. Producing timely publications

2. Work–life balance

3. Preparing promotion packages

4. Guidance on test writing

5. Utilizing technology in the classroom

Bruner goes on to recommend that because of the diversity of roles of the contemporary nursing faculty, a gap analysis must first be conducted to identify mentorship needs. These gaps can be utilized to customize the mentorship program for the faculty (Nick et al., 2012).

Mentoring Throughout the Career Continuum

The NLN's (2008) position paper regarding mentoring of nurse faculty highlights key mentoring activities beneficial at various stages of a nurse educator's career. These include:

- Early-career faculty members: Mentorship targets the faculty member who is new to both the educator role and the institution.
  - Mentoring helps the uninitiated learn the complexities of the faculty role
  - Mentoring provides information about the knowledge, skills, behaviors, and values that comprise the faculty role

* Formal orientation programs often include:
  - An introduction to key personnel and resources
  - A review of the courses and curricula being taught
  - An overview of job benefits and administrative and governance structures
  - An introduction to the culture and political environment of the institution
* Throughout the entire first year an assigned mentor should:
  - Answer questions
  - Interpret situations
  - Provide direct help
  - Share a similar schedule to ensure optimum availability
  - Be friendly and caring

- Midcareer faculty members: Mentorship supports faculty as they identify and test innovative pedagogies, propose new solutions to problems, and evolve as educators or scholars in local, regional, and national arenas. Mentoring is:
  - Eclectic, varied in its content and process
  - Directed more by the mentee than by the mentor
  - Involves reciprocal sharing, learning, and growth
  - Individually focused and takes time to evolve
* Faculty may select a mentor for:
  - Formal and informal mentoring relationships
  - Shared interests inside and outside their academic communities
  - Development of specific aspects in teaching, evaluation of learning, curriculum design, scholarship, service, and leadership
  - Guidance in transitioning into academic leadership positions
* Faculty may develop "multiple mentoring partnerships, where each mentor assists them to grow in a particular area, such as grant-writing or conducting research on a particular topic" or a mentor can "provide guidance in selecting and transitioning into academic leadership positions" (NLN, 2008, p. 6).

- Late-career faculty members: T foundation of mentorship at this level is the responsibility to "identify new faculty members who show potential as leaders in nursing and nursing education and enter into mentor–protégé relationships with them, relationships that extend over long periods of time" (NLN, 2006, p. 4). The mentoring relationship at this level:
  - Is a source of satisfaction derived from guiding another in attaining self-clarity, personal growth, and as the educator continues to develop his or her skills
  - Cultivates a relationship that is situated in common interests and is built upon mutual respect for one another's knowledge and talents
  - Is "characterized by the investment of time, effort, and caring; the identification of mutual goals; and regular, ongoing dialogue designed to ensure the accomplishment of those goals" (NLN, 2006, pp. 7–8)

> In the mentor–protégé relationship, the mentor shares her/his wisdom, knowledge, and expertise; builds connections in multiple communities by introducing personal networks; and keeps open a future of possibilities for someone who is expected to make significant contributions to the profession. Through an extended relationship, the mentor nurtures leadership in the protégé. (NLN, 2006, p. 4)

- The "key variable in the success or failure of the mentoring relationship was the mentor's accessibility, both physical and emotional" (Wasburn, 2007, p. 61).
- It is important to note that mentorship is not limited to a relationship between two faculty members.
- Mentoring, in an ideal sense, involves the entire academic community. Everyone within the organization bears a responsibility to provide a supportive and welcoming environment and to foster a sense of belonging.
- An ongoing commitment to the practice of mentoring requires support from administrators and the entire nursing faculty. "Establishing a healthful work environment where collaborative peer and co-mentoring are an expectation, rather than a possibility, is the responsibility of all involved in nursing education" (Wasburn, 2007, p. 4).

During economic downturns and nursing faculty shortages, mentoring is a retention strategy (Jakubik, 2016). Faculty turnover is costly for educational organizations and disrupts the education process within the program.

Additional information on choosing a mentor in relation to career development is discussed in Chapter 15. Mentorship is so important that it can make or break a person's transition into a role (Goode, 2012).

The NLN recommendations for mentoring at all levels are outlined in Exhibit 13.1.

EVIDENCE-BASED TEACHING PRACTICE

Jakubik (2016) is writing a leadership series about faculty mentoring. The researcher's literature review reveals that mentoring does help retention of faulty but specifics about best practices are lacking.

Ideally, "the teaching of nursing must be evidence-based, with research informing what is taught, how learning is facilitated and evaluated, and how curricula/programs are designed" (NLN, 2002, p. 3). Kalb, O'Conner-Von, Brockway, Rierson, and Sendelbach (2015) report that although evidence-based teaching practice (EBTP) is deemed a professional standard, and most nurse educators are familiar with evidence-based practice, "many were not aware of EBTP or the need to use evidence in their teaching and faculty responsibilities. This lack of awareness has significant implications for the preparation of new nurse faculty and the professional development of current faculty" (p. 217).

EXHIBIT 13.1

The NLN Levels of Mentoring

For nursing faculty
- Contribute to the development of a mentoring program at your institution by identifying the needs of new faculty members and the resources required to meet those needs.
- Actively participate in mentoring relationships.
- Make the teaching done by experienced faculty members more visible to new faculty.
- Be open and friendly to new faculty and identify opportunities to be a "one-minute mentor" through brief, supportive interactions (Oermann, 2001).
- Become sensitive to existing and potential academic community practices that exclude new faculty members.
- Spend time together as a nurse faculty community, talking and listening to one another, and also include the new faculty members.
- Attend professional development workshops and seminars on mentoring.
- Collaborate with the dean/director/chairperson to establish a mentoring program.
- Include content on mentoring in undergraduate and graduate curricula, including how to identify and select caring colleagues with whom to work closely and how to collaborate with colleagues.

For deans/directors/chairpersons
- Initiate and provide support for mentoring initiatives at your institution.
- Engage new, mid career, and seasoned faculty in developing mentoring initiatives at your institution.
- Incorporate innovative strategies for mentoring new faculty members, such as the use of retired nurse educators (Bellack, 2004).
- Value the mentor role and reward faculty who actively serve in mentoring roles.
- Support the development of faculty mentors.
- Model mentoring.

For the NLN
- Support research on mentoring in the academic environment.
- Offer workshops and seminars on mentoring.
- Develop a mentoring toolkit (NLN, 2008).

CRITICAL THINKING QUESTION

Mentoring is a voluntary activity and can extend over a long period of time (Jakubik, 2016). What types of expectations should the mentor have of the protégé?

> **EVIDENCE-BASED TEACHING PRACTICE**
>
> Green and Jackson (2014) explored the negative aspects of mentoring and its effects on mentors and protégés and discussed the ethical boundaries of the relationship and the need to set ground rules so both mentor and protégé can have a positive relationship to promote professional and personal growth.

Kalb et al. (2015) identifies several areas in which faculty can use evidence for teaching:

1. To revise courses
2. To design curriculum
3. To develop course content
4. To guide teaching
5. To answer questions about educational practices
6. To evaluate the effectiveness of teaching
7. To select teaching methods
8. To evaluate the quality of student learning
9. To critique evidence to inform teaching
10. To select evaluation methods

Kalb et al. (2015) emphasize that in order to support EBTP, a deliberate, structured, and sustained approach is required at institutional, administrative, and collegial levels to promote faculty effectiveness and student learning.

MEMBERSHIP IN PROFESSIONAL ORGANIZATIONS

It is important for academic nurse educators to be members of professional organizations. These organizations include, but are not limited to, the following:

- American Nurses Association (ANA)
- State nursing organizations
- NLN
- Sigma Theta Tau International Honor Society for Nursing
- Specialty nursing organizations (American Society of Perianesthesia Nurses, Association of Perioperative Registered Nurses, National Association of Orthopaedic Nurses, Oncology Nursing Society, American Association of Critical Care Nurses, etc.)
- Other related professional organizations (American Pain Society, Society for Critical Care Medicine, American Medical Informatics Association, etc.)

Membership in professional organizations provides the opportunity for knowledge enhancement, networking, and professional activities.

ACTIVE PARTICIPATION IN PROFESSIONAL ORGANIZATIONS

Professional organizational membership and leadership activities are an excellent mechanism for taking an active role in determining the future of nursing. These activities are also important in satisfying the service requirements for nurse educators who can:

- Participate on a committee
- Participate in a special interest group
- Serve as chair of a committee
- Serve as chair of a special interest group
- Run for office or a role on the board of directors at the local, state, or national level
- Participate in a task force
- Volunteer to work on specific initiatives for the organization
- Participate in a strategic work team

COMMITMENT TO LIFELONG LEARNING/FACULTY DEVELOPMENT

According to the ANA's *Scope and Standards for Nursing Professional Development* (2010), the following are some of the beliefs that guided the development of the standards:

- "Lifelong learning is the responsibility of the nurse and is essential to maintain and increase competence in nursing practice" (p. 1).
- "Continuing professional nursing competence is essential to the provision of safe, quality health care to all members of society" (p. 1).
- "The public has a right to expect continuing professional nursing competence throughout the career of the nurse" (p. 1).
- "Self-directed learning is an integral part of continuing education, staff development, and academic education" (p. 2).

The *Scope and Standards* (ANA, 2010) also states that the lifelong professional development of a nurse requires participation in learning activities to assist in the development and maintenance of competence, enhancement of practice, and support for the attainment of career goals. The academic nurse educator has a personal and professional responsibility to:

- Seek continuing-education activities to maintain competency
- Expand knowledge and expertise in a nursing specialty

The NLN's (2001) position statement regarding lifelong learning acknowledges that the "concept of lifelong learning for nursing faculty (or faculty development) is complex and multi-faceted" (p. 1), and that learning starts in a master's and/ or doctoral study program, but continues beyond formal education as a lifelong pursuit. Lifelong learning continues "through self-study and a constant inquisitiveness about the role and all its dimensions" (p. 1). In addition, the NLN (2016b) stresses that concepts of lifelong learning should also be integrated through interprofessional collaborations.

PARTICIPATION IN PROFESSIONAL OPPORTUNITIES TO ENHANCE ONGOING DEVELOPMENT

To maintain high-quality nursing education programs, it is imperative that all faculty remain not only proficient with basic principles but also current with emerging technology and pedagogical trends. There are many different types of professional development opportunities in which the academic nurse educator can participate.

- Provider directed, provider paced
  1. The provider-directed, provider-paced educational opportunity is "an activity in which the provider controls all aspects of the learning activity" (American Nurses Credentialing Center [ANCC], 2015, p. 47).
  2. Examples of provider-directed, provider-paced educational opportunities include seminars, national conferences, and live webcasts.
- Provider directed, learner paced
  1. A provider-directed, learner-paced educational opportunity is "an activity in which the provider controls the content of the learning activity, including the learning outcomes based on a needs assessment, and chooses the content of the learning activity, the method by which it is presented, and the evaluation methods. Learners determine the pace at which they engage in the activity" (ANCC, 2015, p. 47).
  2. Examples of provider-directed, learner-paced educational activities include continuing-education journal articles, online continuing-education modules, and continuing-education programs delivered on CDs or DVDs.
- Learner-directed, learner-paced activities: A learner-directed, learner-paced activity is "a learning activity in which the learner takes the initiative in identifying his or her learning needs, formulating learning goals, identifying human and material resources for learning, choosing and implementing appropriate learning strategies, and evaluating learning outcomes. The learner also determines the pace at which he or she engages in the learning activity. Learner-directed activities may be developed with or without the help of others, but they are undertaken on an individual basis" (ANCC, 2015, p. 46).

Although similarities in learning needs exist, the elements of lifelong learning for the nurse educator vary according to:

- Type of faculty appointment
- Full time, part time, or adjunct
- Tenure track or nontenure track
- Academic or service setting
- Career stages
- Novice faculty

- Mid stage faculty
- Senior faculty
- "The mission of a university affects the nature of expectations for the (NLN, 2001, p. 1):
  * Scope of the role of faculty
  * The educator role"

The NLN (2001) maintains that faculty development programs should be individualized and adaptable and should offer a wide range of topics in multiple modalities. Topics relevant to nurse educators include, but are not limited to:

- Classroom management
- Student advisement
- Student incivility
- Cultural competency
- Informatics competency
- Clinical teaching
- Clinical evaluation
- Test construction
- Developing goal statements and learning objectives
- Outcomes assessment
- Teaching/learning technologies
- Curriculum development and modification
- The accreditation process
- The faculty role as leaders in the university community
- Creative teaching strategies
- Strategies to promote critical thinking
- Strategies to integrate informatics within the curriculum

It is important to note that "no single program or approach will meet the needs of everyone, and even the most senior tenured full professor must never think that she/he has nothing new to learn" (NLN, 2001, p. 2).

CASE STUDY

CASE STUDY 13.1

A nurse educator is mentoring a novice faculty member who was hired to teach the maternal–child health course. The learners in the course are a mixed group of prelicensure students. Fifty percent are traditional and 50% are second-degree learners. What preparation tips would you give to the novice nurse educator about the learners in the class? How would you instruct the novice nurse educator to conduct test reviews?

PRACTICE QUESTIONS

1. A majority of faculty have identified a need for mentorship to accomplish which of the following:
   A. Improvement in classroom teaching
   B. Work–life balance
   C. Preparing for retirement
   D. Identifying venues for professional presentations

2. Mentoring a late-career faculty member may include:
   A. Encouraging and supporting the faculty to identify and test innovative pedagogies
   B. Providing guidance in transitioning into academic leadership positions
   C. Encouraging the faculty to identify new faculty members who show potential as leaders in nursing and nursing education
   D. Encouraging faculty to propose new solutions to problems and to evolve as educators and scholars in local, regional, and national arenas

3. Early-career faculty need mentorship in the following areas:
   A. Help in identifying and testing innovative pedagogies
   B. Help in identifying academic leadership positions
   C. Help navigating political and administrative environment
   D. Help identifying national venues for scholarly presentations

4. The novice nurse educator needs additional mentoring about student boundaries established when he tells his mentor that he:
   A. Shares personal stories that emphasize a content point
   B. Demonstrates a positive attitude with students
   C. Shows enthusiasm for students learning new techniques
   D. Discusses the personnel responsibilities that limit his time

5. Nurse educators understand that one of the main consequences of lack of mentorship is a decrease in:
   A. Understanding of the curriculum
   B. Socialization into the role
   C. Dissatisfaction of faculty
   D. Attrition of faculty

6. A new faculty member is constantly comparing the current teaching methods of the faculty with the methods used by faculty at her previous educational unit. The mentor's best response would be to:
   A. Encourage the new faculty member to return to the previous position
   B. Ask the faculty member to stop comparing
   C. Have the faculty member present ideas in a lunch conference
   D. Explain to the new faculty member that there are many methods that work well

7. The director of an educational unit asks a seasoned faculty mentor to mentor a new hire and the seasoned faculty member objects. The best way to handle this situation would be to:

   A. Document the situation and find someone who is willing

   B. Insist that the faculty mentor do it

   C. Terminate the faculty mentor who refuses

   D. Tell the faculty mentor that it is a professional responsibility

8. A faculty member tells another faculty member, in the hallway, that his skills are out of date because he no longer practices clinically. The director of the educational unit would best respond to this comment by telling:

   A. The faculty member who made the comment that it is incivil

   B. The faculty member who does not work clinically that it would be a good idea to seek out a per diem clinical position

   C. Both faculty members to take their conflict behind closed doors

   D. Both faculty members that competency is not based solely on clinical practice

9. The novice nurse educator understands that faculty role expectations include:

   A. Completing a terminal degree

   B. Concentrating on teaching and not service

   C. Attending conferences in the future

   D. Incorporating ethical and legal principles into teaching practice

10. An important orientation activity for nurse educators is:

    A. Developing a curriculum matrix to follow

    B. Attending departmental meetings

    C. Doing a university-wide scavenger hunt

    D. Socializing with other faculty

REFERENCES

American Nurses Association. (2010). *Scope and standards of practice for nursing professional development* (2nd ed.). Washington, DC: Author.

American Nurses Credentialing Center. (2015). *2015 ANCC primary accreditation provider application manual*. Silver Spring, MD: Author.

Bellack, J. P. (2004). Seasoned faculty: To retire or not? One solution to the faculty shortage—Begin at the end. *Journal of Nursing Education, 43*(6), 243–244.

Billings, D. M., & Halstead, J. A. (2012). *Teaching in nursing: A guide for faculty* (4th ed.). St. Louis, MO: Elsevier Saunders.

Bruner, D. W., Dunbar, S., Higgins, M., & Martyn, K. (2016). Benchmarking and gap analysis of faculty mentorship priorities and how well they are met. *Nursing Outlook*, 321–331. doi:10.1016/j.outlook.2016.02.008

Goode, M. L. (2012). The role of the mentor: A critical analysis. *Journal of Community Nursing, 26*(3), 33–35.

Green, J., & Jackson, D. (2014). Mentoring: Some cautionary notes for the nursing profession. *Contemporary Nurse: A Journal for the Australian Nursing Profession, 47*(1/2), 79–87.

Jakubik, L. D. (2016). Leadership series: "How to" for mentoring. Part 1: An overview of mentoring practices and mentoring benefits. *Pediatric Nursing, 42*(1), 37–38.

Kalb, K. A., O'Conner-Von, S. K., Brockway, C., Rierson, C. L., & Sendelbach, S. (2015) Evidence-based teaching practice in nursing education: Faculty perspectives and practices *Nursing Education Perspectives*, 36(4), 212–219.

National League for Nursing. (2001). Position statement: Lifelong learning for nursing faculty. Retrieved from http://www.nln.org/docs/default-source/about/archived -position-statements/lifelong-learning-for-nursing-faculty-pdf.pdf?sfvrsn=8

National League for Nursing. (2002). The preparation of nurse educators [Position statement]. Retrieved from http://www.nln.org/docs/default-source/about/nln-vision-series -(position-statements)/nlnvision_6.pdf

National League for Nursing. (2006). Position statement: Mentoring of nurse faculty. *Nursing Education Perspectives, 27*(2), 110–113.

National League for Nursing. (2008). Position statement: Preparing the next generation of nurses to practice in a technology-rich environment: An informatics agenda. Retrieved from http://www.nln.org/docs/default-source/professional-development -programs/preparing-the-next-generation-of-nurses.pdf?sfvrsn=6

National League for Nursing. (2016a). Certified nurse educator (CNE) 2016 candidate handbook. Retrieved from http://www.nln.org/docs/default-source/professional -development-programs/certified-nurse-educator-(cne)-examination-candidate -handbook.pdf?sfvrsn=2

National League for Nursing (2016b). NLN research priorities in nursing education 2015–2019. Retrieved from http://www.nln.org/docs/default-source/professional -development-programs/nln-research-priorities-in-nursing-education-single-pages .pdf?sfvrsn=2

Nick, J. M., Delahoyde, T. M., Del Prato, D., Mitchell, C., Ortiz, J., Ottley, C., . . . Siktberg, L. (2012). Best practices in academic mentoring: A model for excellence. *Nursing Research and Practice, 2012*, Article ID 937906. doi:1155/2012/937906

Oermann, M. H. (2001). One minute mentor. *Nursing Management, 32*(4), 12–13.

Wasburn, M. H. (2007). Mentoring women faculty: An instrumental case study of strategic collaboration. *Mentoring & Tutoring: Partnership in Learning, 15*(1), 57–72.

14

Functioning as a Change Agent and Leader

FRANCES H. CORNELIUS

I like a teacher who gives you something to take
home to think about besides homework.
—Edith Ann [Lily Tomlin]

This chapter addresses the Certified Nurse Educator Exam Content Area 6A: Function as a Change Agent and Leader (National League for Nursing [NLN], 2016, p. 5).

- Content Area 6, which includes 6A, 6B, and 6C, make up 21% of the examination
- It is estimated that there will be approximately 31 or 32 questions from Content Area 6

LEARNING OUTCOMES

- Discuss the importance of cultural sensitivity when advocating for change
- Discuss the effect of organizational culture on the climate of innovation within nursing education
- Identify strategies to support a climate of creativity and innovation within nursing education
- Identify measures to evaluate organizational effectiveness in nursing education
- Analyze the nurse educator's leadership role with respect to creating an environment of innovation
- Analyze strategies that drive organizational change
- Elaborate on strategies for integrating a long-term, innovative, and creative perspective into the nurse educator role

This chapter focuses on the nurse educator's role as a leader who interfaces with the larger academic community and administration, the role of the nurse educator within the larger system, and becoming a change agent within a variety of systems.

THE NURSE EDUCATOR'S ROLE AS A LEADER AND CHANGE AGENT

Mahoney (2001) states that the essential qualities of a nurse leader include having competence, confidence, courage, creativity, collaboration, and therapeutic communication skills. In addition, nursing administrators, educators, and clinicians have a responsibility to keep abreast of health care's rapidly changing environment and to make changes proactively. In order for nurses to create change, they must be aware of the key issues affecting the nursing profession.

Opportunities abound for nurses to lead, but few are born leaders: Most nurses must learn effective leadership skills. Effective leadership is enhanced by paying attention, having followers, moving in the right direction, and continually acting and questioning what can be done to make a difference (Dickenson-Hazard, 2004).

The functions of a nurse leader include:

1. Acting as a role model for others
2. Providing expert nursing care based on theory and research findings
3. Demonstrating knowledge about organizational theory to support and influence organizational policies
4. Collaborating with others to provide optimum health care
5. Assuming responsibility for providing information and support to patients
6. Using advocacy to help effect changes that will benefit patients and the health care organization
7. Using the nursing codes of ethics and standards of practice as guidelines for individual and professional accountability (Grant & Massey, 1999, as cited in Mahoney, 2001, p. 270)

Although often *leadership* is often used interchangeably with *management skills*, it is important to note that there is a difference between leadership and management skills.

SKILLS AND ATTRIBUTES OF A LEADER

Carroll (2005) conducted a study to compare the perceptions of female leaders and nurse executives about what skills and attributes would be needed to succeed in the 21st century. Six factors were identified:

1. *Personal integrity*—includes adherence to ethical standards, trustworthiness, and credibility
2. *Strategic vision/action orientation*—related to creating and articulating a vision of a preferred future, managing change, seeing possibilities instead of obstacles, exhibiting a determination to succeed and a commitment to action, being proactive, evaluating, being resilient, promoting excellence, and seeing the big picture
3. *Team building/communication*—skills used to build coalitions, make effective oral presentations, debate and discuss important issues, build a team, and build consensus
4. *Management and technical competence*—ability to make decisions, think critically, solve problems, plan, direct, organize, control, and be technically competent in a field, profession, or discipline

5. *People skills*—ability to empower others, network, value diversity, and work collaboratively

6. *Personal survival skills/attributes*—political sensitivity, self-direction, self-reliance, courage, a competitive and entrepreneurial spirit, and candor

Leadership Protocols

Rubino (2011) discusses the responsibility of the leader to serve as a role model for the organization. He identifies a list of "protocols" that describe certain key behaviors that are essential for effective leaders. These include:

1. Professionalism

2. Reciprocal trust and respect

3. Being confident, optimistic, and passionate

4. Being visible

5. Being an open communicator

6. Taking risks/entrepreneur

7. Admitting fault

Qualities of a Leader

King (2011) identifies key qualities of a leader, which include:

- *Ambition*—having an objective/goal to work toward
- *Knowledge of the business*—a solid understanding of the history and operations of the organization
- *Consistency*—consistent behavior inspires trust and is the foundation for integrity; this is possible only through consistency of thought and action
- *Good listening skills*—essential to build trust and effective working relationships; effective listening contributes to the knowledge and understanding of the leader and provides critical information for decision making
- *Creativity*—a leader will adapt quickly to new information and have the creativity and vision to handle change
- *Ability to own up to mistakes*—a leader who accepts responsibility for his or her mistakes and does not scapegoat others; builds trust among his or her subordinates
- *Decision-making skills*—a strong business leader is decisive, and has the courage to stand by the decision taken

Leadership Activities of Senior Nurses

Frankel (2011) points out that senior nurses, at all levels, should adopt a supportive leadership style and work to develop other staff by providing opportunities for them to "apply theory to practice and encouraging to test new skills in a safe and supportive environment" (p. 4). This style incorporates mentorship, coaching, and supervision as core values.

Leadership Styles

Sims (2009) identifies a variety of different leadership styles. These include being:

- *Task oriented*—For the most part, this leader focuses his or her attention on specific tasks or things to be accomplished. Generally, the communication is one way, from the leader to the subordinate.

- *Relationship oriented*—The leader who is relationship-oriented values open communication and encourages subordinates to give input and participate actively in problem solving. This leader is empathetic and considers the emotional aspects as well as cognitive aspects of situations.

- *Transactional*—The leader who uses a transactional leadership style communicates effectively, particularly in clarifying instructions. This leader will also establish a contractual reward or punishment system for performance outcomes.

- *Transformational*—The transformational leader is empathetic and creates an environment that is intellectually stimulating, inspiring, and challenging to support subordinates' development and maximize performance outcomes.

- *Affiliative*—Ideally, a leader using an affiliative approach to leadership already has a staff who is highly motivated so the objective is to create a friendly workplace and minimize conflict or friction.

- *Coaching*—A leader who uses a coaching leadership style is interested in the professional development of his or her subordinates and strives to "create a team spirit atmosphere in the work setting" (Sims, 2009, p. 273).

The literature abounds with exemplars of leadership skills and practices associated with the transformational leader. Ross, Fitzpatrick, Click, Krouse, and Clavelle (2014) define key transformational leadership practices as:

- *Inspiring a shared vision:* envisioning the future by imagining exciting and ennobling possibilities; enlisting others in a common vision by appealing to shared aspirations

- *Challenging the process:* searching for opportunities by seeking new ways to change, grow, and improve; experimenting and taking risks; generating small wins; and learning from mistakes

- *Enabling others to act:* fostering collaboration by promoting cooperative goals and building trust and strengthening others by sharing power and discretion along the way

- *Encouraging the heart:* recognizing individual contributions, showing appreciation for excellence, and celebrating victories by creating a spirit of community

- *Modeling the way:* finding voice and clarifying personal values by setting an example and aligning actions with the shared values of the team

It is important to note that most effective leaders use a variety of leadership styles—modifying their approach to the context of the situation. An important skill of an effective leader is to be flexible and attuned to the need to adjust one's approach.

> ### EVIDENCE-BASED TEACHING PRACTICE
>
> Delgado and Mitchell (2016) conducted a cross-sectional, online survey to identify nurse faculty leadership qualities that are currently valued and relevant and found the qualities to be integrity, communication clarity, and problem-solving ability.

Pullen (2016) lists the following leadership styles:

1. Servant
2. Transformational
3. Democratic
4. Authoritarian/autocratic
5. Laissez-faire

Pullen states that the "change process is best accomplished using the servant, transformational, and democratic leadership approaches. These three styles often result in people who are motivated through inspiration" (p. 28).

Competencies Associated With Leadership

Dye and Garman (2006) identified 16 essential leadership competencies in health care today. These are organized into four domains called *cornerstones* and include self-awareness, vision, interactions, and executing decisions. Within those four cornerstones are the critical competencies which include:

1. Conviction
2. Emotional intelligence
3. Vision
4. Communication
5. Trust
6. Appropriate power
7. Team development that can build consensus
8. Decision making
9. Openness to creativity
10. Developing outcomes
11. Flexibility or adaptability
12. Mentoring
13. Providing appropriate feedback
14. Actively listening
15. Facilitating functioning teams
16. Energizing team members

Green (2006) also identifies several critical competencies for nurse educators that relate to the role of change agent and leader. These include:

- Collaboration
  - Teamwork—an essential component of the nurse educator's role
  - Developing networks and partnerships to improve nursing's influence within the community
  - Working with faculty and students to support progress toward the achievement of realistic and optimal learning goals
  - Conferring with nursing leadership to make recommendations and develop educational interventions
- Systems thinking
  - Involves the ability of the nurse educator to incorporate the body of knowledge, resources, and tools available within and outside the health care system to optimize learning experiences and teaching opportunities
  - Focuses on interrelationships and how these impact the process of change and are, in turn, affected by this process
  - Identifying the social, economic, political, and institutional forces influencing nursing education
- Advocacy/moral agency
  - Monitor legal and ethical issues relevant to higher education and nursing education, and act to influence, plan, and implement policies and procedures
  - Guide decisions and actions with ethical principles grounded in an appreciation of cultural diversity and individual rights

D. Nelson, Godfrey, and Purdy (2004) studied hospital mentoring programs. They found that hospitals that used a mentorship program spent less and realized great benefits. It was a successful way to recruit and retain the brightest graduate nurses. Hospital-based mentorship programs increase recruitment and retention and are cost-effective (D. Nelson et al., 2004). Mentors are nurses who facilitate learning and model leadership skills.

EVIDENCE-BASED TEACHING PRACTICE

Getha-Taylor, Fowles, Silvia, and Merritt (2015) analyzed data from a local government leadership development program to examine how time affects conceptual and interpersonal leadership skill education and found that skills decline over time. The study indicates a need for consistent and continuous skill reinforcement.

There are three theoretical perspectives that explain how a person can become a leader:

1. *Trait Theory*—A "natural-born" leader possesses natural leadership traits that lead him or her into leadership roles.
2. *Great Events Theory*—An ordinary person responds to a crisis or disastrous event and emerges a leader.

3. *Transformational Leadership*—A person chooses to become a leader by seeking opportunities to develop leadership skills (Clark, 2008).

To develop leadership skills, a nurse educator must assume the responsibility of seeking out opportunities for professional development. It is essential to take the initiative to obtain an accurate assessment of one's current leadership skills and performance.

- This process can be started by creating a list of strengths and weaknesses.
- Typically, it is fairly easy to identify one's strengths, but most people find it difficult to identify their weaknesses.
- The nurse educator must seek out opportunities to develop leadership skills, link with potential leadership mentors and coaches, and actively solicit very specific feedback from a variety of sources.
- It is essential to be receptive to feedback and reflect on it throughout the process.

CRITICAL THINKING QUESTION

Veenema and colleagues (2015) put out a call-for-action paper for nurses as leaders in disaster preparedness and respose. What type of leadership style would you assume in a disaster response situation?

EVIDENCE-BASED TEACHING PRACTICE

Sarros, Cooper, and Santora (2008) found that "transformational leadership is linked with organizational culture primarily through the process of articulating vision, and, to a lesser extent, through setting of high-performance expectations and providing individual support." (p. 155)

Essential Leadership Skills

Sources of influence—Creative and innovative leaders must embody the following traits and abilities:

- "Organizational understanding" and political skills
- Creative thinking skills for idea evaluation
- Self-awareness
- Adaptability is needed in changing environments and to compensate when there are areas that need improvement
- Collaborative thinking—Creative work frequently involves collaboration with other disciplines, as well as with nontraditional partners; looking for partnerships outside one's usual circles can lead to successful, win–win partnerships (Glasgow & Cornelius, 2005)
- Integration minded—Leaders are more effective when using an integrative style that permits them to orchestrate expertise, people, and relationships in such a

way as to bring new ideas into being; there are three critical elements to this integrative style of leadership:

* *Idea generation*—Stresses the role of the leader in facilitating others' idea generation
* *Idea structuring*—Refers to guidance with respect to the technical and organizational merits of the work, setting output expectations, and identifying and integrating the projects to be pursued
* *Idea promotion*—Involves gathering support from the broader organization for the creative enterprise as a whole as well as implementation of a specific idea or project (Mumford, Scott, Gaddis, & Strange, 2002, pp. 738–739)

In other words, making sure resources are available (time, staff, funds, etc.) to complete the project.

EVALUATING ORGANIZATIONAL EFFECTIVENESS

Research has called for organizations to be more flexible, adaptive, entrepreneurial, and innovative to meet the changing demands of today's environment more effectively (Sarros et al., 2008). Additional research has found that organizational performance is linked to participative leadership and an innovative organizational culture (Casida, 2008; Ogbonna & Harris, 2000; Shahzad, Luqman, Khan, & Shabbir, 2012).

Thibodeaux and Favilla (1996) define *organizational effectiveness* as the "extent to which an organization, by the use of certain resources, fulfills its objectives without depleting its resources and without placing undue strain on its members and/or society" (p. 21). There are a number of models that facilitate the evaluation of organizational effectiveness. For the most part, the first step in all approaches to evaluate organizational effectiveness is to identify the criteria for evaluation. Generally, the model selected to approach the organizational assessment will determine which criteria will be utilized, and the model selected is dictated by the type of organization being evaluated. Traditional organizational assessment models include:

1. Goal Model
2. Systems Model
3. Process Model
4. Strategic Constituencies Model
5. Competing Values Framework
6. Baldrige National Quality Program (Martz, 2008)

Many of the models of organizational effectiveness have similar attributes/criteria that demonstrate organizational effectiveness. These include:

* Clear goals that are well communicated
* Resources allocated to innovation and change
* Members (faculty) who are satisfied
* Success is marketed
* Education is rewarded
* A plan for the future exists (Cheng, 1996)

Martz (2008) states that regardless of the organization type, any organization can be assessed by "incorporating an explicit focus on the common functionality innate to all organizations regardless of the organization size, type, structure, design or purpose" (p. 19).

Martz (2010) identifies six steps to use in assessing an organization's effectiveness:

1. Establish the boundaries of the evaluation
2. Conduct a performance needs assessment
3. Define the criteria of merit
4. Plan and implement the evaluation
5. Synthesize performance data with values
6. Communicate and report evaluation findings

Outcomes

Donabedian (2005) conceptualizes evaluation into three dimensions: structure, processes, and outcomes. The outcome of medical care, in terms of recovery, restoration of function, and of survival, has been frequently used as an indicator of the quality of medical care. The most common effectiveness measurements are difficult to define and measure; therefore, a frequent problem is ambiguity and measurement error.

Processes

Leaders understand that outcome is the focus and that micromanagement of the process can lead to limited productivity. They understand that the difference between process and outcome and process management includes:

• Look at "how things are done" versus the outcome.
• Measure work quantity or quality.
• Substituting process criteria for outcome criteria can compromise service. In order for an organization to be effective, the following criteria should be evaluated (Exhibit 14.1).

EXHIBIT 14.1

Outline of the Organizational Effectiveness Checklist

1. Establish the boundaries of the evaluation.
   1.1 Identify the evaluation client, primary liaison, and power brokers.
   1.2 Clarify the organizational domain to be evaluated.
   1.3 Clarify why the evaluation is being requested.
   1.4 Clarify the timeframe to be employed.
   1.5 Clarify the resources available for the evaluation.
   1.6 Identify the primary beneficiaries and organizational participants.
   1.7 Conduct an evaluability assessment.

(continued)

EXHIBIT 14.1

Outline of the Organizational Effectiveness Checklist (*continued*)

2. Conduct a performance needs assessment.
   2.1 Clarify the purpose of the organization.
   2.2 Assess internal knowledge needs.
   2.3 Scan the external environment.
   2.4 Conduct a strength, weakness, opportunity, and threat (SWOT) analysis.
   2.5 Identify the performance-level needs of the organization.
3. Define the criteria to be used for the evaluation.
   3.1 Review the universal criteria of merit for organizational effectiveness.
   3.2 Add contextual criteria identified in the performance needs assessment.
   3.3 Determine the importance ratings for each criterion.
   3.4 Identify performance measures for each criterion.
   3.5 Identify performance standards for each criterion.
   3.6 Create performance matrices for each criterion.
4. Plan and implement the evaluation.
   4.1 Identify data sources.
   4.2 Identify data-collection methods.
   4.3 Collect and analyze data.
5. Synthesize performance data with values.
   5.1 Create a performance profile for each criterion.
   5.2 Create a profile of organizational effectiveness.
   5.3 Identify organizational strengths and weaknesses.
6. Communicate and report evaluation activities.
   6.1 Distribute regular communications about the evaluation progress.
   6.2 Deliver a draft of the written report to client for review and comment.
   6.3 Edit report to include points of clarification or reaction statements.
   6.4 Present written and oral reports to client.
   6.5 Provide follow-on support as requested by client.

Source: Martz (2010).

Structures

- "Concerned with such things as the adequacy of facilities and equipment; the qualifications of medical staff and their organization; the administrative structure and operations of programs and institutions providing care; fiscal organization and the like" (Donabedian, 2005, p. 695).
- Indicators include
  - Organizational features (equipment age or type)
  - Participant characteristics (degree attained, licensing, etc.)

ESTABLISHING A CULTURE OF CHANGE

An organization's climate and culture have a significant impact on the creativity and innovation displayed within it.

- *Climate* is defined as "people's perceptions of organizational interactions and characteristics" (Mumford et al., 2002, p. 732).

- *Culture* is defined as the "normative expectations for desirable behavior," which determines, to a large extent, how people act within that organization (Mumford et al., 2002, p. 732).
- The predominant view is that organizational culture cannot be "managed"; however, there are key events/interventions that can leverage the opportunity to "manage" organizational culture (Willcoxson & Millett, 2000). These include:
  * Recruitment, selection, and replacement—culture management can be affected by ensuring that appointments strengthen the existing culture(s) or support a culture shift.
  * Removal and replacement may be used to dramatically change the culture.
  * Socialization—induction and subsequent development and training can provide for acculturation to an existing or new culture and also for improved interpersonal communication and teamwork, which is especially critical in fragmented organizational cultures.
  * Performance management/reward systems can be used to highlight and encourage desired behaviors, which may (or may not) in turn lead to changed values.
  * Leadership and modeling are needed from executives, managers, and supervisors who can reinforce or assist in the overturning of existing myths, symbols, behavior, and values and demonstrate the universality and integrity of vision, mission, or value statements.
  * Participation of all organization members in cultural reconstruction or maintenance activities and associated input, decision making, and development activities are essential if long-term change in values, and not just behaviors, is to be achieved.
  * Interpersonal communication satisfying interpersonal relationships does much to support an existing organizational culture and to integrate members into a culture; effective teamwork supports either change or development in and communication of culture.
  * Structures, policies, procedures, and allocation of resources need to be congruent with organizational strategy and culture and objectives.

Change may be initiated by a crisis or a shift in leadership, but there are other sources of influence that can drive change. Grenny, Maxfield, and Shimberg (2008) state that effective change agents "drive change by relying on several different sources of influence strategies at the same time. By combining multiple sources of influence, they are up to 10 times more successful at producing substantial and sustainable change" (p. 47). Grenny and colleagues specifically identify six sources of influence that a nurse educator can utilize to influence change. Those sources are divided into motivation and ability under the realms of personal, social, and structural influences. The sources of influence under *motivation* include (a) linking to mission and values, (b) harnessing peer pressure, and (c) aligning rewards and assuring accountability. The sources of influence under *ability* include (a) overinvesting in skill building, (b) creating social support, and (c) changing the environment.

An example of personal motivation to change occurs when the change is valued and the ability for personal change comes with education. Social motivation to change may come in the form of peer pressure, but the social ability to change uses a supportive environment. Structural motivators to change may come in the form of incentives and the ability to change is found in organizational structures that support change. Nurse educators can effect change if they reflect on the motivational aspects of change and the ability to change within the personal, social, and structural systems in which they function. Influencing health care policy is a primary method to effect change (Exhibit 14.2).

EXHIBIT 14.2

Health Care Policy, Finance, and Regulatory Environments

Rationale:

Health care policies, including financial and regulatory policies, directly and indirectly influence nursing practice and the nature and functioning of the health care system.

These policies shape responses to organizational, local, national, and global issues of equity, access, affordability, and social justice in health care. Also, health care policies are central to any discussion about quality and safety in the practice environment.

The baccalaureate-educated graduate will have a solid understanding of the broader context of health care, including how patient care services are organized and financed, and how reimbursement is structured. Regulatory agencies define boundaries of nursing practice, and graduates need to understand the scope and role of these agencies.

Baccalaureate graduates will also understand how health care issues are identified, how health care policy is both developed and changed, and how that process can be influenced through the efforts of nurses and other health care professionals, as well as lay and special advocacy groups.

Health care policy shapes the nature, quality, and safety of the practice environment, and all professional nurses have the responsibility to participate in the political process and advocate for patients, families, communities, the nursing profession, and changes in the health care system, as needed. Advocacy for vulnerable populations with the goal of promoting social justice is also recognized as a moral and ethical responsibility of the nurse.

A baccalaureate program prepares a graduate to:

1. Demonstrate basic knowledge of health care policy, finance, and regulatory environments, including local, state, national, and global health care trends.
2. Describe how health care is organized and financed, including the implications of business principles, such as patient and system cost factors.
3. Compare the benefits and limitations of the major forms of reimbursement on the delivery of health care services.
4. Examine legislative and regulatory processes relevant to the provision of health care.
5. Describe state and national statutes, rules, and regulations that authorize and define professional nursing practice.
6. Explore the impact of sociocultural, economic, legal, and political factors influencing health care delivery and practice.

(continued)

EXHIBIT 14.2
Health Care Policy, Finance, and Regulatory Environments (*continued*)

7. Examine the roles and responsibilities of the regulatory agencies and their effect on patient care quality, workplace safety, and the scope of nursing and other health professionals' practice.
8. Discuss the implications of health care policy on issues of access, equity, affordability, and social justice in health care delivery.
9. Use an ethical framework to evaluate the impact of social policies on health care, especially for vulnerable populations.
10. Articulate, through a nursing perspective, issues concerning health care delivery to decision makers within health care organizations and other policy arenas. Participate as a nursing professional in political processes and grassroots legislative efforts to influence health care policy.
11. Advocate for consumers and the nursing profession.

Sample Content:
- Policy development and the legislative process
- Policy development and the regulatory process
- Licensure and regulation of nursing practice
- Social policy/public policy
- Policy analysis and evaluation
- Health care financing and reimbursement
- Economics of health care
- Consumerism and advocacy
- Political activism and professional organizations
- Disparities in the health care system
- The impact of social trends, such as genetics and genomics, childhood obesity, and aging, on health policy
- Role of nurse as patient advocate
- Ethical and legal issues
- Professional organizations' roles in health care policy, finance, and regulatory environments
- Scope of practice and policy perspectives of other health professionals
- Negligence, malpractice, and risk management
- Nurse Practice Act

Many studies have identified interactional factors that foster an environment of creativity and innovation (Cooper & Jayatilaka, 2006; Denti, 2016; Faber, 2016; Isaksen, 2009; Rowlings, 2016; Sandeen, 2010; Vaidyanathan, 2012). These factors include:

1. Challenge/involvement
2. Freedom
3. Trust/openness
4. Time to brainstorm ideas
5. Playfulness/humor
6. Conflict
7. Idea support

8. Debate

9. Risk taking

The presence of these interacting factors influences the individual's perception of the organization's openness to creativity, and consequently affects his or her willingness to engage in creative efforts and will serve as a catalyst for innovation (Denti, 2016; Faber, 2016; Isaksen, Aerts, & Isaksen, 2009; Isaksen & Akkermans, 2007; Rowlings, 2016).

THE PROCESS OF CHANGE

Nauheimer (2005) states that sustained change requires transformation on three levels: individual, team/unit, and organization or larger system. Successful change can be better understood and facilitated through the lens of change theory.

- In this process, the nurse educator can assist in the identification of positive opportunities for change and strategies to effectively manage change, whether planned or unplanned.

- The nurse educator must not only have skill in applying change theory but also have a keen understanding of which interventions will affect, encourage, and manage the change process.

- It is essential to keep in mind that not all change is improvement, but all improvement is change (White, 2004).

The Nurse Leader as a Change Agent

Acquiring and incorporating the skill sets of effective change agents can help nurse leaders to implement any change successfully. These skills include the ability to:

- Combine ideas from unconnected sources
- Energize others by keeping the interest level up and by demonstrating a high personal energy level
- Develop skill in human relations, such as well-developed interpersonal communication skills, group management, and problem-solving skills
- Retain a big-picture focus while dealing with each part of the system
- Be flexible and willing to modify ideas if the modification will improve the change, but resist nonproductive tampering with the implementation
- Be confident and avoid the tendency to be easily discouraged
- Think realistically regarding how quickly staff will accept and perform new processes competently
- Be trustworthy, with a track record of integrity and success through other systemic changes
- Articulate a vision through insights and versatile thinking to instill confidence in others
- Be able to handle resistance to a new process (White, 2004)

Change Theories

The predominant models of change include:

1. Lewin's Three-Step Change Theory
2. Lippitt's Phases of Change Theory
3. Prochaska and DiClemente's Change Theory
4. Social Cognitive Theory
5. Theory of Reasoned Action
6. Theory of Planned Behavior

Characteristics of Various Change Theories

Lewin's Three-Step Change Theory

Lewin's Three-Step Change Theory (unfreeze, change, refreeze) sees change as a dynamic balance of forces working in opposing directions.

- Driving forces:
  * Facilitate change
  * Push individuals/organizations in the desired direction for change
- Restraining forces:
  * Hinder change
  * Push individuals/organizations in the opposite direction of the desired change
  * Forces must be analyzed and manipulated to shift the balance in the direction of the planned change

Lewin's model is very rational and goal and plan oriented. It does not take into account personal factors that can affect change.

Lippitt's Phases of Change Theory

- Lippitt's Phases of Change Theory is an extension of Lewin's Three-Step Change Theory and focuses on the *change agent*, rather than the change itself.
- Lippitt's theory includes seven steps:
  1. Diagnose the problem.
  2. Assess the motivation and capacity for change.
  3. Assess the resources and motivation of the change agent. This includes the change agent's commitment to change, power, and stamina.
  4. Choose progressive change objects. In this step, action plans are developed and strategies are established.
  5. The role of the change agents should be selected and clearly understood by all parties so that expectations are clear. Examples of roles are cheerleader, facilitator, and expert.
  6. Maintain the change. Communication, feedback, and group coordination are essential elements in this step of the change process.

7. Gradually withdraw from the helping relationship. "The change agent should gradually withdraw from their role over time. This will occur when the change becomes part of the organizational culture" (Lippitt, Watson, & Westley, 1960, pp. 58–59, as cited in Kritsonis, 2004–2005).

Prochaska and DiClemente's Change Theory

Prochaska and DiClemente's Change Theory considers change from the perspective that a person moves through stages of change. The stages are:

1. Precontemplation
2. Contemplation
3. Preparation
4. Action
5. Maintenance

Prochaska and DiClemente's model is cyclical, not linear. It takes relapses or failures into account. Individuals who relapse can revisit the contemplation stage and make plans for action in the future (Kritsonis, 2004–2005).

Social Cognitive Theory (Social Learning Theory)

- In social cognitive theory, self-efficacy is the most important characteristic and must be present for successful change. "Self-efficacy is defined as having the confidence in the ability to take action and persist in the action" (Kritsonis, 2004–2005, p. 6).
- Social cognitive theory proposes that behavioral change is affected by environmental influences and personal factors.
- This theory takes into account both external and internal environmental conditions (Grizzell, 2007; Kritsonis, 2004–2005).

Theory of Reasoned Action

- The theory of reasoned action states that a person's actions are determined by his or her intention to perform that action.
- Intention is determined by two major factors:
    1. The person's attitude toward the behavior or change (i.e., beliefs about the outcomes of the behavior and the value of these outcomes).
    2. The influence of the person's social environment or subjective norms (i.e., beliefs about what other people think the person should do, as well as the person's motivation to comply with the opinions of others (Grizzell, 2007; Kritsonis, 2004–2005).

Theory of Planned Behavior

- The theory of planned behavior expands upon the theory of reasoned action by including the concept of the individual's perceived control over the opportunities, resources, and skills necessary to perform a behavior or change. This perception of control is believed to be a critical facet of behavior change processes (Grizzell, 2007).
- As with the social cognitive theory, self-efficacy is an important characteristic and must be present for successful change.

Diffusion of Innovation Theory

Rogers's diffusion of innovation theory provides insight into the process by which new ideas are disseminated and integrated. It can be both spontaneous and planned. "The main elements in the diffusion are

1. An innovation
2. That is *communicated* through certain *channels*
3. *Over time*
4. Among the members of a *social system*" (Rogers, 2003, p. 35)

In order for diffusion to be successful, it is absolutely essential to have key people and policy makers interested in the innovation and committed to its implementation. This theory further identifies the five steps in the process of innovation diffusion as:

1. *Knowledge*: The decision-making unit is introduced to the innovation and begins to understand it.
2. *Persuasion*: An attitude, favorable or unfavorable, forms toward the innovation.
3. *Decision*: Activities lead to a decision to adopt or reject the innovation.
4. *Implementation*: The innovation is put to use, and reinvention or alterations may occur.
5. *Confirmation:* "The individual or decision-making unit seeks reinforcement that the decision was correct. If there are conflicting messages or experiences, the original decision may be reversed" (White, 2004, pp. 50–51).

Rogers (2003) describes diffusion as a "kind of *social change*, defined as the process by which alteration occurs in the structure and function of a social system. When new ideas are invented, diffused, and adopted or rejected, leading to certain consequences, social change occurs" (p. 6). Berwick (2003) uses Rogers's theory to explain the rate of change and states that the rate correlates to the following:

1. Perceptions of the innovation/change
   * Perceived benefit of the change.
   * Compatibility with the values, beliefs, history, and current needs of individuals.
   * Level of complexity of the proposed innovation or change. The rate of change for simpler changes is generally faster than those that are more complex.
   * "Re-invention" of the innovation or change (the adaptability of the change). The capability of making local (or point of use) modifications, which often involve simplification, is a common characteristic of successful dissemination.
   * Changes spread faster when they have these five perceived attributes: benefit, compatibility, simplicity, trialability (ability to "test the waters"), and observability.
2. Characteristics of the people who either adopt the innovation or do not:
   * The curve of adoption of the innovation or change over time generally takes an S-shape, characterized with an early slow phase affecting a very few

individuals (early adopters), a rapid middle phase with widespread adoption, followed by a slow third phase, typically ending with incomplete adoption. It has been described as being similar to the epidemic curve of a contagious disease.

* Rogers's (2003) diffusion of innovation theory includes five levels of adoption (for more information, see Figure 14.1):

  1. Innovators
  2. Early adopters
  3. Early majority
  4. Late majority
  5. Laggards

Contextual factors include situational/environmental factors associated with a particular organization or social system, such as management, leadership, communication, or incentives that can either "encourage and support, or discourage and impede, the actual processes" of diffusion (Berwick, 2003, p. 1972).

Davis's Technology Acceptance Model

Davis's technology acceptance model (TAM) is an extension of the theory of reasoned action (described earlier in the chapter). The TAM model provides a mechanism to view how external factors influence the intention to use technology. Specifically, the model considers the external factors that influence (a) perceived usefulness and (b) perceived ease of use as key factors influencing an individual's attitude toward use and in turn, how that influences the actual use (Figure 14.2).

Chaos theory of change or diffusion is a theory that deals with dynamic instability of complex systems such as nursing educational units. The basic premise is that one small change can affect, over time, many larger changes in a system because they are sensitive or dependent on the initial condition. An often-used illustration of chaos theory is that the flap of butterfly wings in one part of the world can cause a random effect that may eventually turn out to be a tornado in another part of the world (Gleick, 1987).

FIGURE 14.1 Rogers's (2003) adopter areas.

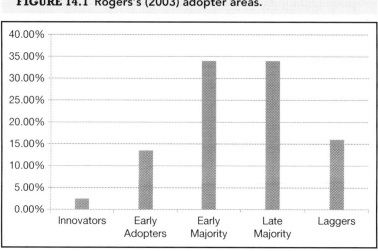

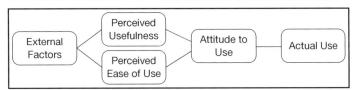

FIGURE 14.2 Davis's technology acceptance model.

Complexity theory is also discussed in nursing as a change process that has its roots in the physical sciences. Similar to chaos theory, the organization structure must be viewed as a whole that is composed of multiple systems. Decisions are made in relation to human-to-human interactions and may appear random and unrelated, but in the larger scheme of things, make sense within the context in which they were made. It expands the theoretical notions that changes have causes and effects that can always be predetermined (Yoder-Wise, 2011).

CRITICAL THINKING QUESTION

Using chaos theory, what may happen to the learners by their senior year if a change was made in the fundamentals class to include a simulation scenario on communication?

CULTURAL SENSITIVITY WHEN ADVOCATING FOR CHANGE

Individuals' ethnic identities and cultural backgrounds strongly influence their attitudes, values, and practices. When advocating for change, it is essential that the nurse educator consider these factors and act in a culturally sensitive manner. Cultural considerations must be incorporated in any efforts to influence change. Rationales for including higher level cultural competence skills/strategies in health organization policies include:

1. Response to current and projected demographic changes
2. Elimination of long-standing health disparities among people from diverse racial, ethnic, and cultural backgrounds
3. Improvement of the quality of and access to health services (National Center for Cultural Competence, n.d.)

Saha, Beach, and Cooper (2008) observe that cultural competence has become an "all-encompassing approach to address interpersonal and institutional sources of racial and ethnic disparities in health care. Though the concept of cultural competence has changed over time and continues to evolve, it has always contained at its core the principles of patient-centered health care delivery" (pp. 6–7). When applying these concepts broadly to efforts to influence change, key considerations would include:

- Sensitivity to others' beliefs and values
- Sensitivity to individual/group needs, preferences, and experiences
- Tailoring communication/materials to the appropriate level, language, and literacy
- Openness and flexibility

> **Teaching Gem:** A transformative teacher is one who models caring to his or her students at all times in order for the students to reflect on themselves as caring people (Diekelmann, 1995).

A. Nelson, Anis-Abdellatif, Larson, Mulder, and Wolff (2016) acknowledge that a diverse classroom has significant benefits in education—providing multiple perspectives to the learning experience—but point out that there are often gaps in new faculty orientation as well as ongoing faculty development that leave them unprepared to function effectively in the diverse classroom. The authors advocate for ongoing diversity and inclusiveness training within higher education to ensure cultural competency.

The essential cultural competencies relevant to the process of advocating for change include:

- Awareness and sensitivity to the differences that individuals, groups, and organizations may have in their experiences and responses to the change
- Ability to recognize differences and to identify similar patterns of responses to change among individuals, groups, and organizations
- Avoidance of stereotyping by acknowledging variations among individuals, groups, and organizations
- Awareness that communication is inextricably interwoven with culture
- Awareness of how language (preference, level of comfort, and proficiency) influences an individual's perception and ability to understand, develop meanings, and make sense out of the world
- "Knowledge of diversity in communication patterns, styles, and protocols, and of how language and communication may influence the development of trust in relationships" (Meleis, 1999, p. 12)

Strategies for Planned Change

Successful change involves making a compelling case for the change and then putting into place measures to manage change risk to protect the organization and its stakeholders (Kee & Newcomer, 2008). Strategies for leading change include:

1. Diagnosing change risk and organizational capacity
2. Strategizing and making the case for change
3. Implementing and sustaining change
4. Reinforcing change by creating a change-centric learning organization (p. 5)

Strom (2001) identifies the top eight effective change implementation strategies:

1. *Multiple interventions*—Comprehensive interventions that take into account the many characteristics of the organization as well as the external environment

2. *Outreach visits*—Intensive support by a change agent who provides education, feedback, practical support, reminders, and praise for progress

3. *Opinion leaders*—Recruit individuals who are recognized by peers as influential educators to promote the change

4. *Reminders*—Prompt health care professionals to perform a patient-specific clinical action (behavioral approach), which is generally effective across a range of clinical behaviors; this is less effective if used for routine items of care or if too many prompts are presented at the same time

5. *Feedback*—Auditing and providing feedback of summarized clinical performance

6. *Interactive* (computer based)—Using computer information systems to support practice, such as teleconferencing, chat-room techniques, and information sharing through listservs

7. *Interactive* (educational)—Customized, phased, educational interventions designed specifically to mitigate potential barriers, including user resistance and teaching new skills

8. *Administrative intervention*—Clinical effectiveness and successful change can be achieved by using a continuous quality-improvement (CQI) or quality-management approach, focusing on the core processes as the centerpiece of the initiative.

POLITICAL ACTION

The nurse educator has an obligation to function as a role model to others in active engagement in the political processes on a local, regional, national, and global level. By virtue of the role of educator, the nurse educator is uniquely positioned to influence other nurses (and aspiring nurses) to become politically active. Opollo, Bond, Gray, and Lail-Davis (2012) stress the importance of this involvement by pointing out that "both the ANA and the ICN [International Council of Nurses] call on nurses to collaborate with other health professionals and the public to promote community, national, and international efforts to meet health needs" (pp. 77–78). The authors identify four key rationales for nursing involvement:

1. The successful attainment of the United Nations Millennium Development Goals will require strong global partnerships and collaborations.

2. Equipping nurses with culturally relevant competencies is important for promoting the delivery of effective, culturally appropriate health care globally.

3. Key tools for engaging in global health efforts include partnerships, education, media outreach, and grassroots and grasstops approaches.

4. Nurses are strategically positioned to influence global health research, education, policy, and practice by participating in continuing-education programs, interprofessional exchanges, and volunteerism with a global health focus (Opollo et al., 2012, p. 79).

Political Action Resources

- Professional organizations (e.g., AACN, and NLN)
- Political organizations (e.g., American Civil Liberties Union [ACLU])
- Federal, state, and local government agencies (e.g., Occupational Safety and Health Administration [OSHA])
- Electronic political information organizations (e.g., Electronic News Media, Political Information Search Engine: www.politicalinformation.com)
- Government representatives (e.g., contact federal, state, and local representatives via USA.gov websites such as www.usa.gov/Contact/Elected.shtml)

CASE STUDIES

CASE STUDY 14.1

St. Mary's Hospital, a midsized community hospital, initiated a hospital-wide clinical improvement project. An interdisciplinary team of health care professionals was recruited to serve on the clinical improvement project panel. One area identified for improvement was to reduce the number of patient falls. A comprehensive, 40-page clinical guideline published by the U.S. Agency for Health Care Research and Quality (AHRQ) was selected for implementation. However, the project team determined that full implementation of these guidelines was too complex and time-consuming for the staff, and therefore would not likely be successful. The panel identified two changes that could be easily implemented and would likely have a significant impact on fall incident rates. A nurse representative from each inpatient unit was recruited to serve as unit leader for the implementation of these changes. A targeted information campaign was designed, and staff in-services were conducted on all units for all shifts. Those two simple innovations, not the larger, more detailed and complex guidelines, reduced the rate of falls in vulnerable patients by 75%.

What strategies for change were utilized by the panel to implement this clinical improvement project? How was Rogers's theory of diffusion applied? How would the principles of leadership support the process? How can evaluation criteria for organizational effectiveness be applied in this scenario? Which criteria would be relevant?

> **CASE STUDY 14.2**
>
> The nursing programs of Drexel University, the Community College of Philadelphia, Bloomsburg University of Pennsylvania, and Howard University entered into a collaborative agreement to incorporate the use of technology in their respective undergraduate and graduate nursing programs. Drexel University, College of Nursing and Health Professions (DUCNHP), with Dr. Linda Wilson as the project director, will be the lead school and will share its technology expertise and resources by working jointly with the faculty of the collaborating schools to ensure faculty competence in selected technologies used by DUCNHP to enhance nursing education curricula and teaching processes. Topics that fall under this initiative include the following: "incorporation of the personal digital assistant into didactic courses and in clinical, development, and implementation of cases and evaluation methods for human simulation including the use of standardized patients and patient simulators, the use of web-based courseware, and the development of a server repository/portal for various interactive learning modules for use by the collaborating nursing programs" (Wilson, 2007, p. 1).
>
> How can the principles of good community–campus partnerships be applied to this initiative to increase the likelihood of success? What strategies for change must be considered? Discuss this initiative from the perspective of organizational culture. What factors must be considered?

PRACTICE QUESTIONS

1. Davis's technology acceptance model involves consideration of which of the following:

   A. External factors

   B. Early majority

   C. Thought leaders

   D. Community members

2. Strom (2001) identifies which of the following strategies for successful change implementation:

   A. Use only one intervention to support change

   B. Keep site visits at minimum

   C. Send frequent reminders

   D. Communicate a shared vision

3. Donabedian (2005) conceptualizes evaluation into three dimensions that include:

   A. People

   B. Places

   C. Processes

   D. Constructs

4. Which of the following practices is likely to be utilized by the transactional leader?

   A. Enlisting others in a common vision by appealing to shared aspirations

   B. Using a rewards/punishment system

   C. Experimenting and taking risks

   D. Sharing power

5. Under the realm of motivation, Grenny and colleagues' (2008) sources of influence include:

   A. Creating social support

   B. Linking to mission and values

   C. Overinvesting in skill building

   D. Changing the environment

6. There are things that a manager can do to "manage" organizational culture. These include which of the following?

   A. Purposeful recruitment, selection, and replacement

   B. Conduct a performance needs assessment

   C. Establish partnerships outside one's usual circles

   D. Plan and implement policies and procedures

7. The theory that describes change as a dynamic balance of forces working in opposing directions is:

   A. Lippitt's Phases of Change Theory

   B. Prochaska and DiClemente's Change Theory

   C. Theory of planned behavior

   D. Lewin's Three-Step Change Theory

8. The theory that describes change from the perspective of the person moving through stages of change is:

   A. Social cognitive theory

   B. Prochaska and DiClemente's Change Theory

   C. Theory of reasoned action

   D. Theory of planned behavior

9. Contextual factors of the change process include all of the following except:

   A. Situational/environmental factors

   B. Leadership

   C. Communication or incentives

   D. Personal traits

10. The National Center for Cultural Competence states that the integration of high-level cultural competence skills/strategies is a priority for health organizational policies because nurses must do which of the following?

   A. Be sensitive to others' beliefs and values

   B. Eliminate health disparities among people from diverse racial, ethnic, and cultural backgrounds

   C. Consider individual/group needs, preferences, or experiences

   D. Be able to develop communications/materials at the appropriate level, language, and literacy

REFERENCES

Berwick, D. M. (2003). Disseminating innovations in health care. *Journal of the American Medical Association, 289*(15), 1969–1975.

Carroll, T. L. (2005). Leadership skills and attributes of women and nurse executives. *Nurse Administrator, 29*(2), 146–153.

Casida, J. (2008). Linking nursing unit's culture to organizational effectiveness: A measurement tool. *Nursing Economic$, 26*(2), 106–110.

Cheng, Y. C. (1996). *School effectiveness and school-based management: A mechanism for development.* London, UK: Routledge.

Clark, D. R. (2008). Concepts of leadership. Retrieved from http://www.nwlink.com/~donclark/leader/leadcon.html

Cooper, R. B., & Jayatilaka, B. (2006). Group creativity: The effects of extrinsic, intrinsic, and obligation motivations. *Creativity Research Journal, 18*(2), 153–172. doi:10.1207/s15326934crj1802_3

Delgado, C., & Mitchell, M. M. (2016). A survey of current valued academic leadership qualities in nursing. *Nursing Education Perspectives, 37*(1), 10–15. doi:10.5480/14-1496

Denti, L. (2016). Top six components of a creative climate, innovation psychology. Retrieved from http://www.innovationmanagement.se/2013/05/22/top-six-components-of-a-creative-climate/

Dickenson-Hazard, N. (2004). Notes from the chief executive officer. "I have experienced this before." *Reflections on Nursing Leadership, 30*(2), 4, 38.

Diekelmann, N. L. (1995). Reawakening thinking: Is traditional pedagogy nearing completion? *Journal of Nursing Education, 34*(5), 195–196.

Donabedian, A. (2005). Evaluating the quality of medical care. *Millbank Quarterly, 83*(4), 691–729.

Dye, C. F., & Garman, A. N. (2006). *Exceptional leadership: 16 critical competencies for health care executives.* Chicago, IL: Health Administration Press.

Faber, H. (2016). Three box solution for sustainable innovation, innovation psychology. Retrieved from http://www.innovationmanagement.se/2016/04/21/three-box-solution-for-sustainable-innovation

Frankel, A. (2011). What leadership styles should senior nurses develop? *Nursing Times, 104*(35), 23–24.

Getha-Taylor, H., Fowles, J., Silvia, C., & Merritt, C. C. (2015). Considering the effects of time on leadership development. *Public Personnel Management, 44*(3), 295–316. doi:10.1177/0091026015586265

Glasgow, M. E. S., & Cornelius, F. H. (2005). Benefits and costs of integration of technology into an undergraduate nursing program. *Nursing Leadership Forum, 9*(4), 175.

Gleick, J. (1987). *Chaos: Making a new science.* New York, NY: Penguin Books.

Grant, A. B., & Massey, V. H. (1999). *Nursing leadership, management & research.* Springhouse, PA: Springhouse Corporation.

Green, D. A. (2006). A synergy model of nursing education. *Journal for Nurses in Staff Development, 22*(6), 277–283.

Grenny, J., Maxfield, D., & Shimberg, A. (2008). How to have influence. *MIT Sloan Management Review, 50*(1), 47–52. Retrieved from http://sloanreview.mit.edu/article/how-to-have-influence

Grizzell, J. (2007). Behavior change theories and models. Retrieved from http://www.csupomona.edu/%7Ejvgrizzell/best_practices/bctheory.html#Reasoned%20Action

Isaksen, S. G. (2009). Exploring the relationship between problem-solving style and creative psychological climate. In J. Funke, P. Meusburger, & E. Wunder (Eds.), *Knowledge and space: Milieus of creativity* (pp. 169–188). Dordrecht, Netherlands: Springer Science+Business Media.

Isaksen, S. G., Aerts, W. S., & Isaksen, E. J. (2009). *Creating more innovative workplaces: Linking problem-solving style and organizational climate.* Orchard Park, NY: The Creative Problem Solving Group. Retrieved from http://www.cpsb.com/research/articles/featuredarticles/Creating-Innovative-Workplaces.pdf

Isaksen, S. G., & Akkermans, H. J. (2007). *An introduction to climate.* Orchard Park, NY: Creative Problem Solving Group.

Kee, J. E., & Newcomer, K. E. (2008). Why do change efforts fail? *Public Manager, 37*(3), 5–12.

King, W. (2011). What qualities must a leader have? *National Driller, 32*(2), 56.

Kritsonis, A. (2004–2005). Comparison of change theories. *International Journal of Scholarly Academic Intellectual Diversity, 8*(1), 1–7. Retrieved from http://www.nationalforum .com/Electronic%20Journal%20Volumes/Kritsonis,%20Alicia%20Comparison%20 of%20Change%20Theories.pdf

Mahoney, J. (2001). Leadership skills for the 21st century. *Nursing Management, 9*(5), 269–271.

Martz, W. (2008). Evaluating organizational effectiveness. *Dissertation Abstracts International, 69*(07). Publication No. ATT3323530.

Martz, W. (2010). Validating evaluation checklists using a mixed method design. *Evaluation and Program Planning, 33*, 215–222. doi:10.1016/j.evalprogplan.2009.10.005

Meleis, A. I. (1999). Culturally competent care. *Journal of Transcultural Nursing, 10*(1), 12.

Mumford, M. D., Scott, G. M., Gaddis, B., & Strange, J. M. (2002). Leading creative people: Orchestrating expertise and relationships. *Leadership Quarterly, 13*, 705–750.

National Center for Cultural Competence. (n.d.). The compelling need for cultural and linguistic competence. Retrieved from http://nccc.georgetown.edu/foundations/need.html

Nauheimer, H. (2005). *Taking stock: A survey on the practice and future of change management.* Johannesburg, South Africa: Change Source.

Nelson, A., Anis-Abdellatif, M., Larson, J., Mulder, C., & Wolff, B. (2016). New faculty orientation: Discussion of cultural competency, sexual victimization, and student behaviors. *Journal of Continuing Education in Nursing, 47*(5), 228–233.

Nelson, D., Godfrey, L., & Purdy, J. (2004). Using a mentorship program to recruit and retain student nurses. *Journal of Nursing Administration, 34*(12), 551–553.

Ogbonna, E., & Harris, L. C. (2000). Leadership style, organizational culture and performance: Empirical evidence from UK companies. *International Journal of Human Resource Management, 11*(4), 766–788.

Opollo, J. G., Bond, M. L., Gray, J., & Lail-Davis, V. J. (2012). Meeting tomorrow's health care needs through local and global involvement. *Journal of Continuing Education in Nursing, 43*(2), 75–80.

Pullen, R. L. (2016). Leadership in nursing practice. *Nursing Made Incredibly Easy, 14*(3), 26–31.

Rogers, E. M. (2003). *Diffusion of innovations* (5th ed.). New York, NY: Free Press.

Ross, E. J., Fitzpatrick, J. J., Click, E. R., Krouse, H. J., & Clavelle, J. T. (2014). Transformational leadership practices of nurse leaders in professional nursing associations. *Journal of Nursing Administration, 44*(4), 201–206.

Rowlings, M. (2016). Innovative workplace benefits: Perks employees look for, innovation psychology. Retrieved from http://www.innovationmanagement.se/2016/03/15/ innovative-workplace-benefits-perks-employees-look-for

Rubino, L. (2011). Leadership. In S. B. Buchbinder & N. H. Shanks (Eds.), *Leadership, in introduction to health care management* (2nd ed.). Sudbury, MA: Jones & Bartlett.

Saha, S., Beach, M., & Cooper, L. (2008). Patient centeredness, cultural competence and health care quality. *Journal of the National Medical Association, 100*(11), 1275–1285.

Sandeen, C. A. (2010). Fostering creativity and innovation in the workforce: An annotated bibliography. *Continuing Higher Education Review, 74*, 93–100.

Sarros, J. C., Cooper, B. K., & Santora, J. C. (2008). Building a climate for innovation through transformational leadership and organizational culture. *Journal of Leadership & Organizational Studies, 15*(2), 145. Retrieved from http://www.pogc.ir/Portals/0/ maghalat/890724-2.pdf

Shahzad, F., Luqman, R. A., Khan, A. R., & Shabbir, L. (2012). Impact of organizational culture on organizational performance: An overview. *Interdisciplinary Journal of Contemporary Research in Business, 3*(9), 975–985.

Sims, J. M. (2009). Styles and qualities of effective leaders. *Dimensions of Critical Care Nursing, 28*(6), 272–274.

Strom, K. (2001). Quality improvement interventions: What works? *Journal for Health Care Quality, 23*(5), 4–14.

Thibodeaux, M. S., & Favilla, E. (1996). Organizational effectiveness and commitment through strategic management. *Industrial Management & Data Systems, 96*(5), 21–25.

Vaidyanathan, S. (2012). Fostering creativity and innovation through technology. *Learning & Leading With Technology, 39*(6), 24–27.

Veenema, T. G., Griffin, A., Gable, A. R., MacIntyre, L., Simons, N., Couig, M. P., . . . Larson, E. (2015). Nurses as leaders in disaster preparedness and response: A call to action. *Journal of Nursing Scholarship, 48*(2), 187–200. doi:10.1111/jnu.12198

White, A. (2004). Change strategies make for smooth transitions. *Nursing Management, 35*(2), 49–52.

Willcoxson, L., & Millett, B. (2000). The management of organisational culture. *Australian Journal of Management & Organisational Behaviour, 3*(2), 100–106.

Wilson, L. (2007). 2229-Wilson-PADCNETC_Abstract. Retrieved from grants.hrsa.gov via https://www.google.com/url?sa=t&rct=j&q=&esrc=s&source=web&cd=3&ved=0a hUKEwi_9OfTrL3QAhUn44MKHZ8uDd4QFggiMAI&url=https%3A%2F%2Fgrants .hrsa.gov%2F2010%2Fweb2Internal%2FInterface%2FCommon%2FPublicWebLinkCo ntroller.aspx%3FGrantNumber%3DU1KHP09542%26WL_WEBLINK_ID%3D1&usg= AFQjCNH93vnTW60vyypAzoWqwh49JyepTg

Yoder-Wise, P. S. (2011). *Leading and managing in nursing* (5th ed.). St. Louis, MO: Elsevier.

15

Engaging in the Scholarship of Teaching

DIANE M. BILLINGS

Education is the most powerful weapon which
you can use to change the world.
—Nelson Mandela

This chapter addresses the Certified Nurse Educator Exam Content Area 6B: Engage in the Scholarship of Teaching (National League for Nursing [NLN], 2016, p. 5).

- Content Area 6, which includes 6A, 6B, and 6C, makes up 21% of the examination
- It is estimated that there will be approximately 31 to 32 questions from Content Area 6

LEARNING OUTCOMES

- Discuss the meaning of scholarship in the nurse educator role
- Identify the types of scholarship outlined by Boyer
- Differentiate between the scholarship of teaching and the scholarship of teaching–learning and being a scholar
- Exhibit a spirit of inquiry about teaching, learning, and evaluation
- Identify the attributes of the science of nursing education
- Learn how to participate in research activities related to nursing education
- Appreciate the knowledge developed from evidence in education
- Demonstrate integrity as a scholar

Being a scholar and engaging in scholarship is an important aspect of the role of nurse educator. This chapter defines Boyer's model of scholarship and the Carnegie Foundation's work in promoting the scholarship of teaching and learning (SoTL). This chapter also discusses the ways nurse educators can engage in scholarship and develop the science of nursing education by participating in research activities and demonstrating integrity as a scholar.

SCHOLARSHIP IN NURSING AND NURSING EDUCATION

A *scholar* is a person who has particular knowledge in an area of specialization. A scholar has a spirit of inquiry and is able to think logically and communicate effectively. Scholarship is a hallmark of nursing, and is an expectation of all nurse educators. The American Association of Colleges of Nursing (AACN; 1999) defined *scholarship in nursing* as those activities that systematically advance the teaching, research, and practice of nursing through rigorous inquiry that (a) is significant to the profession, (b) is creative, (c) can be documented, (d) can be replicated or elaborated, and (e) can be peer reviewed through various methods. *Scholarship* in nursing education is an inquiry process that results in outcomes; for example, innovations in teaching–learning strategies; the development of courses, course materials, and curricula; and the development of measures to assess and evaluate student learning. Scholarship in nursing education is recognized by peer reviews of the outcomes of teaching–learning practices, awards for teaching excellence, receipt of grants, and invitations to consult or share the scholarly work with others. Scholarship is also recognized by presentations, publications, and citation of the scholarly work by others.

THE SCHOLAR'S ROLE

The role of the nursing scholar is to develop and disseminate evidence for best practices in nursing education. The scholarly role is expected of nurse educators who work in schools of nursing. The scholar's role is demonstrated by:

- Critiquing evidence for practice in nursing education
- Using evidence for teaching and learning in one's own practice
- Identifying issues for research
- Conducting research
- Disseminating findings
- Serving on committees of professional organizations
- Serving on editorial boards of journals related to teaching and learning

BOYER'S MODEL OF SCHOLARSHIP

Boyer's model of scholarship is a model that is used in many schools of nursing and institutions of higher learning to guide the work of faculty. This model, proposed by Ernest Boyer (1990), describes four types of scholarship that form the basis of scholarly work and contribute to effective teaching and learning. Although distinct, in practice the four types of scholarship are integrated. Boyer's four types of scholarship are:

- *Scholarship of discovery*—Research or discovery of new knowledge, systematic inquiry, use of methods to develop a strong basis for practice-related knowledge

Example: A nurse educator is using podcasting with senior baccalaureate students. The nurse educator conducts a study to determine whether the use of podcasting is appropriate for students with specific types of learning styles.

- *Scholarship of integration*—Interpretation and synthesis of knowledge; may cross the disciplinary boundaries

   Example: A nurse educator reviews the health sciences literature about using simulations for teaching students to manage a diabetic crisis. He or she then uses the information to develop a multidisciplinary simulation for nursing students in an undergraduate nursing program.

- *Scholarship of application*—Connects theory and practice; seeks to apply knowledge to significant problems; is a translational work, which assists end users to integrate the findings into their practices; application is also evident in service to the profession

   Example: A nurse educator who has an area of expertise in team-based learning presents the outcomes of the work at a national meeting and then consults with schools to help them integrate the method into their own academic programs and classrooms.

- *Scholarship of teaching*—The use of evidence to facilitate learning; the scholarship of teaching also involves identifying a problem, testing strategies, and making teaching and learning public through self-reflection, peer review, and the dissemination of work in appropriate disciplinary journals

   Example: A nurse educator developed a method of peer testing and has used the method in the classroom with outcomes of improved deep learning and higher test scores; students rate the method highly. The nurse educator develops a manuscript to share the findings of this approach to testing. The manuscript is accepted for publication for wider dissemination and the potential to further test method in other classrooms (see Figure 15.1).

FIGURE 15.1 Boyer's four dimensions of scholarship.

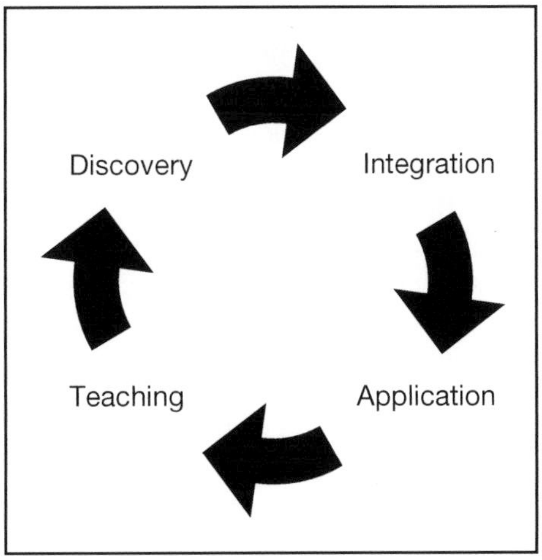

THE USE OF BOYER'S MODEL

Boyer's model is used in nursing education as a framework for:

- Appointment
- Performance evaluation

    Demonstration of merit for awards and pay increases

- Promotion and tenure guidelines
- Organizing the professional portfolio

EVIDENCE-BASED TEACHING PRACTICE

Baker, Fitzpatrick, and Griffin (2011) studied 139 nurse educators who worked in associate degree programs and found that psychological empowerment was positively correlated with job satisfaction regardless of the educator's educational degree, tenure status, rank, or scholarship accomplishments.

SCHOLARLY TEACHING, SCHOLARSHIP OF TEACHING, SoTL, AND BEING A SCHOLAR

Educators make a distinction among good teaching, scholarly teaching, scholarship of teaching, SoTL, and being a scholar.

- *Good teaching*—Good teaching is typically defined by student satisfaction and positive student ratings of teaching (Allen & Field, 2005). It involves understanding the students and using effective teaching–learning practices.

- *Scholarly teaching*—Scholarly teaching refers to nurse educators' use of practice wisdom, reflections on the effectiveness of one's own approach to teaching and evaluation, and the use of evidence to guide teaching practice (Allen & Field, 2005). Scholarly teaching involves a systematic study of teaching and learning practices and may result in the dissemination of knowledge through presentations and publications.

- *Scholarship of teaching*—Scholarship of teaching refers to teaching that extends beyond the classroom (Allen & Field, 2005). Scholarship of teaching may include the development of products (simulations, books, games, and podcasts) that can be used by learners and others, development of teaching models that can be shared and replicated, or development of innovative curricula that are implemented statewide or serve as examples of curriculum development for others. Scholarship of teaching also involves using evidence-based teaching practices (EBTPs) and conducting research about teaching and learning. Nurse educators demonstrate scholarship of teaching when they publish their work in peer-reviewed journals; disseminate their work in poster or podium presentations at local, national, and international meetings; obtain peer review from colleagues; and are recipients of grants.

- *The SoTL*—The SoTL is an initiative of the Carnegie Foundation (2013) that builds on Boyer's model of scholarship to enhance the value of teaching, advocate for student learning, and bring recognition to teaching as scholarly work. Many campuses have communities of faculty who collaborate to explore, share, and recognize each other's work to develop the SoTL.
- *Being a scholar*—Being a scholar involves developing habits of inquiry and intellectual persistence. Scholars seek truth, challenge assumptions, demonstrate integrity, continually learn, and seek review of their work. Being a scholar is a prerequisite for scholarly teaching, using evidence-based teaching, and developing the science of nursing education.

DEVELOPING A SPIRIT OF INQUIRY ABOUT TEACHING, LEARNING, AND EVALUATION

Nurse educators develop a spirit of inquiry by reflecting on their own practice; being open to new ideas; reviewing the literature for evidence of best practices in teaching, learning, and evaluation; and determining whether the use of evidence warrants changes in their own teaching practices. Nurse educators also demonstrate a spirit of inquiry when they identify gaps in the literature and conduct or participate in research that will seek answers to problems related to teaching, learning, and evacuation. Nurse educators are lifelong learners who strive to improve their teaching practice by seeking evidence for their practice.

THE SCIENCE OF NURSING EDUCATION

The *science of nursing education* refers to the research-based foundation on which the best practices for teaching nursing are developed and tested. Building the science of nursing education involves:

- Defining a significant problem
- Critiquing the literature and identifying gaps
- Developing or using a framework to guide research
- Designing studies (classroom studies, multisite studies, and multimethod studies)
- Conducting studies
- Disseminating findings by sharing effective teaching or evaluation strategies and summaries of surveys about classroom practices. Dissemination also takes place when nurse educators present findings from research studies. Evidence of dissemination includes publications and presentations. Publications in peer-reviewed and indexed journals are more highly valued than publications in journals with limited circulation or abstracts in conference proceedings and newsletters; the publication of scholarly work is preferred to presentations at scientific meetings. Publication is a learned skill that can be assisted through mentorship of experts (Oermann & Hayes, 2011).
- Using evidence in scholarship and research: The cycle of scholarship and research is complete when nurse educators base their curriculum development, teaching, evaluation, and use of technology on evidence. Evidence can be found in nursing

journals that report study findings, at conferences where papers are presented, and at school and university scholarship days where the results of pilot studies and classroom research are presented. Increasingly, nursing education scholarship and research are interdisciplinary, and evidence for nursing education practice is available in a variety of venues. All nurse educators must read the evidence, test it in their classrooms, and then determine the best practices for their own students.

EVIDENCE-BASED TEACHING PRACTICE

Heinrich (2016) discusses how to turn your teaching into scholarship by focusing on the SoTL and a three-step process that includes (a) framing a researchable question; (b) designing a systematic inquiry; and (c) planning for public, peer-reviewed products.

DEVELOPING THE SCIENCE OF NURSING EDUCATION

Nurse educators also have responsibilities for developing the science of nursing education by conducting or participating in research and scholarly work. Developing the science of nursing education:

> **Teaching Gem:** Conard and Pape (2014) relate Boyer's model of scholarship to practice and state: "Boyer's Model of Scholarship includes four interrelated and overlapping domains of discovery, integration, application, and teaching. Each domain is explained with examples for the pediatric nurse scholar, which includes roles in academia as well as in the practice setting" (p. 87).

- Can be conducted by educators, regardless of educational preparation, who participate in the research process as leaders or members of a research team
- Requires the researcher and research team to maintain integrity as scholars by ensuring the protection of human subjects, safeguarding data, using ethical approaches to inquiry, and collaborating with others
- Can involve collaboration with colleagues at the same and other institutions (multisite research) and with colleagues in other disciplines (interdisciplinary research)

DEMONSTRATING INTEGRITY AS A SCHOLAR

Scholarly integrity involves the observance of ethical principles in teaching, service, and the conduct of research while working as an individual faculty member, member of a research team, and while supervising the scholarly work and research conducted by students. Most colleges and universities have policies about maintaining scholarly integrity, procedures for monitoring integrity of faculty and students, and consequences for misconduct. Nurse educators maintain integrity as scholars by:

- Assuming responsibility for the intellectual quality of their work
- Recognizing and citing works of others to avoid misrepresenting it as their own work

- Protecting human subjects when conducting research by seeking approval of an institutional review board (IRB) before conducting and publishing studies
- Safeguarding data when conducting research
- Safeguarding students when implementing or testing new strategies for teaching, learning, or evaluation
- Observing principles of ethics when serving on research teams
- Establishing clear guidelines for ownership of data or products and publication credit prior to initiating a study or project (Oermann & Hayes, 2011)
- Following publication guidelines for authorship credit
- Serving as a role model for students in the use of evidence and conduct of research
  - Being a mentor and role model for students and colleagues
  - Conducting peer review of teaching, manuscripts, publications
  - Observing codes of civility in communications with others

FUNDING THE SCIENCE OF NURSING EDUCATION

Funding for nursing education research comes from a variety of sources. Professional nursing education organizations, such as the NLN (2007), AACN, Sigma Theta Tau International, and a variety of specialty organizations, have grant programs to fund nursing education research. Also, most colleges and universities have small funds for classroom research. Funding for projects and research that involves educational reform may be sought from foundations, such as the Robert Wood Johnson Foundation or the Macy Foundation, or federal sources such as the Health Resources and Service Administration (HRSA) or the Department of Education. Nurse educators who are involved in interprofessional research can also seek funding from agencies that are funding collaborative research.

EVIDENCE-BASED TEACHING PRACTICE

Malik, McKenna, and Plummer (2015) conducted a study of nurse educators (academic and clinical; $N = 135$) using a mixed-method questionnaire and found that nurse educators relied heavily on personal experience, organizational policies, and protocols as formal sources of knowledge. Participants reported positive attitudes toward evidence-based practice but did not have the skills to appraise and utilizing evidence into practice.

EVIDENCE-BASED TEACHING PRACTICE

EBTP in nursing is the use of evidence to make decisions about developing educational programs, choosing the best teaching–learning strategies to achieve outcomes for a particular group of students in a particular setting, and selecting appropriate methods for evaluation. EBTP:

- Draws on research in nursing education, higher education, psychology, and allied health disciplines

- Uses wisdom and accepted practices and is guided by theory and empirical testing
- Questions existing teaching–learning practices that are unfounded, based in tradition, and have not been tested

---

EVIDENCE-BASED TEACHING PRACTICE

Josephsen (2013) studied evidence-based reflective teaching practice based on a nursing process framework to develop, implement, and evaluate assignment efficacy directly related to course objectives through four assignments. Participation in evidence-based reflective teaching practice enhanced reflective practice that can advance the discipline of nursing education.

SUMMARY

Teaching Gem: If a nurse educator is notified by a nurse educator graduate student or established researcher who would like to use his or her learners as subjects, the researcher should be advised to contact the IRB of the university and the departmental chair or dean. IRB approval from the researcher's institution does not automatically translate to IRB approval in the institution of the planned study site.

Scholarship and producing scholarly work is one of the expectations of the role of the nurse educator. Boyer's model describes four aspects of scholarship for guiding the appointment, retention, and promotion of nurse educators. Nurse educators conduct research and develop the science of nursing education. Much more research is needed in nursing education to build a solid body of evidence and knowledge. Promoting the science of nursing education through evidence is imperative to guide our future in nursing. Without curricula that are evidence based and grounded in up-to-date science, the scholarship of education cannot survive. All four areas of Boyer's model of scholarship are intertwined; each is dependent on the others, as pictured in Figure 15.1.

CASE STUDIES

CASE STUDY 15.1

A team of three nurse educators teaches a nursing skills course in a learning resources center, and each has the responsibility for clinical supervision of 10 students on a medical–surgical nursing unit at the local hospital. One of the educators, an associate professor, has a doctorate in clinical nursing; two of the nurses have MSN degrees in nursing and are clinical instructors. Scholarship is included in the appointment requirements for all faculty at the school

---

(continued)

CASE STUDY 15.1 (*continued*)

of nursing. The teaching team has noticed that students frequently break the sterile field when changing a sterile dressing. The nurse educators would like to conduct a study to determine whether using simulation with a low-fidelity manikin versus using return demonstration would improve the students' ability to change a sterile dressing correctly.

1. What is the evidence that needs to be obtained to determine the best practices for teaching students to change a sterile dressing?
2. What steps are needed to design the study?
3. What resources will the faculty need to conduct this study?
4. Will conducting the study fulfill requirements for producing "scholarly work" to meet the criteria for their rank?
5. What will be the most appropriate roles on the research team for each of the nurse educators?

CASE STUDY 15.2

A nurse educator with a doctorate is appointed as an assistant professor of nursing. The nurse educator will have to teach nine credits of undergraduate courses each semester and is expected to develop a program of research and provide service to the school. The school uses Boyer's model of scholarship, and within 5 years, the nurse educator will be expected to have published several articles, obtained excellent ratings in the area of teaching, and provided leadership to the school in the nurse educator's area of expertise. The nurse educator's mentor asks the nurse educator to identify an area of expertise for the program of research.

1. What factors should the nurse educator consider when identifying an area of expertise for developing a program of research?
2. How can the nurse educator best work with a mentor?
3. What strategies should the nurse educator consider when attempting to meet the expectations for excellence in the three primary areas noted in Boyer's model?
4. What goals and priorities should the nurse educator set for the first year?
5. Is teaching nine credits each semester a reasonable workload, given the other expectations for productivity?

PRACTICE QUESTIONS

1. A nurse educator's area of expertise is mentoring. Which of the following indicates the educator is meeting expectations for scholarship of discovery?

A. Serves as a mentor in a mentoring program of a national organization

B. Conducts research about the characteristics of a mentor

C. Offers workshops about being a mentor

D. Serves on a national committee to develop mentoring guidelines

2. The promotion and tenure committee at a school of nursing is reviewing a nurse educator's dossier for promotion to associate professor. Which of the following indicates the nurse educator is demonstrating the scholarship of teaching? The dossier indicates that the nurse educator:

   A. Has received consistently excellent student reviews of teaching over six semesters

   B. Has created and implemented a scenario to be used in a simulation

   C. Has improved her teaching following a peer review

   D. Has published three articles about innovative teaching in peer-reviewed journals

3. Which of the following indicates a nurse educator is developing in the role of a scholar?

   A. Identifies the need for evidence about best practices for clinical placement of students

   B. Participates in a "journal club" at the school of nursing

   C. Is asked to be a mentor for new faculty

   D. Teaches a research course in a graduate program

4. Which is a characteristic of scholarship?

   A. Funding from a federal organization

   B. Peer review

   C. Implementing a new teaching strategy

   D. Reporting the use of a teaching strategy on a curriculum vitae (CV)

5. Boyer's model of scholarship is most appropriately used to guide which of the following decisions?

   A. Determining an area of research to pursue

   B. Awarding promotion and tenure

   C. Selecting a nursing organization to join

   D. Choosing a mentor

6. Which indicates a nurse educator is demonstrating integrity as a scholar?

   A. Publishes results of an attitude survey administered to students

   B. Includes only recent publications in the reference list of a manuscript

   C. Ensures that all persons who contributed to the writing and reviewing of the manuscript are listed as authors

   D. Tells a student that she or he cannot be considered as an author on a manuscript because the work was done in his or her role as student

7. A nurse educator is seeking funding to conduct a pilot study of the effects of peer testing in the educator's classroom. The nurse educator should first seek funding from:

   A. The university's research fund for teaching and learning

   B. Health Resources and Services Administration (HRSA)

   C. National Institutes of Health (NIH)

   D. Robert Wood Johnson Foundation

8. A nurse educator administers a standardized learning-style inventory to incoming students and is planning to correlate the findings with the students' grade point average (GPA). The nurse educator should first:

   A. Administer the learning-style inventory and request the GPA for each student from the student services office

   B. Administer the learning-style inventory and ask each student to self-report his GPA

   C. Seek review and approval from the Institutional Review Board (IRB) to conduct this study

   D. Find a colleague with research skills to be a coinvestigator for this project

9. A faculty member who is a full professor is collaborating with a faculty member who is an assistant professor, a nursing doctoral student, and a doctorally prepared statistician who is not a nurse to conduct research that will result in a paper to be submitted for publication. The group agrees that each member will write a significant component of the paper according to his or her expertise. Who should be listed as author on the paper?

   A. The full professor

   B. The two faculty members

   C. Only the nurses

   D. All members of the team

10. A nurse educator who has a DNP degree and is a psychiatric nurse practitioner with an appointment as clinical assistant professor is receiving an annual review from the department chair following the first year of teaching. Which of the following provides the best evidence that the nurse educator has met the requirement for continued employment in the area of scholarship of teaching? The nurse educator:

   A. Received student reviews of teaching of 4.8 on a 5-point scale

   B. Attended two conferences related to using simulations

   C. Presented the findings from a study of student response to stress during clinical assignments

   D. Has received the outstanding teacher award presented by the student nurses association at the school

REFERENCES

Allen, M. N., & Field, P. A. (2005). Scholarly teaching and scholarship of teaching: Noting the difference. *International Journal of Nursing Education Scholarship, 2*(1), Article 12. Retrieved from https://www.ncbi.nlm.nih.gov/pubmed/16646906

American Association of Colleges of Nursing. (1999). Defining scholarship for the profession of nursing. Retrieved from http://www.aacn.nche.edu/publications/position/defining-scholarship

Baker, S. L., Fitzpatrick, J. J., & Griffin, M. Q. (2011). Empowerment and job satisfaction in associate degree nurse educators. *Nursing Education Perspectives, 32*(4), 234–239.

Boyer, E. (1990). *Scholarship reconsidered: Priorities of the professoriate.* San Francisco, CA: Jossey-Bass.

Carnegie Foundation. (2013). Carnegie Academy for the Scholarship of Teaching and Learning. Retrieved from http://www.carnegiefoundation.org/scholarship-teaching-learning

Conard, P. L., & Pape. T. (2014). Roles and responsibilities of the nursing scholar. *Pediatric Nursing, 40*(2), 87–90.

Heinrich, K. (2016). Turn your teaching into scholarship. *Reflections on Nursing Leadership, 42*(1), 1–3.

Josephsen, J. M. (2013). Evidence-based reflective teaching practice: A preceptorship course example. *Nursing Education Perspectives, 34*(1), 8–11.

Malik, G., McKenna, L., & Plummer, V. (2015). Perceived knowledge, skills, attitude and contextual factors affecting evidence-based practice among nurse educators, clinical coaches and nurse specialists. *International Journal of Nursing Practice,* (Suppl. 21), 46–57. doi: 10.1111/ijn.12366

National League for Nursing. (2007). Position statement on funding nursing education research. Retrieved from http://www.nln.org/docs/default-source/about/archived-position-statements/nursingedresearch_051807.pdf?sfvrsn=6

National League for Nursing. (2016). Certified nurse educator (CNE) 2016 candidate handbook. Retrieved from http://www.nln.org/docs/default-source/professional-development-programs/certified-nurse-educator-(cne)-examination-candidate-handbook.pdf?sfvrsn=2

Oermann, M. H., & Hayes, J. C. (2011). *Writing for publication in nursing* (2nd ed.). New York, NY: Springer Publishing.

Functioning Effectively Within the Institutional Environment and Academic Community

MARY ELLEN SMITH GLASGOW

> *Courage is the most important of all the virtues*
> *because without courage, you can't practice any*
> *other virtue consistently.*
> —Maya Angelou

This chapter addresses the Certified Nurse Educator Exam Content Area 6C: Function Effectively Within the Institutional Environment and the Academic Community (National League for Nursing [NLN], 2016, p. 5).

- Content Area 6, which includes 6A, 6B, and 6C, makes up 21% of the examination
- It is estimated that there will be approximately 31 or 32 questions from Content Area 6

LEARNING OUTCOMES

- Identify internal and external factors influencing nursing education
- Describe the relationship of the mission of the parent institution with that of the nursing curriculum
- Discuss the impact of the organizational climate on the development of the nurse educator
- Elaborate on the importance of a professional career development trajectory for nurse educators
- Investigate the concepts of *mentorship* and *protégé* as they relate to the educator role
- Analyze the nurse educator's leadership role with respect to institutional governance

This chapter focuses on the nurse educator's roles and responsibilities within the institutional environment and academic community, with particular emphasis on teaching, research/scholarship, and service requirements, as well as internal and external forces affecting nursing education.

INTERNAL AND EXTERNAL FORCES INFLUENCING NURSING AND HIGHER EDUCATION

The faculty role in higher education has changed from that of a single-focused mission of teaching to a triad of teaching, scholarship, and service. Nursing education has changed dramatically from being housed in the service sector setting to the college and university setting (Finke, 2012). As nursing education entered the university setting, nursing faculty were held to the same research and scholarship standards as their nonnursing academic colleagues. The emphasis on research and scholarship continues to be a benchmark for nursing faculty productivity in most university settings, particularly at research and comprehensive universities. There are many other internal and external forces influencing both nursing education and higher education today. These driving forces include:

- Multiculturalism of society
- Expanding technology, including distance education
- Limited financial resources
- Nursing faculty shortage
- Nursing shortage
- Aging population
- Health disparities
- Knowledge explosion
- Emphasis on the "learner" instead of the "teacher" in relation to pedagogy
- Increased demand for accountability
- Outcomes assessment
- Accreditation requirements
- Federal funding
- General economy
- Political landscape
- Health care reform

External landmark reports have made strong recommendations to nursing education and the nursing profession in general. Among these, *The Future of Nursing Report: Leading Change, Advancing Health*, (Institute of Medicine, 2010) recommended that "nurses should achieve higher levels of education and training through an improved education system that promotes seamless academic progression" (p. 4-1). Such education needs to provide learners with "a better understanding of and experience in care management, quality improvement methods, systems-level change management, and the reconceptualized roles of nurses in a reformed health care system" (p. 4-1). Nursing educators need to create academic programs that are competency based and interdisciplinary in nature, inspiring lifelong learning, and promoting the diversity of the student population. The report proposes "strategies to shape the future of health care by creating models of nursing education focused not only on curriculum changes, but also, on transforming the student population, integrating the science and research in the curriculum and influencing health care policy" (Smith Glasgow, Dunphy, & Mainous, 2010, p. G9).

The 2010 Carnegie Foundation study (Benner, Sutphen, Leonard, & Day, 2010) called for educators to transform nursing education. This report noted that "nursing education needs teachers with a deep nursing knowledge who also know how to teach and conduct research on nursing education" (p. 6).

Enrollment, curriculum design, pedagogy, faculty expectations, faculty competencies, and scholarly productivity are all shaped by social, political, and economic forces. For example, societal multiculturalism will continue to shape curricula, and faculty will need to teach students to understand and respond effectively to the cultural needs of patients they meet in health care encounters (Giger et al., 2007). Today, changing demographics, culture, and linguistic diversity need to be emphasized in nursing curricula at all levels. Curricula need to be continually reexamined in light of these internal and external forces.

Preparation for the Faculty Role

The nurse educator role requires specialized preparation. It is critical that nurse educators are cognizant of teaching, learning, and evaluation and have knowledge and skill in curriculum development, assessment of program outcomes, and being an effective member of an academic community (National League for Nursing, n.d). Just as one would never be allowed to practice as a nurse practitioner without formal course work and supervised clinical practice, one should not be allowed to practice as an educator without formal course work and supervised teaching practice. Nursing faculty need specialized course work on teaching/learning, learning styles, how the brain works in relation to learning, curriculum development, program evaluation, the multiple demands of the educator role, the dynamics of academe, resolution of student-related issues, course development, effective student advisement, innovative teaching strategies, online pedagogy, and relevant educational research. Nurse educators should be knowledgeable about the nationally endorsed nurse educator competencies (Halstead, 2007) and certification (NLN's Certified Nurse Educator) available to document one's expertise as an educator (NLN, n.d.; Valiga, 2016).

EVIDENCE-BASED TEACHING PRACTICE

The current nursing faculty shortage has prompted research into why faculty stay or leave academia. A wealth of literature exists on reasons nursing faculty leave academia; however, little research exists on reasons nursing faculty stay in academia. Garbee and Killacky (2008) examined predictor

(continued)

EVIDENCE-BASED TEACHING PRACTICE (*continued*)

variables for *intent to stay* in nursing education. An online survey was conducted over 6 weeks using four instruments: Index of Job Satisfaction, Mentoring Scale, Organizational Commitment Questionnaire, and Leadership Behavior Description Questionnaire. A random cluster sample of schools of nursing in states within the Southern Regional Education Board resulted in a sample of 39 nursing schools with 316 responses from nursing faculty.

Findings indicated that levels of job satisfaction and organizational commitment were within the range for normative means. Intent-to-stay scores for 1 and 3 years were high. Although scores were lower for intent to stay 5 years, there was more variability in scores. Job satisfaction had a significant positive correlation with intent to stay in 1 and 5 years. Slightly over half, 55.7% (176), reported having a mentor; however, mentoring scores alone were not found to significantly predict intent to stay. Organizational commitment scores alone significantly predicted intent to stay for 1 and 5 years, explaining 19.3% and 20.6% of the variance, respectively. *Mentored faculty scored significantly higher than nonmentored faculty on organizational commitment.* Leadership behaviors measuring consideration significantly predicted intent to stay 1 and 5 years, but explained a small amount of variance, 6.8% and 8.5%, respectively.

Accreditation

- There are three national professional nursing organizations that currently accredit nursing education programs: the Commission for Nursing Education Accreditation (CNEA), the Accreditation Commission for Education in Nursing (ACEN), and the Commission for Collegiate Nursing Education (CCNE). The NLN's accreditation services, represented by the NLN CNEA, accredits all nursing programs, including licensed practical nursing, nursing diploma, associate degree, baccalaureate degree, master's degree, and doctor of nursing practice (DNP) programs. The ACEN was originally the National League for Nursing Accreditation Commission (NLNAC) but split off from the NLN in 2013 and is now a separate legal entity. ACEN accreditation includes practical, diploma, associate, baccalaureate, master's/post master's certificate, and clinical doctorate programs of nursing education. The American Association of Colleges of Nursing (AACN) represented by the CCNE accredits baccalaureate, master's, and DNP degree programs.

- CCNE accredits DNP programs that focus on advanced practice nursing, nursing leadership/administration, and health policy. In addition, it must be noted that all BSN to DNP programs that require new licensure (certified nurse midwife, nurse practitioner, and nurse anesthetist) require accreditation.

- Currently, CCNE will not accredit DNP programs that have an educator track as part of their core curriculum. Since 2004, the AACN has been clear that the educator role is not an advanced nursing practice role and requires a research-focused doctorate; they underscored the point with the 2006 publication of

The Essentials of Doctoral Education for Advanced Nursing Practice (AACN, 2004, 2006). ACEN will accredit DNP program options with a clinical focus; therefore, if the DNP is an educational track, it still needs to have a clinical focus (N. Ard, personal communication, May 2, 2016).

- Research-focused doctoral programs (PhD, EdD, DNS, and DNSc) are not subject to accreditation.

- Baccalaureate nursing education programs or higher can choose to be accredited by CNEA, ACEN, or CCNE; some programs elect to be accredited by more than one organization. Associate degree or diploma programs are accredited by CNEA.

- The accreditation process provides an evaluative review of all components of the education program with an emphasis on program outcomes. Substantive components considered for accreditation include curriculum, institutional and program governance, fiscal resources, instructional learning resources, student support services, faculty qualifications, student qualifications, faculty and student accomplishments, and a program evaluation plan that guides faculty program reviews and decision making.

- The process for CNEA, ACEN, and CCNE accreditation requires an onsite visit from faculty colleagues or peer reviewers from similar institutions.

- Prior to the onsite visit, faculty members prepare a written self-study report addressing each accreditation standard. It is important for faculty to have a clear understanding of the accreditation standards that guide the nature and execution of their nursing program.

- The CNEA accreditation standards can be found online at www.nln.org/accreditation-services/overview, the CCNE accreditation standards can be found at www.aacn.nche.edu/Accreditation/index.htm, and the ACEN standards can be located at www.acenursing.org.

THE ACADEMIC SETTING

College/University

The organizational structures of American colleges and universities vary depending on institutional type, culture, and history, yet they also have much in common. Although a private liberal arts and public research university in a state system may differ in terms of mission and focus, the majority of public and private universities are overseen by an institutional or system-wide governing board. Faculty self-governance is common in academia, and faculty members are involved in their campuses' strategic planning, fiscal oversight, curriculum planning, and student affairs.

Historically, the majority of American colleges and universities are nonprofit; however, there is a burgeoning of for-profit universities that deliver predominantly online academic programs. University norms, such as faculty self-governance, are less common in these new for-profit academic organizations as a result of different business and organizational models; however, these institutions needs to meet the same accreditation requirements as their nonprofit colleagues if they seek accreditation.

School of Nursing

- The school of nursing or nursing program's mission, philosophy, program outcomes, and curriculum are based on the college's and university's mission.
- The expectations of the internal and external stakeholders need to be considered during program development or evaluation (Sauter, Gillespie, & Knepp, 2012).

Mission

- According to Csokasy (2009), a mission statement is a public statement of what an institution is about and why it exists.
- A mission statement provides direction for the planning of educational activities and provides clarity related to the target constituencies' goals for the institution related to teaching, research, and practice, and the level to which the institution aspires.
- The nursing educational mission is derived from the institution's mission statement, and the two mission statements need to be congruent with one another (Valiga, 2012).
- The nursing educational mission statement describes the unique attributes of the program and provides direction for curriculum development.
- Curricular and structural changes need to consider the missions of both the university and its nursing program.

Faculty Governance

- Finke (2012) describes how faculty have traditionally enjoyed the right of self-governance within the university setting.
- Self-governance includes developing policies related to student affairs, faculty expectations; faculty tenure and promotion guidelines; serving on faculty search committees; and developing, revising, and evaluating the curriculum.
- Faculty in partnership with academic administrators, who also hold a faculty rank in many instances, work collaboratively to address issues facing the university and larger academic community.

Organizational Climate

- The organizational climate, or culture, is critical to the retention of nursing faculty, enthusiasm for innovation and learning, scholarly productivity, and clinical excellence.
- An organizational culture that encompasses the values and beliefs that the organization wants to promote is integral to any organization's success.
- Reports on faculty cite great stress and burnout as a result of high job expectations for combining teaching, research, and service. Heavy workloads often preclude having a meaningful life outside of work, pressures to maintain clinical competence are high, and frustrations emerge with demands from multiple constituencies (Shirey, 2006). Promoting a healthy workplace in academic nursing settings is vital to recruiting and retaining faculty and enhancing the

work life of faculty for optimism and happiness. Renewed attention is needed to focus on the importance of adopting standards to combat incivility, to stay optimistic despite challenges, and use the tenets of appreciative inquiry (Fontaine, Koh, & Carroll, 2012).

- Leaders need to effect change, promote a positive organizational culture, articulate a vision, implement strategic plans, garner resources, network, and adapt to changing landscapes.

- The requisite leadership skills needed to oversee an academic program include aptitude, emotional intelligence, self-awareness, self-regulation, motivation, empathy, risk taking, creativity, and social skills (Goleman, 2002; Grossman & Valiga, 2005).

- The importance of promoting a healthy environment in academic schools of nursing where faculty can flourish cannot be overstated. It is time in nursing's history to focus on a collegial, healthy educational environment given the increase in retirements of senior faculty. New faculty are seeking a supportive, fulfilling work environment as they learn the nurse educator role (Fontaine et al., 2012).

Community of Inquiry

As online learning becomes a leading pedagogy resulting from access and convenience factors, Garrison, Anderson, and Archer's Community of Inquiry (CoI) Framework (2000) has been instrumental in understanding online learner engagement and has generated great interest among educational researchers. The CoI framework has been used extensively in the research and practice of online and blended learning, identifying the core elements associated with role adjustment to online learning, namely, cognitive, social, and teaching presence in an online environment. Garrison, Anderson, and Archer (2000) define *cognitive*, *social*, and *teaching presence* as:

- "Cognitive presence relates to the design and development of instructional materials, enabling students to construct and confirm meaning through related reflection and discourse" (p. 93).

- "Social presence relates to the establishment of a supportive learning community, providing a venue for communication within a trusted environment where students can express individual identities and establish social relationships. Social presence is defined as the ability of participants in a community of inquiry to project themselves socially and emotionally, as 'real' people (i.e., their full personality), through the medium of 'communication being used'" (p. 94).

- "Teaching presence relates to the process of design, facilitation, and direction throughout the learning experience in order to realize desired learning outcomes. The three major categories under teaching presence are instructional design and management, building understanding, and direct instruction. Establishing teaching presence means, creating a learning experience for students to progress through with instructor facilitation, support, and guidance" (p. 101).

Five areas of adjustment characterize the move toward competence in online learning: (a) interaction, (b) self-identity, (c) instructor role, (d) course design, and (e) technology (Garrison, Cleveland-Innes, & Fung, 2004). Faculty preparation in online pedagogies is a crucial prerequisite for a successful higher educational experience (Figure 16.1).

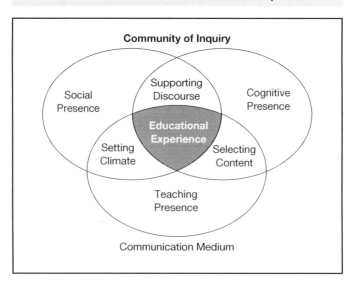

FIGURE 16.1 Elements of an educational experience.

Source: Garrison et al. (2000).

Collaboration, Partnerships, and Innovation

- To develop and maintain an innovative curriculum, nurse educators need to lead a cultural paradigm shift in nursing education that welcomes innovation, embraces creativity, and designs novel curricula and pedagogy that will ultimately improve the health and welfare of patients and professional nurses (Smith Glasgow et al., 2010).

- Strategic partnerships are one example of innovation as nurse leaders devise ways to manage the nursing shortage and the nurse faculty shortage and to increase the number of BSN-prepared nurses. Innovative curricular models, such as the Oregon Consortium for Nursing Education, provide a model to facilitate the movement of students through associate degree to baccalaureate degree programs in a seamless fashion, which eliminates duplication and prepares graduates with the competencies needed to meet the needs of the state's aging and ethnically diverse population.

- These strategic models of synergistic collaboration are being used to address issues of both nursing and nursing faculty shortages. Dedicated education units offer a new way to conceptualize the roles of nurse educators, students, and clinical staff during clinical learning experiences. "This new model of education is broader, more inclusive, and seeks to find commonalities in the culture of both service and academe, and may provide the best site for faculty practice as well" (Smith Glasgow et al., 2010, p. G9).

- Collaborative arrangements between academic and health care institutions allow partners to combine their respective strengths in achieving their mutual goals of increasing the registered nurse and nursing faculty workforce (Oermann, 2007; Smith Glasgow et al., 2010).

- Typically, the master's prepared nurse clinician or DNP-prepared advanced practice nurse is selected by the academic and health care institution to teach students in the clinical area based on his or her educational preparation, clinical expertise, and desire to teach (Danzey et al., 2011; Tanner, 2005).

- Leaders need to create a safe, inclusive environment where faculty can feel comfortable regarding the adoption of innovative learning experiences.

> **Teaching Gem:** Nurse educators should keep an ongoing electronic file and record each activity that adds to the portfolio as soon as the activity is completed. For helpful tips on preparing a portfolio, nurse educators should consider reading *The Academic Portfolio: A Practical Guide to Documenting Teaching, Research, and Service* (Seldin & Miller, 2009).

- Visionary leaders are successful in developing partnerships in the organization while leading faculty and anticipating the effects of innovation by:
  - Staying focused on the educational program's core mission and values while being responsive to trends in the profession
  - Identifying innovations of use to the institution

EVIDENCE-BASED TEACHING PRACTICE

Laurencelle, Scanlan, and Brett (2016) explored nurse eductors' (*N* = 15) meaning for being in academia and used a phenolmological approach. They found six subthemes, which included (a) opportunities, (b) wanting to teach, (c) seeing students learn, (d) contributing to the profession, (e) the unattractive career choices, and (f) flexibility.

ACADEMIC RESPONSIBILITIES

Teaching

Elements of faculty participation in the teaching mission of an institution include (Finke, 2012):

- Effectiveness in undergraduate and graduate teaching in the classroom and/or clinical area
- Contributions to the curriculum, such as substantial revisions of existing courses, and the development of new courses and techniques for teaching
- Development of student evaluation methods
- Publications related to teaching, such as textbooks, manuals, and articles
- Effectiveness as an undergraduate and/or graduate adviser and/or mentor, including dissertation, thesis, or independent study advisement
- Teaching is evaluated based on student evaluations of teaching strategies, peer reviews of teaching strategies, evaluation of a teaching dossier, and assessment of student learning (Sauter et al., 2012)

EVIDENCE-BASED TEACHING PRACTICE

Beckmann, Cannella, and Wantland (2013) conducted a study to determine the prevalence of bullying among faculty members in schools or colleges of nursing. Bullying of nursing faculty in the academic setting is of interest in terms of recruitment, retention, job satisfaction, and the overall quality of the work environment. The cross-sectional, descriptive study of faculty was conducted in three northeastern states of the United States. The Negative Acts Questionnaire-Revised (NAQ-R) was used to survey faculty members in schools of nursing that award a baccalaureate degree (or higher) in nursing. Four-hundred and seventy-three (473) faculty members met the inclusion criteria and responded to the NAQ-R. An iterative exploratory principal-components analysis with orthogonal rotation was performed. Thirteen of the original 22 items were retained to measure the experiences of negative acts in the nursing faculty workplaces. The mean total score for the 13-item instrument was 17.90 (SD = 6.07) and ranged from 13 to 56. The resulting components structure produced three clear subscales identifying the experiences of Verbal abuse, Physical abuse, and Devaluing. The revised 13-item instrument had a Cronbach's alpha value of 0.88. Experiences of bullying were reported in 169 of the 473 (36%) respondents. A significant correlation was found between meeting frequency and the report of bullying (r = 0.18, $p \le .001$). Administrators and senior faculty were more likely than expected to be the perpetrators of bullying. If the leaders are identified as bullies, the environment cannot be perceived as supportive and healthy. These unhealthy environments may have serious consequences related to retaining nursing faculty.

Research/Scholarship

Elements of faculty participation, particularly for tenure-track and tenured faculty, in a continuing program of research or other scholarship, include:

- Quantity and quality of research or scholarship, as evidenced by publications, presentations of papers (including invited presentations nationally and internationally), and peer-reviewed scholarship
- Publications related to the advancement of pedagogical theory
- Success in securing intramural (internal or institutional) funding
- Success in securing extramural funding (external federal funding or private funding)
- Effectiveness in directing the research of students
- Originating, participating in, and/or directing research projects (Sauter et al., 2012)

Service

Elements of faculty participation in service to the program, department, school or college, and university, and to the profession at the national and/or international level include:

- Leadership and/or participation in faculty elective bodies and service on committees at the program, department, college or school, and university levels

- Faculty mentoring
- Service to individual students and/or student organizations
- Promotion of the university through extramural activities, such as recruitment events, alumni affairs, and so on
- Other forms of service to the profession and society, such as serving on editorial boards, national organizations, and grant-review panels (Finke, 2012)

APPOINTMENT, PROMOTION, AND TENURE

Faculty Appointment

- Potential faculty candidates are invited to interview by a faculty search committee appointed by a dean or other university administrator. Faculty candidates may be asked to conduct a presentation about their research agenda or to demonstrate teaching competency during the interview process. Potential faculty candidates may also be interviewed by the department chair, associate dean for research, and dean, depending on the academic rank.
- Once considered for appointment, the faculty candidate's vita is reviewed by the appointment, promotion, and tenure committee or another appropriate committee for the recommendation of faculty rank to the dean. The academic ranks of instructor, assistant professor, associate professor, and professor are typically appointed based on the faculty candidate's teaching, research, and service experience and expertise.
- More recently, there has been an increase in the number of faculty appointed to clinical-track positions. These faculty members may enjoy the same promotion in rank as their tenure-track and tenured colleagues but are usually not eligible for tenure. Faculty who are hired into a clinical-track position typically have the designation *clinical* before their academic rank and are hired for their clinical knowledge and expertise. Many of these clinical faculty members may have joint appointments with a health care institution, which involves an adjustment and negotiation in workload.

Academic Ranks

- Finke (2012) noted that appointment ranks, or tracks, have been developed to specify the responsibilities of faculty members in relation to teaching, scholarship, and service.
- Ranks include *tenure, clinical,* or *research scientist*. Clinical and research faculty have a designation before their academic rank (e.g., clinical assistant professor or research associate professor). Tenure-track and tenured faculty titles have no prefix.
- Tenure-track faculty are considered tenure probationary until they achieve tenure. The tenure track is established for faculty whose primary responsibilities are teaching and research.
- The clinical faculty track was developed for those faculty members whose primary responsibilities are clinical practice or clinical supervision of students.
- The research scientist track is for faculty whose primary responsibilities are generating new knowledge and disseminating research findings.

Nontenure Appointments

Clinical and research faculty are generally nontenured positions and are considered contracted faculty. Faculty members receive contracts on an annual or multiyear basis.

The Appointment, Promotion, and Tenure Process

- The contemporary concept of tenure in U.S. colleges and universities can be traced to the "Statement of Principles of Academic Freedom and Tenure," which was adopted in 1940 by the American Association of University Professors (AAUPs) and the Association of American Colleges, where the basic principles of tenure as a system to protect the academic freedom of faculty members were first articulated.

- Criteria for promotion and tenure are based on a university's overall mission and the Carnegie Foundation's university classification system; therefore, requirements vary among institutions from tribal colleges to doctoral universities. Doctoral universities are assigned to one of three categories based on a measure of research activity. Nurse educators should evaluate their research productivity/skills in lieu of these categories when seeking tenure and promotion.

- *Promotion* refers to advancement in rank. To be considered for promotion, a faculty member must submit a dossier as evidence of excellence in teaching, scholarship, and service.

- The criteria for tenure and/or promotion are established by the school/college and are evaluated by a committee of peers, school and university administrators, and the university board of trustees or other governing body.

- In most schools of nursing, a tenure-track faculty member is appointed as an assistant professor and can expect to be promoted to the rank of associate professor at the time when tenure is granted.

- The AAUP can serve as a resource related to faculty rights pertaining to tenure and promotion. Their website is www.aaup.org/aaup.

CAREER DEVELOPMENT FOR NURSE EDUCATORS

Both new and experienced faculty need clear guidelines on career development and advancement in their respective academic institutions (Seldin & Associates, 2006; Seldin & Miller, 2009; Seldin, Miller, Seldin, & McKeachie, 2010).

Portfolio Development

- The professional portfolio/dossier is typically used to display one's work when applying for appointments, promotions, and tenure. A portfolio or dossier should include sample publications, grant submissions, awards, syllabi, teaching evaluations, and recommendation letters. A portfolio or dossier is a practical way to reflect on and document one's teaching, research, and service (Seldin & Associates, 2006; Seldin & Miller, 2009; Seldin et al., 2010; Wittmann-Price, 2012).

- In recent years, electronic portfolios have come into use in academic institutions as a means for students to display their work and demonstrate competency related to writing, clinical objectives, and so on.
- Some academic institutions are also using electronic portfolios for faculty to construct and display their promotion and tenure dossiers.

Developing a Career Trajectory

Successful faculty members have often developed a career development plan for themselves. Such a plan may include the following elements:

- Developing career goals
- Short-term career goals
- Long-term career goals
- Using effective time management
- Identify the most productive intellectual time and protect it
- Maximize the value of scholarship and research time
- Understanding of the trajectory and stages of an academic career and the goals at each stage
- Mastery of negotiation and conflict-resolution skills
- Developing a teaching portfolio
- Developing collaboration skills and the ability to maximize the benefits of collaboration while maintaining autonomy and boundaries
- Valuing the benefits of being mentored
- Developing a primary mentor–protégé relationship
- Appreciation for the need for lifelong learning
- Consulting a coach to deal with any issues and barriers effectively (Doucette, 2008; Weinstock & Smith Glasgow, 2016)

Career Stages

Distinct academic accomplishments are associated with various levels of faculty appointments during progressive career stages. These can generally be described for each faculty level as follows:

1. Instructor
   - Develop skills in the scholarship of discovery (research or discovery of new knowledge)
   - Develop skills in the scholarship of teaching
   - Develop skills in scholarship of integration (interpretation and synthesis of knowledge across discipline boundaries in a manner that provides new insights)

* Develop skills in the scholarship of application of knowledge (connects theory and practice; Boyer, 1997)
* Understand the responsibilities of protégé and mentor

2. Assistant Professor
   * Develop an area of expertise
   * Pose and address an important question or focus in that area that has the potential for significant findings or impact (scholarship or research)
   * Develop oneself autonomously within this area or develop an interdisciplinary research team and bring your area of expertise to the team
   * Develop one's own laboratory for evaluating these questions, whether the laboratory is a wet-bench laboratory; the skills, staff, and resources for clinical, population-based, or teaching investigation; or another setting (i.e., demonstrating the ability to function scientifically as an "independent" investigator or "collaborative" investigator)
   * Lead or collaborate in the development and evaluation of an innovative educational program
   * Present findings from this work at appropriate national meetings and/or publish the results of this work in peer-reviewed journals
   * Obtain external, peer-reviewed funding to support this work
   * Become nationally recognized for this body of work, whether it be clinical research or education
   * Initiate or continue to compile the teaching portfolio (Seldin & Miller, 2009)
   * Provide faculty teaching and service to the nursing department (Wittmann-Price, 2012)

3. Associate Professor
   * Continue research/scholarship in one's area of expertise as an autonomous investigator and in publication productivity
   * Become an interdependent investigator and/or leader
   * Continue with the activity of developing and evaluating innovative educational programs
   * Establish a body of contributions that one can make in one's defined area; become nationally and internationally recognized for this work
   * Take on responsibility for an area important to one's own institution, becoming a resource and leader recognized beyond one's department
   * Mentor junior faculty in a productive manner
   * Demonstrate peer-reviewed awards, honors, or other indications of excellence
   * Demonstrate peer-reviewed support for research or program development
   * Become involved at the national level through involvement in societies reflective of one's expertise
   * Serve on national committees such as study sections
   * Serve on departmental and university functions, particularly some time-consuming committees

4. Professor

- Continue to demonstrate leadership in research, teaching, and service at a national and international level
- Become internationally recognized for this body of work, whether it be clinical research or educational research
- Function as a role model and enhance the mentoring role and, in particular, assist junior faculty in their career development

Choosing a Mentor

- A faculty mentor either can be assigned to the protégé, or the mentor and protégé can mutually agree upon the relationship. The mentoring relationship is generally consultative and constructive in most institutions; however, some schools have a more prescriptive approach (Sauter et al., 2012).
- Grossman and Valiga (2005) define a *mentor* as an individual who assists his or her protégé as he or she works to establish a professional reputation. The mentor provides support and guidance during times of stress while assisting in the development and enhancement of the protégé's professional skills.

Some organizations have more formalized mentoring programs for junior faculty such as Sigma Theta Tau International Nurse Faculty Leadership Academy (NFLA). The Sigma Theta Tau NFLA, is an intense international leadership development experience designed to (a) facilitate personal leadership development; (b) foster academic career success; (c) promote nurse faculty retention and satisfaction; and (d) cultivate high-performing, supportive work environments in academe (Sigma Theta Tau International Inc., 2016).

- The mentor helps the protégé learn the political landscape, expand his or her network, gain professional insight, and foster personal and professional growth.
- An authentic mentor invests a great deal of time and effort into the advancement of his or her protégé. The mentor–protégé relationship is conscious, purposeful, and typically lasts for a number of years.
- It is important for the protégé to set goals, track progress, and obtain feedback from the mentor on his or her development plan.
- A mentor looks for the following attributes in the protégé:
  - Intelligence
  - Strong work ethic
  - Initiative
  - Integrity
  - Professional demeanor
  - Commitment
  - Ability to accept feedback
  - Intellectual curiosity

- A protégé looks for the following attributes in the mentor:
  - Intelligence
  - Someone who is willing to invest in him or her
  - Willingness to give feedback
  - Strong networking capabilities
  - Professional contacts
  - Ability to motivate
  - Integrity

Faculty Orientation and Development

New nursing faculty members struggle to meet the individual needs of an increasingly diverse and growing population of nursing students, while simultaneously attempting to balance the research, scholarship, and stewardship requirements of their institutions. To meet these demands, a formal, robust faculty orientation is essential. During a faculty orientation, new nursing faculty members begin the process of socialization into the academy. Novice faculty need to understand the expectations for tenure and promotion and the sociopolitical issues of the institution upon assuming their new role as educators (Sauter et al., 2012; Suplee & Gardner, 2009).

- Nurse educators need to understand the mission and goals of the institution, the nature of the curriculum, academic policies and procedures, the organization of the program, the school and how it fits into the university, and the structure and charges of the various nursing and university committees.

> **Teaching Gem:** It is important for the novice nurse faculty member to keep continuous track of accomplishments and maintain a current, comprehensive curriculum vitae (CV) in addition to uploading teaching evaluations, publications, continuing education certificates, and so forth in an electronic portfolio for tenure and/or promotion.

- Seasoned nurse educators should be involved in these orientation and development sessions to facilitate collegial relationships, impart knowledge and expertise, and encourage mentor–protégé relationships.
- The use of travel monies to attend conferences, seminars, and research colloquia is critical to faculty development.
- Nurse educators who need to maintain clinical certification as an advanced practice nurse should negotiate practice time as part of their faculty role.
- It is essential that the novice faculty member have an "action plan" to develop his or her career that is realistic and is congruent with the promotion and tenure guidelines of the institution.

Finke (2012) stated that ongoing support and professional development are needed for nurse educators throughout their careers in the following areas:

- Curriculum development, teaching, using teaching, learning, information resources, and evaluating student outcomes

- Professional practice
- Relationships with learners and colleagues
- Service and faculty governance
- Scholarship
- Mentoring

The Curriculum Vitae

- A curriculum vitae—often called a CV or vita—is used for academic positions. Thus, vitae tend to provide great detail about academic and research experiences. Although résumés tend toward brevity, vitae lean toward detail (Seldin et al., 2010). A sample CV format can be found in Exhibit 16.1.

EXHIBIT 16.1

Sample Curriculum Vitae

A curriculum vitae should include the following items:
1. Name in full
2. Current home and mailing address, telephone number, fax number, and e-mail address
3. Education
    A. List of degrees, with the last degree listed first
    B. For each degree, include the name of the college/university, year degree was granted, major(s)/concentration(s), minor(s), title of dissertation/thesis, if applicable
    C. Postgraduate training
    i. List chronologically, starting with most recent position
    ii. Give years, institutions, and type of training
4. Employment history
    A. List chronologically, starting with the most recent position held and including consulting positions, if applicable
    B. Indicate each place of employment and years employed
5. Certification and licensure (including recertification)
6. Military service
7. Honors and awards
    A. Starting with the most recent, list chronologically by name of the award
    B. Include each awarding institution and/or organization
    C. Indicate the nature of each award if not apparent
8. Memberships and offices in professional societies
9. Professional committees and administrative service
    A. Institutional: Committees on which you have served or chaired, including years of membership
    B. Extramural (local, regional, national, and international). Include:
    i. Membership on editorial boards
    ii. Editorship of symposia volumes, texts, or journals
    iii. Service as an examiner for a professional organization

---

(continued)

EXHIBIT 16.1

Sample Curriculum Vitae (*continued*)

    iv. Reviewer of grants for extramural funding sources

    v. Reviewer of manuscripts for journal publications

    vi. Convener of symposia, conferences, or workshop in one's field and/or profession

    C. Name of each organization or publication, your role, and years of service

10. Community service (service not related to the institution but provided by you, either in your profession or in some other capacity)

    A. List chronologically, earliest first

    B. Give your role and the organization

11. Educational activities

    A. Courses/clerkships/programs taught, coordinated, or developed

    B. Advising/mentoring/tutoring: For each of the aforementioned areas, include course title, audience, and years of involvement

    C. Educational materials: List texts, atlases, manuals, evaluation tools, and so on, developed that were used only within the institution

12. Clinical activities

    A. Outline of major clinical activities, including rounds, clinics, development and/or implementation of clinical programs and quality assessment of programs

    B. Health care education in the lay community

13. Support

    A. List past and present extramural support received

    B. List past and present intramural support received. Include role in the project, title of study, funding agencies, including appropriate ID number, effective dates, and total amount of award

    C. List grant applications already submitted and still pending, with the same information as aforementioned

14. Graduate students, postdoctoral fellows, and postgraduate trainees

    A. List the graduate students who have received advanced degrees (master's, PhD) with you as their supervisor; give the name of each student and years of study, thesis title, date when degree was awarded, program/department in which study was done, and institution awarding degree

    B. List postdoctoral fellows and postgraduate trainees and visiting scientists who have been under your direct supervision for their training; give names, years, research or clinical study, and means of support (if training grant or NRSA)

15. Publications in the lay press

    A. Published full-length papers

        1. Provide a chronological list with complete citations, including:

            i. Names and initials of all authors

            ii. Titles of the articles

            iii. Name of journal, volume, page numbers, year

        2. Indicate whether peer reviewed by using an asterisk before the citation

    B. Books and chapters in books, including page numbers; provide complete citations, including press and city of printing

    C. Communications, such as videotapes, disks, slide atlases, and computer programs, and so on, used by others outside the institution

(continued)

EXHIBIT 16.1

Sample Curriculum Vitae (*continued*)

    D. Book reviews, letters to editors (if these are not articles, which they can be, as in Nature [London] or *Journal of Molecular Biology*); provide complete citations

    E. Abstracts (optional, but if included, provide complete citations). Indicate by asterisk whether peer reviewed

16. Presentations

    A. By invitation: May include invited seminar presentations (except those for job interviews) and presentations at conferences, society meetings, and professional boards

    B. By competition or peer review

    For each presentation, provide type, full title, date and place presented, and the auspices presented under (program, department, college, university, society, etc.); wherever possible, use American Psychological Association (APA) style

17. Bibliography

    To be listed under the following separate headings and according to APA style

    N.B.: Items "accepted for publication" and/or "submitted for publication" should be so indicated and should include, together with the following information, the expected date of publication and/or date of submission

CASE STUDY

CASE STUDY 16.1

A new DNP graduate, with a strong clinical background but limited teaching experience, is interviewing at a *very high-activity research* university. What questions would you want to ask this faculty candidate regarding her career trajectory plan? What is important to convey to this faculty member given her early developmental stage as a nurse educator? Should you advise this faculty member to apply for a tenure track or nontenure track position?

PRACTICE QUESTIONS

1. Learners of nursing understand the mandate of today's health care society best when they are taught:

    A. Interprofessional collaboration

    B. Fundamental skills

    C. Information technology

    D. Triage management

2. Developing a curriculum based on current demographics would best include which of the following?

    A. Complementary therapies

    B. Childbearing choices for women with previous cesarean births

    C. Health issues of HIV-positive patients

    D. Geriatric concepts of aging

3. The nurse educator is putting together an academic portfolio for review and includes a curriculum vitae (CV). In what order should the information appear?

   A. Education, work history, courses taught, references

   B. Education, work history, honors, licensure

   C. Licensure, education, work history, references

   D. Work history, education, licensure, honors

4. When designing a curriculum, which answer would meet the criteria needed for today's health care system? It would be a curriculum that:

   A. Develops a concept-based curriculum

   B. Includes combined classes with junior and senior nursing students for role modeling

   C. Builds on standardized skills that are practiced and then demonstrated back, in order to pass

   D. Delivers a community-based curriculum concept throughout the program

5. The 2010 Carnegie Foundation study calls for nurse educators to increase:

   A. Rehabilitation content

   B. Psychomotor domain learning

   C. Research on nursing education

   D. Scholarship related to active learning strategies

6. Sigma Theta Tau International Nurse Faculty Leadership Academy (NFLA) was founded as a result of data that nurse educators stay in academia because of:

   A. A research degree versus a practice degree

   B. Mentoring

   C. Faculty practice

   D. Salary

7. Programs of nursing use an accreditation agency in order to:

   A. Tell the public that standards are met

   B. Ensure faculty governance

   C. Establish NCLEX-RN® scores above the national average

   D. Increase student satisfaction

8. Tenure criteria differ from institution to institution and are mostly dependent on:

   A. The professional department of the faculty applicant

   B. The current governance system

   C. The faculty applicant's years of service

   D. The Carnegie Classification of the institution

9. The Community of Inquiry Framework identifies three core elements associated with role adjustment to online learning, which include all of the following except:

   A. Discourse presence

   B. Teaching presence

   C. Social presence

   D. Cognitive presence

10. Teaching portfolios should include all of the following items except:

A. CV

B. Current student support letters

C. Examples of syllabi

D. Teaching philosophy

REFERENCES

American Association of Colleges of Nursing. (2004). AACN position statement on the practice doctorate in nursing. Retrieved from http://www.aacn.nche.edu/DNP/pdf/DNP.pdf

American Association of Colleges of Nursing. (2006). Essentials of doctoral education for advanced nursing practice. Received from http://www.aacn.nche.edu/DNP/pdf/Essentials.pdf

Beckmann, C. A., Cannella, B. L., & Wantland, D. (2013). Faculty perception of bullying in schools of nursing. *Journal of Professional Nursing, 29*(5), 287–294.

Benner, P., Sutphen, M., Leonard, V., & Day, L. (2010). *Educating nurses: A call for radical transformation.* San Francisco, CA: Jossey-Bass/Carnegie Foundation for the Advancement of Teaching.

Boyer, E. L. (1997). *Scholarship reconsidered: Priorities of the professoriate.* New York, NY: Jossey-Bass.

Csokasy, J. (2009). Philosophical foundations of the curriculum. In D. M. Billings & J. A. Halstead (Eds.), *Teaching in nursing: A guide for faculty* (3rd ed., pp. 105–118). St. Louis, MO: Elsevier Saunders.

Danzey, I. M., Ea, E., Fitzpatrick, J. J., Garbutt, S. J., Rafferty, M., & Zychowicz, M. E. (2011). The doctor of nursing practice and nursing education: Highlights, potential and promise. *Journal of Professional Nursing, 27*(5), 311–314.

Doucette, J. N. (2008). Coaching nurses. In H. Feldman (Ed.), *Nursing leadership: A concise encyclopedia* (pp. 114–115). New York, NY: Springer Publishing.

Finke, L. M. (2012). Teaching in nursing: The faculty role. In D. Billings & J. Halstead (Eds.), *Teaching in nursing: A guide for faculty* (4th ed., pp. 1–14). St. Louis, MO: Elsevier Saunders.

Fontaine, D., Koh, E., & Carroll, T. (2012). Promoting a healthy workplace for nursing faculty and staff. *Nursing Clinics of North America, 47*(4), 557–566. Retrieved from http://www.aana.com/resources2/professionalpractice/Pages/Promoting-a-Culture-of-Safety-and-Healthy-Work-Environment.aspx

Garbee, D., & Killacky, J. (2008). Factors influencing intent to stay in academia for nursing faculty in the Southern United States of America. *International Journal of Nursing Education Scholarship, 5*(1), 1–15.

Garrison, D. R., Anderson, T., & Archer, W. (2000). Critical inquiry in a text-based environment: Computer conferencing in higher education. *Internet and Higher Education, 2*(2–3), 87–105.

Garrison, D. R., Cleveland-Innes, M., & Fung, T. (2004). Student role adjustment in online communities of inquiry: Model and instrument validation. *Journal of Asynchronous Learning Network, 8*(2), 61–74.

Giger, J., Davidhizar, R., Purnell, L., Harden, T., Phillips, J., & Strickland, O. (2007). American Academy of Nursing expert panel report: Developing cultural competencies to eliminate health disparities in ethnic minorities and other vulnerable populations. *Journal of Transcultural Nursing, 18*(2), 100.

Goleman, D. (2002). *Primal leadership.* Boston, MA: Harvard Business School Press.

Grossman, S. C., & Valiga, T. M. (2005). *The new leadership challenge: Creating the future of nursing.* Philadelphia, PA: F. A. Davis.

Halstead, J. A. (2007). *Nurse educator competencies: Creating an evidence-based practice for nurse educators.* New York, NY: National League for Nursing.

Institute of Medicine. (2010). *The future of nursing: Leading change, advancing health*. Washington, DC: National Academies Press.

Laurencelle, F. L., Scanlan, J. M., & Brett, A. L. (2016). The meaning of being a nurse educator and nurse educators' attraction to academia: A phenomenological study. *Nurse Education Today, 39*, 135–140. doi:10.1016/j.nedt.2016.01.029

National League for Nursing. (2016). Certified nurse educator (CNE) candidate handbook. Retrieved from http://www.nln.org/professional-development-programs/Certification-for-Nurse-Educators/handbook

National League for Nursing. (2016). Certification for nurse educators (CNE). Retrieved from http://www.nln.org/docs/default-source/professionaldevelopment-programs/certified-nurse-educator-%28cne%29-examination-candidate-handbook.pdf?sfvrsn=2

Noble, K. A., Miller, S. M., & Heckman, J. (2008). The cognitive style of nursing students: Educational implications for teaching and learning. *Journal of Nursing Education, 47*(6), 245–253.

Oermann, M. H. (2007). *Annual review of nursing education: Clinical nursing education* (Vol. 6). New York, NY: Springer Publishing.

Sauter, M. K., Gillespie, N. N., & Knepp, A. (2012). Educational program evaluation. In D. Billings & J. Halstead (Eds.), *Teaching in nursing: A guide for faculty* (4th ed., pp. 503–549). St. Louis, MO: Elsevier Saunders.

Seldin, P., & Associates. (2006). *Evaluating faculty performance: A practical guide to assessing teaching, research, and service*. Boston, MA: Anker Publishing.

Seldin, P., & Miller, E. J. (2009). *The academic portfolio: A practical guide to documenting teaching, research, and service*. San Francisco, CA: Jossey-Bass.

Seldin, P., Miller, J. E., Seldin, C. A., & McKeachie, W. (2010). *The teaching portfolio: A practical guide to improved performance and promotion/tenure decisions*. San Francisco, CA: Jossey-Bass.

Shirey, M. R. (2006). Stress and burnout in nursing faculty. *Nurse Educator, 31*, 95–97.

Sigma Theta Tau International. Honor Society of Nursing. (2016). Sigma Theta Tau Internaitonal Nurse Faculty Leadership Academy (NFLA). Retrieved from http://www.nursingsociety.org/learn-grow/leadership-institute/nurse-faculty-leadership-academy-%28nfla%29

Smith Glasgow, M. E., Dunphy, L. M., & Mainous, R. O. (2010). Innovative nursing educational curriculum for the 21st century. Transformational models of nursing across different settings. In *Institute of medicine report on the future of nursing: Leading change, advancing health* (G8–G12). Washington, DC: National Academies Press.

Smith Glasgow, M. E., Niederhauser, V., Dunphy, L. M., & Mainous, R. O. (2010). Supporting innovation in nursing education: Regulatory issues. *Journal of Nursing Regulation, 1*(3), 23–27.

Suplee, P. D., & Gardner, M. (2009). Fostering a smooth transition to the faculty role. *Journal of Continuing Education in Nursing, 40*(11), 514–520.

Tanner, C. A. (2005). What are our priorities? Addressing the looming shortage of nurse faculty. *Journal of Nursing Education, 44*, 247–248.

Valiga, T. (2016). The role of the educator: Reflective response. In H. M. Dreher & M. E. Smith. Glasgow (Eds.), *DNP role development for doctoral advanced nursing practice*. New York, NY: Springer Publishing.

Valiga, T. M. (2012). Philosophical foundations of the curriculum. In D. Billings & J. Halstead (Eds.), *Teaching in nursing: A guide for faculty* (4th ed., pp. 107–118). St. Louis, MO: Elsevier Saunders.

Weinstock, B., & Smith Glasgow, M. E. (2016). Executive coaching to support doctoral role-transitions and promote leadership consciousness. In H. M. Dreher & M. E. Smith Glasgow (Eds.), *DNP role development for doctoral advanced nursing practice*. New York, NY: Springer Publishing.

Wittmann-Price, R. A. (2012). *Fast facts for developing a nursing academic portfolio*. New York, NY: Springer Publishing.

17

Comprehensive Exam and Answer Rationales

1. The novice nurse educator understands the job market correctly when she states:
   A. "The job I choose should depend on my degree and organizational fit"
   B. "I should choose a job as soon as possible because a lot of people are graduating"
   C. "The job I choose may not be secure because of the current market"
   D. "The education of nurses is moving back into the hospital setting as a result of residencies"

2. Certification in a specialty is done by professionals in order to:
   A. Be compliant with regulatory bodies
   B. Establish licensure
   C. Develop better consumer outcomes
   D. Verify continuing education

3. An educational unit is interviewing candidates for nurse administrator. In order to enact a shared governance system the recruitment committee should include:
   A. Several administrators and faculty from various departments
   B. A community person along with nursing faculty
   C. Tenured nurse faculty and faculty who teach prerequisite courses
   D. Students and faculty from various disciplines

4. A student discusses his test anxiety with the nurse educator and the student expresses understanding when he states:
   A. My anxiety is not bad because I can sleep most of the night
   B. A little anxiety is a motivation to study
   C. Many students have palpitations during the test
   D. If I take a double dose of my anxiety medication I can think better on the test

5. Boyer's model of scholarship includes all of the following scholarship EXCEPT:
   A. Research based
   B. Peer reviewed
   C. Manuscript development
   D. Teaching innovation

6. The novice nurse educator needs more understanding when he states:
   A. "I will categorize my test questions according to the NCLEX® test plan"
   B. "My test questions should reflect the content that is discussed in class"
   C. "My test questions can be mapped to the Quality and Safety Education for Nurses (QSEN) criteria"
   D. "I should use test bank questions because they will be more reliable than ones I make"

7. A new academic nurse educator needs further understanding of execution of the role when she states:
   A. "I should use the syllabus to write down all my expectations"
   B. "If I do not care for the textbook I will change it next semester"
   C. "I think it is better to use a red pen to correct care plans for effect"
   D. "I provide the class with breaks every hour"

8. The nurse administrator notices that the attrition rate is rising each year. The admission criteria are the same. The only difference is that the biology department has made the anatomy and physiology course specific for prenursing students. The best way to approach this dilemma in an academic setting would be to:
   A. Meet with the chair of the biology department and explain that biology faculty are not rigorous
   B. Ask the nursing admissions committee to raise the overall admission grade point average
   C. Ask the college administrator to take the specialty biology courses off the books
   D. Review the trend and increase the science grade point average needed

9. A nurse educator is in the planning stages for teaching his first online course. He is concerned that students may not understand the course requirements and assignments. One strategy he can use that is interactive and would permit discussion is:
   A. Voice-over PowerPoints
   B. Webinars
   C. Podcasts
   D. YouTube videos

10. An experienced faculty member is explaining to a novice why she still uses lecture as her primary teaching strategy. What statement by the faculty member would require the novice's mentor to intervene?
    A. "I am able to cover all my content when using this strategy"
    B. "Learners generally prefer lecture over other methods"
    C. "Lecture allows me to identify important concepts for the learners"
    D. "The learners develop higher level thinking when listening to lectures"

11. A graduate nurse educator student has written a discussion board post about the benefits of assigning readings for students. What statement indicates that she is accurate with her post?

    A. "Reading assignments are necessary for learners to identify important concepts"
    B. "Students may have difficulty learning from reading assignments"
    C. "Reading is an active learning strategy with many benefits"
    D. "Most learners prefer reading assignments to sitting in lecture"

12. An educator is planning her course assignments for the semester. When deciding whether to make a research paper a small-group assignment or an individual assignment, it is important to consider that:

    A. Learners generally prefer group assignments
    B. Group assignments allow each learner to be graded individually
    C. Research papers can be very time consuming to read and grade
    D. Written assignments are the best measure of student learning

13. A nurse educator is planning to have a skills check-off day for her fundamental students. What method would best lend itself to use with a large number of learners?

    A. Return demonstration
    B. Simulation
    C. Case studies
    D. Games

14. A faculty group interviews four candidates for an instructor position. The group decides to hire the person with intensive care unit (ICU) experience. After the new faculty member is there for a while she tells them that she is really not comfortable doing clinical in the medical ICU because she has just worked at a step-down care facility. The nurse administrator discusses the misrepresentation with her and classifies it as:

    A. Incivility
    B. Slander
    C. Tort
    D. Perjury

15. A program learning outcome states that the learner will demonstrate cultural competence. The best assessment of the learner meeting this program learning outcome would be:

    A. A paper on the fundamentals of nursing course describing pain reactions of a patient in a different culture
    B. A concept map in the first adult health course integrating cultural preferences
    C. An interview with a childbearing woman of another culture or living an alternative lifestyle in the women's health course
    D. A clinical evaluation in the senior capstone course that is satisfactory for cultural competence

16. The curriculum committee members are leveling student learning outcomes (SLOs) for interprofessional collaboration. An appropriate first-level SLO would be:

    A. Understand the importance of interprofessional collaboration
    B. Discuss interprofessional collaboration with another health professional
    C. Interact with a different disciplined health professional about a patient issue
    D. Analyze scope of practice for different health professionals in a case study

17. The curriculum committee members are leveling student learning outcomes (SLOs) for cultural competence. An appropriate second-level SLO would be:

    A. Interact with a person from a different culture
    B. Describe the health care mores of another culture
    C. Critique the differences between two Latino cultures
    D. Analyze a different culture through an unfolding case study

18. A novice nurse educator needs additional knowledge in curriculum development when he states:

    A. "Developing student learning outcomes (SLOs) assists in the evaluative process"
    B. "SLOs are needed to direct the teaching–learning strategies"
    C. "I should also address affective behavior in the clinical course's SLOs"
    D. "SLOs assist students to construct knowledge based on expectations"

19. An experienced nurse educator is assessing a novice nurse educator's classroom teaching. The novice nurse educator uses PowerPoint, automated response system questions, and a short interactive group activity. The novice nurse educator is asked a question by the student and states, "I think that happens because of the fluid overload." A suggestion the expert nurse educator should make on her appraisal form is:

    A. Do not use so many different strategies in a 2-hour class
    B. Try not to use PowerPoint at all, if possible
    C. For questions for which you are unsure of the answer, tell students you will look it up
    D. Have students write their questions down on paper and submit them at break

20. An experienced nurse educator is asking senior nursing students to write their own student learning outcomes (SLOs) for an independent study course. All the students must complete some type of quality-improvement project. By asking the student to write the SLOs, the nurse educator is advocating which educational philosophy:

    A. Emancipatory
    B. Realism
    C. Behaviorism
    D. Constructivism

21. Some of the considerations against predetermining student learning outcomes (SLOs) include:

    A. Students may be overwhelmed by them initially and become discouraged
    B. SLOs normally set the learning achievements at minimal competencies
    C. SLOs restrict learning and all learning cannot be observed
    D. Students do not understand their purpose and therefore do not use them

22. A nurse educator is having difficulty communicating with the nurse administrator and asks a seasoned nurse educator for assistance. The senior nurse educator should advise her peer to:

    A. Attend a leadership conference so she better understands the nurse administrator's role
    B. Have an alternative career plan in case it is needed
    C. Address the nurse administrator directly about the issue
    D. Use a personality-type indicator to better understands her reaction

23. A novice nurse educator states that she does not go over the pathophysiology of an illness because the students had a pathophysiology course as a prerequisite. The seasoned nurse educator explains that by providing a short review the novice is actually enacting which step of Gagne's conditions of learning?

    A. Gaining attention
    B. Providing feedback
    C. Activating past learning
    D. Enhancing retention

24. A new nurse educator indicates that cannot seem to "cover" all his material in class. A suggestion that may help would be to:

    A. See whether the other medical–surgical courses teach similar information
    B. Look at the educational unit's curriculum matrix to identify a place where more content could be added and move content
    C. Instruct the students to read the book for information that was not covered
    D. Develop a lesson plan with times and content that match your student learning outcomes

25. A student comes for a test review and states that he now understands that listening to recorded lectures assists him better than just taking notes in class. The student is demonstrating:

    A. Critical thinking
    B. Decision making
    C. Self-efficacy
    D. Metacognition

26. A student is developing a concept map for a patient and explains that the medication that the patient has been given is linked to the observed manifestation and is not part of disease process. The student is demonstrating:

    A. Critical thinking
    B. Decision making
    C. Self-efficacy
    D. Metacognition

27. Which assignment is most likely to elicit critical thinking in students?
    A. Participating in a Jeopardy game about ethical concepts
    B. Developing a group project about a case study
    C. Participating in a debate
    D. Do a literature review about a clinical issue

28. The nurse educator who teaches mental health nursing reads a student's journal, which describes a fictitious terrorist attack on a nursing school that supposedly was relayed to her by a patient. The nurse educator recalls that the patient whom the student was with was depressed and catatonic, and it is unlikely the patient relayed such a vivid, lengthy description of an event. The nurse educator should:
    A. Call the student in and question her about the meaning of the description
    B. Hold the journal in confidence
    C. Call the police about a possible upcoming event
    D. Notify campus administrators of the unusual description

29. A student in the back of the class is disturbing the others by fidgeting, trying to talk with them, and moving constantly. Last week the nurse educator spoke to the student about this behavior and it has continued. The next step should be:
    A. Give the student a warning for unprofessional behavior
    B. Address it in class
    C. Move the student
    D. Ask the student to leave class

30. The novice educator states that after her course is over she will fix all the things that she would like fixed for the following semester. Good advice to provide her would be to:
    A. Trend things for more than one semester, then fix them
    B. Fix things as you go
    C. Things that need to be fixed can be done at the semester's end
    D. Do not fix too much, students adjust

31. The nurse educator has heard that students have the test banks to all the books. The class grades reflect an increase in scores over the past two tests. The best action for the nurse educator is to:
    A. Give all the tests over
    B. Tell the students she is aware of the stolen test
    C. Make a faculty-made test for the next one
    D. Consult the college grade appeal committee

32. A good example of evidence-based teaching practice would be:
    A. Using an automated response system for answering questions
    B. Using high-stakes test results to remediate at-risk students
    C. Providing students with test plans based on the NCLEX-RN plan
    D. Use repeated simulation events for concept learning

33. A nurse educator is trying to adapt her teaching style to promote deep learning. A good method to use to do this would be to incorporate:

A. Using drug cards to categorize medications
B. Playing Jeopardy to understand nursing's historical figures
C. Reviewing the pathophysiology of a disease before the symptomology using a task trainer
D. Providing a vignette about a patient and asking for the top three nursing interventions

34. A clinical nurse educator demonstrates poor professional boundaries when he:

A. Assists the students in the clinical learning environment to prioritize their tasks
B. Tells the students that "book way" is what they should follow
C. Takes them to the cafeteria to study when the census is low
D. Gives the students his cell phone number for emergency use only

35. A nurse educator is up for her midpoint review and is marginally satisfactory. The nurse administrator provides her with constructive advice when she states:

A. "Do not write any more grants because the two that you wrote were not funded"
B. "Submit publications to local newspapers"
C. "Try to just get elected to departmental committees and do not worry about university committees"
D. "Decrease the overload that you are teaching and concentrate that time on scholarship"

36. The best method for a nurse faculty member to demonstrate Boyer's scholarship of integration is to:

A. Develop an interprofessional simulation experience about cultural competence
B. Become a consultant for schools applying for National League of Nursing's Center of Excellence Award
C. Examine whether grouping test questions in a content area increases medical–surgical student's test scores
D. Develop a value-clarification exercise that can be used with large class groups

37. The best method for a nurse faculty member to demonstrate Boyer's scholarship of application is:

A. Develop an interprofessional simulation experience about cultural competence
B. Become a consultant for schools applying for National League of Nursing's Center of Excellence Award
C. Examine whether grouping test questions in a content area increases medical–surgical student's test scores
D. Develop a value-clarification exercise that can be used with large class groups

38. The best method for a nurse faculty member to demonstrate Boyer's scholarship of discovery is:

    A. Develop an interprofessional simulation experience about cultural competence
    B. Become a consultant for schools applying for National League of Nursing's Center of Excellence Award
    C. Examine whether grouping test questions in a content area increases medical–surgical student's test scores
    D. Develop a value-clarification exercise that can be used with large class groups

39. The best method for a nurse faculty member to demonstrate Boyer's scholarship of teaching is:

    A. Develop an interprofessional simulation experience about cultural competence
    B. Become a consultant for schools applying for National League of Nursing's Center of Excellence Award
    C. Examine whether grouping test questions in a content area increases medical–surgical student's test scores
    D. Develop a value-clarification exercise that can be used with large class groups

40. A test item had the following statistics:

    $p = 55\%$. The correct answer is B.

	A	B	C	D
Point biserial	−0.7	0.32	0.09	−0.12
Percentage	6	31	14	7

    The nurse educator should:

    A. Revise distractor A
    B. Revise distractor B
    C. Revise distractor C
    D. Revise distractor D

41. Which of the following best demonstrates a nurse educator using role modeling in a practice setting?

    A. Sharing how many years she has been a nurse and how to maintain a "thick skin"
    B. Determining whether one student's medication calculations are correct on a whiteboard for the clinical group to see
    C. Sharing in postconference a medication error the nurse educator made as a novice nurse
    D. Sharing an example of a practice error a colleague had made while providing patient care

42. Which of the following verbs should be used when writing instructional objectives at the comprehension level of Bloom's taxonomy?

    A. Compare, contrast, and critique
    B. Design, create, and implement
    C. Examine, comprehend, and analyze
    D. Review, summarize, and explain

43. Which of the following activities is an example of active learning?

    A. Attend a lecture at a local conference
    B. Answer NCLEX-style alternative-format questions on the computer
    C. Have the educator demonstrate the correct way to perform a psychomotor skill
    D. Debrief a simulation experience of a small clinical group

44. It has been brought to the nurse educator's attention that a student is performing questionable safe nursing practice in clinical. Which of the following would be a priority for the nurse educator to do?

    A. Notify the program administrator for the student's immediate dismissal from the program
    B. Document the pattern of marginal performance or unsatisfactory behavior in a formative evaluation and tell the student quite clearly what he or she needs to do to improve
    C. Ascertain whether the student has passed the basic clinical competency skills
    D. Ask the student's friends whether something is going on in clinical you should know about

45. Which of the following is an example of a well-written student learning outcome?

    A. Discussing various methods of implementing and prioritizing care of a group of people
    B. Identifying nursing diagnosis to prevent disease transmission
    C. Summarizing key points of a PowerPoint presentation on respiratory distress
    D. Utilizing selected aspects of the nursing process to provide care to the geriatric population

46. A novice nurse educator is discussing how to measure his teaching effectiveness with his mentor. Which of the following statements indicates that the novice nurse educator understands this concept?

    A. "If the learners met the course objectives, my teaching was effective"
    B. "Anonymous computer evaluations are biased and are an unreliable assessment of my teaching effectiveness"
    C. "All the students passed NCLEX and my course; my teaching was effective"
    D. "Multiple methods will be needed to determine whether my teaching was effective"

47. A new educator was texting her boyfriend in class while presenting her lecture to the students. This is an example of:

    A. Incivility
    B. Bullying
    C. Good use of time
    D. Multitasking

48. Which of the following demonstrates the best way to facilitate learning for a diverse group of learners?

    A. Utilize a variety of teaching techniques to best meet the needs of the learners
    B. Use a teaching strategy that best meets the instructor's style
    C. Match instructors with learners from the same culture
    D. Use YouTube videos

49. Which of the following is an example of role-playing in the classroom?

    A. Have the students perform a song that demonstrates blood flow through the heart
    B. Give students a question and have them act out the answer
    C. Have a student demonstrate a therapeutic communication response to another student who is exhibiting signs of depression
    D. Have the faculty member name a disease process and have the students choose responses that are consistent with that disease process

50. Which of the following statements are true about utilizing a flipped classroom and its purpose in education?

    A. It enables the faculty member to have a day off
    B. It cuts down on the faculty member's prep work and shifts it to the student
    C. It enables the student to take charge of his or her learning by researching a clinical situation and presenting it to the class
    D. It is like postconference when students find an interesting case and present it to the class for credit

51. Which of the following statements is true about using "gaming" in the classroom?

    A. It is effective for affective and cognitive learning
    B. It makes the classroom fun and more course content will get covered
    C. The students don't like it, it makes them feel juvenile
    D. It enables the faculty member to keep better control of all students in the classroom

52. Which of the following statements is correct about problems with the use of simulation experiences? (Select all that apply.)

    A. It is very expensive to implement
    B. Simulation works best when a small group of learners is involved in the simulation experience
    C. It doesn't really help prepare the students for the "real world"
    D. Learners can practice in a safe environment

53. The chair of the education committee is known as a transformational leader. This indicates that the leader:

    A. Develops criteria within the committee to accomplish a task
    B. Provides opportunities for the committee to make choices
    C. Directs the flow of the committee to complete objectives and tasks
    D. Energizes the committee to perform with his or her vision and guides change through inspiration

54. Which of the following is the best way to increase the facilitation of knowledge when building learning experiences into a curriculum?

   A. Experiential learning
   B. Reviewing procedural knowledge
   C. Presenting information from simple to complex methods
   D. Provide exemplars

55. A nurse educator is teaching an online course. One of the learners has posted a response to a discussion board question that reflects a negative opinion about the profession of nursing. Other learners in the class post comments agreeing with the first opinion. What should the nurse educator do?

   A. Do nothing and let all the learners "speak their piece" and vent their feelings
   B. Courteously question the first learner's post and open further dialogue about the topic giving illustrations of other possible conclusions
   C. Post evidence-based research to prove the learner is grossly misinformed
   D. Remind the learner that negative posts are inappropriate and will be deleted

56. A nurse educator understands that a visual leaner would prefer which of the following activities?

   A. Read a book, then write an essay
   B. Perform a skill in the simulation laboratory
   C. Listen to a book on CD and write a report
   D. Watch a movie and then discuss it with the class

57. Which of the following objectives is written at Bloom's highest taxonomy level?

   A. Define *homeostasis* in the body
   B. Explain how the body tries to maintain homeostasis
   C. Contrast homeostasis intracellularly and extracellularly
   D. Demonstrate how homeostasis in the renin–angiotensin system works

58. Which of the following behaviors exhibited by faculty might be considered uncivil by student learners in the classroom?

   A. Supporting and valuing content taught by other faculty
   B. Telling the students you do not know the answer to their question but will find it out by next class
   C. Coming unprepared for class and "winging" the content since you taught the course before
   D. Starting class late to answer student questions about an upcoming exam

59. Which of the following statements is true about the role of mentoring?

   A. Mentors should be mandated to new educators upon hiring into a new faculty role
   B. Sending new faculty to conferences in the hopes of their networking and finding a mentor is a great way to pair up novice faculty with mentors
   C. A mentor should attend the mentee's classes regular and provide critiques of the novice educator's teaching style
   D. A key component in mentoring is that the mentor should be accessible both physically and emotionally for the novice educator

60. A learner reports that another learner cheated by writing the arterial blood gas values on her desk before the test. The best action for the nurse educator to take first would be:

    A. Verify the story with another learner who was sitting close by
    B. Take a picture of the desk in question
    C. Ask the learner who was being accused
    D. Tell the learner who is reporting that there is no proof

61. The admission and progression committee in the nursing educational unit is revising the progression standards to improve program outcomes. Which of the following is not a criterion for progression in the nursing program?

    A. A minimum grade of 80% is required for nursing and science courses
    B. Learners may repeat a nursing course one time
    C. Junior-level status must be achieved to begin the nursing program
    D. Learners must achieve the national standard average on the standardized test

62. A novice nurse educator states that she evaluated a learner doing a procedure for the second time and the learner corrected her first mistakes but took a long time to do the procedure. The nurse educator states, "By the performance of this learner I am not sure learning has taken place." From this statement, one can deduce that the novice nurse educator subscribes to the learning theory of:

    A. Behaviorism
    B. Cognitivism
    C. Constructivism
    D. Realism

63. Social forces are increasing the accountability of institutions of higher education. One of the main social forces that propels this change, which is demanding accountability in outcomes achieved, is:

    A. Increase in college-educated citizens
    B. Funding
    C. Accessibility
    D. Legal sanctions

64. After administering an exam, the nurse educator is reviewing the item analysis for each of the multiple-choice questions. One question yielded the following statistics for the items:

Point Biserial = 0. 43	Correct Answer = A		Total Group = 57%	
Distractor Analysis	A	B	C	D
Point Biserial	0.43	−0.15	0.00	−0.48
Frequency	57%	23%	0%	20%

Based on this analysis, what action should be taken by the nurse educator?

    A. Revise distractor A
    B. Revise distractor B
    C. Revise distractor C
    D. Revise distractor D

65. The nurse educator intentionally involves the learners in a group activity without providing them with specific directions for accomplishing the task. The learners are left to their own ingenuity and creativity to reach the learning outcome. This type of learning is referred to as:

    A. Inquiry-based learning
    B. Critical thinking activity
    C. Goal-directed learning
    D. Problem-based learning

66. When considering level outcomes, the educators must ensure that they progress logically to eventually reflect the:

    A. Philosophy of the parent institution
    B. Outcomes of the program
    C. Demographics of the community
    D. Beliefs of the faculty

67. Review of an item on a test reveals the following statistics:

Point Biserial = −0.13	Correct Answer = D		Total Group = 82%	
Distractor Analysis	A	B	C	D
Point Biserial	0.02	0.19	0.01	−0.13
Frequency	12%	5%	1%	82%

The likely cause for this frequency distribution is:

    A. Higher scoring learners answered the question correctly
    B. Higher scoring learners answered the question incorrectly
    C. Lower scoring learners answered the question incorrectly
    D. The distractors show clear discrimination

68. One phase of service learning is reflection. Use of reflection is important for learners because it fosters the development of:

    A. Cultural competency
    B. Cognitive interpretation
    C. Kinesthetic learning
    D. Inductive reasoning

69. An example of learner misconduct that can be considered an annoying act and should be addressed as soon as possible is:

    A. Stealing a test
    B. Watching YouTube videos in class and laughing out loud
    C. Cheating on an exam
    D. Cyberbullying

70. The chair of the nursing department has had complaints from learners that a novice instructor does not finish the material because she is using too many slides. The best initial response by the leader would be:
    A. Speak to the novice educator about the complaints
    B. Observe the instructor delivering a lecture
    C. Ask the learners to speak directly to the instructor
    D. Show the novice educator how to cut down the information for each class

71. Item analysis of an exam question revealed the following statistics:

Point Biserial = 0. 40	Correct Answer = A		Total Group = 72%	
Distractor Analysis	A	B	C	D
Point Biserial	0.40	0.03	0.04	0.12
Frequency	72%	6%	15%	7%

How should the nurse educator interpret these results?
    A. This question needs to be revised as too many learners answered it correctly
    B. High-scoring learners answered the question correctly
    C. Lower scoring learners answered the question correctly
    D. There is inadequate discrimination of the distractors

72. The novice educator is asking her mentor for an example of experiential learning. The best example to illustrate the concept of experiential learning is when learners:
    A. Develop a community needs assessment related to chronic conditions
    B. Practice taking blood pressures on shoppers at the mall one Saturday
    C. Develop an in-service presentation for a grammar school class about hypertension
    D. Develop a group project about hypertension

73. A novice educator is asking her mentor what would be the best learning strategy to use to teach diabetes in her adult health course. The mentor should tell the mentee that the best learning strategies are those that:
    A. Keep the learners involved
    B. Relate to the desired outcomes
    C. Can be easily evaluated
    D. Are comfortable for a novice educator

74. When developing or changing the curriculum, the leader's most appropriate action is to:
    A. Usher the faculty through the process, handing out tasks so that resistance is decreased and time is saved
    B. Set up a meeting with each faculty member in order to decrease group resistance
    C. Give individuals the opportunity to express their opinions and concerns in ongoing meetings
    D. Remember to remain positive in all communications about the proposed new curriculum

75. The nurse educator is arranging a promotional dossier and wants to include an exemplar of the scholarship of teaching. The best evidence to include would be to use:

    A. The class standardized testing scores that are above normal
    B. Individual learner projects that received an A
    C. Course evaluations in which the educator scored above normal
    D. The syllabus of a newly developed course that integrates the faculty's research into the course

76. The following statistics were recorded on an item analysis of a test question:

Point Biserial = 0. 04	Correct Answer = C		Total Group = 61%	
Distractor Analysis	A	B	C	D
Point Biserial	−0.26	0.18	0.04	0.02
Frequency	18%	20%	61%	1%

    These statistics indicate which of the following?

    A. There was high discrimination of the distractors
    B. Lower scoring learners answered the question correctly
    C. The distractors are too difficult
    D. There is inadequate discrimination and one of the items is flawed

77. A learning activity that promotes positive interdependence among learners is:

    A. Clicker response questions
    B. Debates
    C. Peer evaluations
    D. A cooperative learning project

78. An experienced nurse educator who has been teaching traditional under-graduate nursing students is now assigned to teach second-degree learners. Her evaluations are much lower than usual. Which of the following syllabus modifications would be appropriate to tailor her teaching toward this group of learners?

    A. Increase observation clinical hours
    B. Decrease objective testing
    C. Increase reflective journaling
    D. Decrease number of care plan assignments

79. Which of the following objectives is written at Bloom's highest taxonomy level?

    A. Define *homeostasis* in the body
    B. Explain how the body tries to maintain homeostasis
    C. Contrast homeostasis intracellularly and extracellularly
    D. Demonstrate how homeostasis in the renin–angiotensin system works

80. The novice nurse educator would like to change a course in the curriculum. The best question to be asked by the members of the curriculum committee is:

    A. "Does the new course duplicate any material in other courses?"
    B. "Who will teach the new course?"
    C. "What are the student expectations for the course?"
    D. "Was this change based on trended data?"

81. Newly hired nurse educators should expect their orientations to include all of the following EXCEPT:

    A. The rights and responsibilities of faculty
    B. The organization's role in creating an enhancing environment
    C. Teaching methodologies to be used in the classroom
    D. Overview of the curriculum

82. An item analysis of an exam question revealed the following statistics:

Point Biserial = 0. 31	Correct Answer = C		Total Group = 35%	
Distractor Analysis	A	B	C	D
Point Biserial	0.31	−0.41	0.26	−0.02
Frequency	35%	58%	6%	1%

    The nurse educator interprets these results to mean which of the following?

    A. Learners who scored lower on the exam chose the correct answer
    B. Learners who scored higher on the exam chose the incorrect answer
    C. The point biserial indicates good discrimination among the distractors
    D. The item difficulty for the correct answer indicates the question should be revised

83. A clinical nurse educator asks her mentor what she should do about a clinical issue that is occurring in the simulation laboratory during the exam time. Learners are asking clinical questions when they are being evaluated for skill performance. The advice of the mentor that is most helpful is:

    A. "Tell learners they can ask questions when they are done"
    B. "Allow learners to take a break during the activity to ask questions and then resume"
    C. "Review the expectations with the learners and the outcomes that are being evaluated"
    D. "Tell the learners that they will fail if they continue to ask questions"

84. Nurse educators are undertaking a curriculum revision. The nurse educators want to align the curriculum with current practice issues. The most effective method to keep up to date with practice issues is to:

   A. Buy a subscription to a peer-reviewed clinical journal for each curriculum committee member
   B. Do a practice analysis every 3 years at the clinical facilities used for learner experiences
   C. Survey alumni of the program about their transition to work and identify deficits.
   D. Have a faculty liaison who participates in the practice counsel at each affiliate clinical facility

85. A nurse educator is developing a professional nursing role course for second-degree learners and is deciding on a learning activity to meet the outcome of professional socialization. The best learning activity for this outcome would be:

   A. Incorporate a guest speaker who is in a specialist nursing role
   B. Develop a group project about nursing roles
   C. Increase clinical hours so the learners can observe nurses
   D. Have the learners join the student nurse organization

86. An item analysis for a 50-item test showed these statistics:

   Mean score = 77

   KR-20 = 0.68

   Standard deviation (SD) = 2.9

   These findings indicate which of the following?

   A. There were not enough items on the test
   B. Items were poorly written and do not discriminate
   C. The test is reliable and shows clear discrimination
   D. There were too many easy questions on the test

87. An example of a provider-directed, provider-paced educational activity is a(n):

   A. Seminar
   B. Journal article
   C. On-demand video
   D. All of the above

88. An example of a provider-directed, learner-paced educational activity is a(n):

   A. Live webcast
   B. On-demand video
   C. Seminar
   D. All of the above

89. An academic nursing unit is interviewing for a medical–surgical instructor and is having difficulty finding applicants because of all of the following reasons EXCEPT:

   A. Salary
   B. Overqualification
   C. Lack of scholarly production
   D. Demands of academia

90. Lewin's change theory is characterized by the presence of:
    A. The motivation and capacity for change
    B. Driving and restraining forces
    C. Self-efficacy
    D. Perceived control over opportunities

91. The department chair of nursing is aware that the percentage of tenured nursing faculty is lower than in many other academic departments. To increase the number of tenured faculty, the most effective thing the department chair should do is:
    A. Establish faculty classes on academic progression and leadership
    B. Assist faculty to develop long-term and short-term goals
    C. Encourage faculty to shadow a tenured professor in another department
    D. Mentor faculty about developing an effective academic portfolio

92. An item analysis for a 25-item multiple-choice test administered to 60 learners showed these statistics:

    Mean score = 20.32

    KR-20 = 0.29

    $SD = 5.67$

    The findings indicate this about the test:
    A. The test is reliable and shows clear discrimination
    B. More questions should be added to the test
    C. The questions were most likely of average difficulty
    D. Scoring was subjective

93. The item analysis revealed the following statistics for a multiple-choice question:

Point Biserial = 0. 22	Correct Answer = C		Total Group = 81%	
Distractor Analysis	A	B	C	D
Point Biserial	−0.45	−0.01	0.22	0.26
Frequency	12%	1%	81%	6%

    On the basis of these statistics, the nurse educator should do which of the following when using this item on future exams?
    A. Nothing, as the point biserial is just a little low but within acceptable range
    B. Revise distractor A
    C. Revise distractor B
    D. Revise distractor D

94. A clinical nurse educator tells the department chair that a learner may fail for consistent low-level clinical performance and it is 1 week before the end of the semester. A priority inquiry question from the department chair to the clinical nurse educator should be:
    A. "Would you like another faculty member to assess the learner?"
    B. "Do you have formative evaluations completed?"
    C. "What does the learner do that is below expected competency?"
    D. "Is this the learner's second course failure?"

95. Which statement by a learner should alert the nurse educator to a possible learning disability?

 A. "I have never been given such low grades before and I study the same way"
 B. "I read the book and PowerPoint slides before class as I am told to do"
 C. "I do extra questions every night to practice and it helps"
 D. "I understand the material in class but cannot pick the right test answer"

96. The members of a curriculum committee discuss the manner in which learners address the faculty and respond to learning experiences. This type of value-laden discussion of behavior is part of the program's:

 A. Operational curriculum
 B. Illegitimate curriculum
 C. Hidden curriculum
 D. Null curriculum

97. Which of the following are not protected under copyright law?

 A. Literary works
 B. Sound recordings
 C. Recorded choreographic works
 D. Nonrecorded choreographic works

98. A nurse educator has completed a funded study about the effectiveness of the use of podcasts for nursing students with an auditory learning style preference. Which of the following is the most effective way to share results of this study?

 A. Publish in a nursing education journal
 B. Present at national meeting of nurse educators
 C. Present at statewide meeting of educators in higher education
 D. Send the report of the findings to the funding agency

99. Review of an item on a test reveals the following statistics:

Point Biserial = –0.04	Correct Answer = B		Total Group = 82%	
Distractor Analysis	A	B	C	D
Point Biserial	0.02	–0.04	–0.01	0.04
Frequency	1%	82%	1%	16%

The report indicates item D should be reviewed. The likely rationale for this suggestion is:

 A. Higher scoring learners answered the question correctly
 B. The distractor was not clear
 C. Lower scoring learners answered the question incorrectly
 D. The distractors show clear discrimination

100. The following multiple-choice question is written at which level of Bloom's taxonomy?

The nurse understands that the patient needs more teaching when the patient states:

1. "I should take two of my hypertensive pills if I forget one the day before"
2. "I should rest if I feel lightheaded"
3. "I should call my primary care practitioner if I feel too weak to walk"
4. "I should increase my fluids to 8 to 10 glasses of water each day"

A. Understanding
B. Comprehension
C. Application
D. Evaluation

COMPREHENSIVE EXAM ANSWERS AND RATIONALES

1. The novice nurse educator understands the job market correctly when she states:

A. **"The job I choose should depend on my degree and organizational fit"—YES, this should be the highest consideration for a career choice.**
B. "I should choose a job as as soon as possible because a lot of people are graduating"—NO, nurse educators are in demand.
C. "The job I choose may not be secure because of the current market"—NO, nurse educators are in demand.
D. "The education of nurses is moving back into the hospital setting as a result of residencies"—NO, residency programs supplement academic education not replace it.

2. Certification in a specialty is done by professionals in order to:

A. Be compliant with regulatory bodies—NO, this is not always needed.
B. Establish licensure—NO, certification and licensure are many times different and come from different regulatory agencies.
C. **Develop better consumer outcomes—YES, expert practitioners are more likely to facilitate better outcomes.**
D. Verify continuing education—NO, certifications may add to educational compliances but that is not their intent.

3. An educational unit is interviewing candidates for nurse administrator. In order to enact a shared governance system the recruitment committee should include:

A. Several administrators and faculty from various departments—NO, this is a hierarchical committee.
B. A community person along with nursing faculty—NO, interviews are usually not public.
C. Tenured nurse faculty and faculty who teach prerequisite courses—NO, nontenured faculty should have a voice.
D. **Students and faculty from various disciplines—YES, students are an important factor in shared governance.**

4. A student discusses his test anxiety with the nurse educator and the student expresses understanding when he states:

A. My anxiety is not bad because I can sleep most of the night—NO, anxiety does not always manifest in insomnia.

B. **A little anxiety is a motivation to study—YES, excessive anxiety is not beneficial but a little can be motivating.**

C. Many students have palpitations during the test—NO, this is not normal.

D. If I take a double dose of my anxiety medication I can think better on the test—NO, self-medicating is never a good idea.

5. Boyer's model of scholarship includes all of the following in the scholarship of discovery EXCEPT:

A. Research based—NO, scholarship can be research.

B. Peer reviewed—NO, it should include peer-reviewed publications.

C. Manuscript development—NO, it should include manuscript development.

D. **Teaching innovation—YES, this comes under teaching scholarship.**

6. The novice nurse educator needs more understanding when he states:

A. "I will categorize my test questions according to the NCLEX test plan"—NO, this is a correct planning technique.

B. "My test questions should reflect the content that is discussed in class"—NO, this is correct.

C. "My test questions can be mapped to the Quality and Safety Education for Nurses (QSEN) criteria"—NO, this is a good technique to use.

D. **"I should use test bank questions because they will be more reliable than ones I make"—YES, this is not necessarily true.**

7. A new academic nurse educator needs further understanding of execution of the role when she states:

A. "I should use the syllabus to write down all my expectations"—NO, this is correct, the syllabus should be clear about expectations.

B. "If I do not care for the textbook I will change it next semester"—NO, this is correct, textbooks should not be changed during the semester.

C. **"I think it is better to use a red pen to correct care plans for effect"—YES, red marks are not recommended, they can be demeaning.**

D. "I provide the class with breaks every hour"—NO, this is correct, frequent breaks help learning.

8. The nurse administrator notices that the attrition rate is rising each year. The admission criteria are the same. The only difference is that the biology department has made the anatomy and physiology course specific for prenursing students. The best way to approach this dilemma in an academic setting would be to:

   A. Meet with the chair of the biology department and explain that biology faculty are not rigorous—NO, this will cause friction between departments.
   B. Ask the nursing admissions committee to raise the overall admission grade point average—NO, this will include all prerequisite courses and other disciplines have not changed.
   C. Ask the college administrator to take the specialty biology courses off the books—NO, this will cause friction.
   D. **Review the trend and increase the science grade point average needed— YES, this will focus the change where it is needed.**

9. A nurse educator is in the planning stages for teaching his first online course. He is concerned that students may not understand the course requirements and assignments. One strategy he can use that is interactive and would permit discussion is:

   A. Voice-over PowerPoints—NO, this is not interactive.
   B. **Webinars—YES, this would allow interaction and discussion between the learners and educator.**
   C. Podcasts—NO, this is not interactive.
   D. YouTube videos—NO, this is not interactive.

10. An experienced faculty member is explaining to a novice why she still uses lecture as her primary teaching strategy. What statement by the faculty member would require the novice's mentor to intervene?

    A. "I am able to cover all my content when using this strategy"—NO, this is correct.
    B. "Learners generally prefer lecture over other methods"—NO, this is correct; most learners are used to lecture from previous experience.
    C. "Lecture allows me to identify important concepts for the learners"—NO, this is correct.
    D. **"The learners develop higher level thinking when listening to lectures"—YES, lecture is a passive teaching strategy that does not promote higher level learning.**

11. A graduate nurse educator student has written a discussion board post about the benefits of assigning readings for students. What statement indicates that she is accurate with her post?

    A. "Reading assignments are necessary for learners to identify important concepts"—NO, educators can assist learners to identify important concepts during lecture or other active learning strategies.
    B. **"Students may have difficulty learning from reading assignments"— YES, many students are unable to complete all readings and have difficulty identifying key points.**
    C. "Reading is an active learning strategy with many benefits"—NO, reading is a passive strategy.
    D. "Most learners prefer reading assignments to sitting in lecture"—NO, there is no evidence to this effect.

12. An educator is planning her course assignments for the semester. When deciding whether to make a research paper a small-group assignment or an individual assignment, it is important to consider that:

    A. Learners generally prefer group assignments—NO, this is not correct.
    B. Group assignments allow each learner to be graded individually—NO, with group assignments, learners usually receive a group grade.
    C. **Research papers can be very time consuming to read and grade—YES, papers are a significant time commitment for the learners to write and educators to read and grade; individual paper assignments do not lend themselves well to use in larger classes.**
    D. Written assignments are the best measure of student learning—NO, there is no evidence to this effect.

13. A nurse educator is planning to have a skills check-off day for her fundamental students. What method would best lend itself to use with a large number of learners?

    A. **Return demonstration—YES, this is most effective for evaluating skills acquisition, but it is still time consuming.**
    B. Simulation—NO, this works best with small groups of learners.
    C. Case studies—NO, this is not effective in evaluating skills acquisition.
    D. Games—NO, it may be difficult to evaluate individual student learning with games.

14. A faculty group interviews four candidates for an instructor position. The group decides to hire the person with intensive care unit (ICU) experience. After the new faculty member is there for a while she tells them that she is really not comfortable doing clinical in the medical ICU because she has just worked at a step-down care facility. The nurse administrator discusses the misrepresentation with her and classifies it as:

    A. **Incivility—YES, misrepresentating yourself is a form of incivility.**
    B. Slander—NO, this is not against another person.
    C. Tort—NO, this is not a criminal act.
    D. Perjury—NO, this is not lying under oath.

15. A program learning outcome states that the learner will demonstrate cultural competence. The best assessment of the learner meeting this program learning outcome would be:

    A. A paper on the fundamentals of nursing course describing pain reactions of a patient in a different culture—NO, this may assess a course outcome in a beginning course.
    B. A concept map in the first adult health course integrating cultural preferences—NO, this assesses cultural knowledge in a course that is not at an upper level.
    C. An interview with a childbearing woman of another culture or living an alternative lifestyle in the women's health course—NO, this assignment does not deal with a generalized population.
    D. **A clinical evaluation in the senior capstone course that is satisfactory for cultural competence—YES, this is an end assessment and cultural competence is demonstrated.**

16. The curriculum committee members are leveling student learning outcomes (SLOs) for interprofessional collaboration. An appropriate first-level SLO would be:

    A. **Understand the importance of interprofessional collaboration—YES, in Bloom's taxonomy this is the lowest level verb.**
    B. Discuss interprofessional collaboration with another health professional—NO, this is a higher level verb on Bloom's taxonomy and often placed under analysis.
    C. Interact with a different disciplined health professional about a patient issue—NO, this is application.
    D. Analyze scope of practice for different health professionals in a case study—NO, this is analysis.

17. The curriculum committee members are levelling student learning outcomes (SLOs) for cultural competence. An appropriate second-level SLO would be:

    A. **Interact with a person from a different culture—YES, this is application.**
    B. Describe the health care mores of another culture—NO, this is remembering.
    C. Critique the differences between two Latino cultures—NO, this is evaluating.
    D. Analyze a different culture through an unfolding case study—NO, this is analyzing.

18. A novice nurse educator needs additional knowledge in curriculum development when he states:

    A. "Developing student learning outcomes (SLOs) assists in the evaluative process"—NO, this is true, evaluative mechanisms should relate back to the SLOs.
    B. "SLOs are needed to direct the teaching–learning strategies"—NO, this is true, the SLOs should direct the strategies used.
    C. "I should also address affective behavior in the clinical course's SLOs"—NO, this is true; affective behavior and professionalism are important elements in nursing.
    D. **"SLOs assist students to construct knowledge based on expectations"—YES, SLOs represent behavioralism, not constructivism, because learning is preset.**

19. An experienced nurse educator is assessing a novice nurse educator's classroom teaching. The novice nurse educator uses PowerPoint, automated response system questions, and a short interactive group activity. The novice nurse educator is asked a question by the student and states, "I think that happens because of the fluid overload." A suggestion the expert nurse educator should make on her appraisal form is:

    A. Do not use so many different strategies in a 2-hour class—NO, this is appropriate.
    B. Try not to use PowerPoint at all, if possible—NO, PowerPoint is a useful tool.
    C. **For questions for which you are unsure of the answer, tell students you will look it up—YES, do not guess or pretend knowledge.**
    D. Have students write their questions down on paper and submit them at break—NO, when possible, questions should be answered when asked.

20. An experienced nurse educator is asking senior nursing students to write their own student learning outcomes (SLOs) for an independent study course. All the students must complete some type of quality-improvement project. By asking the student to write the SLOs, the nurse educator is advocating which educational philosophy:

    A. Emancipatory—NO, this has to do with learning environment equality.
    B. Realism—NO, this has to do with empirical knowledge development.
    C. Behaviorism—NO, this has to do with predetermining the learning objectives.
    D. **Constructivism—YES, students construct their own knowledge.**

21. Some of the considerations against predetermining student learning outcomes (SLOs) include:

    A. Students may be overwhelmed by them initially and become discouraged— NO, students should not be overwhelmed if SLOs are explained.
    B. SLOs normally set the learning achievements at minimal competencies— NO, SLOs set the benchmark at the expected level of achievement.
    C. **SLOs restrict learning and all learning cannot be observed—YES.**
    D. Students do not understand their purpose and therefore do not use them—NO, students are acclimated to SLOs and their purpose in higher education.

22. A nurse educator is having difficulty communicating with the nurse administrator and asks a seasoned nurse educator for assistance. The senior nurse educator should advise her peer to:

    A. Attend a leadership conference so she better understands the nurse administrator's role—NO, this is not useful for her nurse educator position.
    B. Have an alternative career plan in case it is needed—NO, this is not a good resolution.
    C. Address the nurse administrator directly about the issue—NO, this may not be comfortable for her personality type.
    D. **Use a personality-type indicator to better understands her reaction— YES, knowing personality type may assist with communication and conflict resolution.**

23. A novice nurse educator states that she does not go over the pathophysiology of an illness because the students had a pathophysiology course as a prerequisite. The seasoned nurse educator explains that by providing a short review the novice is actually enacting which step of Gagne's conditions of learning?

    A. Gaining attention—NO, this is the first step of Gagne's conditions of learning.
    B. Providing feedback—NO, this takes place after content is presented.
    C. **Activating past learning—YES.**
    D. Enhancing retention—NO, this is the last step in the process.

24. A new nurse educator indicates that he cannot seem to "cover" all his material in class. A suggestion that may help would be to:

    A. See whether the other medical–surgical courses teach similar information—NO, the information may be at a different level.
    B. Look at the educational unit's curriculum matrix to identify a place where more content could be added and move content—NO, this may overload another course.
    C. Instruct the students to read the book for information that was not covered—NO, content should be included in an active environment so students can ask questions.
    D. **Develop a lesson plan with times and content that match your student learning outcomes—YES, this may help the new nurse educator to stay on track with time.**

25. A student comes for a test review and states that he now understands that listening to recorded lectures assists him better than just taking notes in class. The student is demonstrating:

    A. Critical thinking—NO, critical thinking is more about acquiring and linking new knowledge.
    B. Decision making—NO, this has to do with having options to choose from.
    C. Self-efficacy—NO, this demonstrates the ability to complete tasks.
    D. **Metacognition—YES, this executive function enables students to change their learning styles to make themselves successful.**

26. A student is developing a concept map for a patient and explains that the medication that the patient has been given is linked to the observed manifestation and it is not part of disease process. The student is demonstrating:

    A. **Critical thinking—YES, this demonstrates logical reasoning.**
    B. Decision making—NO, this has to do with having options.
    C. Self-efficacy—NO, this has to do with being successful in skill attainment.
    D. Metacognition—NO, this has to do with executive functioning.

27. Which assignment is most likely to elicit critical thinking in students?

    A. Participating in a Jeopardy game about ethical concepts—NO, this is a knowledge-based activity.
    B. Developing a group project about a case study—NO, this does not necessarily use critical thinking skills.
    C. **Participating in a debate—YES, this prompts students to make a logical argument about an issue.**
    D. Do a literature review about a clinical issue—NO, this does not necessarily use critical thinking skills.

28. The nurse educator who teaches mental health nursing reads a student's journal, which describes a fictitious terrorist attack on a nursing school that supposedly was relayed to her by a patient. The nurse educator recalls that the patient whom the student was with was depressed and catatonic, and it is unlikely the patient relayed such a vivid, lengthy description of an event. The nurse educator should:

A. Call the student in and question her about the meaning of the description—NO, the student will probably deny that it is connected to her.

B. Hold the journal in confidence—NO, this is a public threat.

C. **Call the police about a possible upcoming event—YES, the police should investigate the student for any past violations and gun or knife purchases.**

D. Notify campus administrators of the unusual description—NO, this can be done, but the police need to know first.

29. A student in the back of the class is disturbing the others by fidgeting, trying to talk with them, and moving constantly. Last week the nurse educator spoke to the student about this behavior and it has continued. The next step should be:

A. Give the student a warning for unprofessional behavior—NO, this may happen, but changing the environment is first.

B. Address it in class—NO, behaviors should always be corrected privately.

C. **Move the student—YES, fix the environment.**

D. Ask the student to leave class—NO, this will embarrass the student and that is not the goal.

30. The novice educator states that after her course is over she will fix all the things that she would like fixed for the following semester. Good advice to provide her would be to:

A. Trend things for more than one semester, then fix them—NO, things that need to be fixed should be fixed.

B. **Fix things as you go—YES, this way they are fresh in your mind.**

C. Things that need to be fixed can be done at the semester's end—NO, it is easy to forget what needs to be fixed.

D. Do not fix too much, students adjust—NO, they should be fixed if they need to be.

31. The nurse educator has heard that students have the test banks to all the books. The class grades reflect an increase in scores over the past two tests. The best action for the nurse educator is to:

A. Give all the tests over—NO, this will put students who didn't cheat in jeopardy.

B. Tell the students she is aware of the stolen test—NO, this is unprofessional.

C. **Make a faculty-made test for the next one—YES.**

D. Consult the college grade appeal committee—NO, they hear student's appeals.

32. A good example of evidence-based teaching practice would be:

    A. Using an automated response system for answering questions—NO, this is a teaching activity.

    B. Using high-stakes test results to remediate at-risk students—NO, this is an identification of high-risk students.

    C. Providing students with test plans based on the NCLEX-RN plan—NO, this is something that is done to direct the curriculum.

    D. **Use repeated simulation events for concept learning—YES, there is evidence that multiple simulation experiences improve learning.**

33. A nurse educator is trying to adapt her teaching style to promote deep learning. A good method to use to do this would be to incorporate:

    A. Using drug cards to categorize medications—NO, this promotes surface learning and memorization.

    B. Playing Jeopardy to understand nursing's historical figures—NO, this is just factual learning.

    C. **Reviewing the pathophysiology of a disease before the symptomology using a task trainer—YES, this provides past knowledge to link with new knowledge.**

    D. Providing a vignette about a patient and asking for the top three nursing interventions—NO, this is application knowledge.

34. A clinical nurse educator demonstrates poor professional boundaries when he:

    A. Assists the students in the clinical learning environment to prioritize their tasks—NO, this is an appropriate teaching activity.

    B. Tells the students that "book way" is what they should follow—NO, this is an appropriate teaching activity.

    C. **Takes them to the cafeteria to study when the census is low—YES, his job is not didactic and he is impinging on another faculty's responsibility and overstepping his boundaries with the students.**

    D. Gives the students his cell phone number for emergency use only—NO, this is appropriate.

35. A nurse educator is up for her midpoint review and is marginally satisfactory. The nurse administrator provides her with constructive advice when she states:

    A. "Do not write any more grants because the two that you wrote were not funded"—NO, the faculty member should continue to write grants for scholarship.

    B. "Submit publications to local newspapers"—NO, the faculty member should be submitting to peer-reviewed professional journals.

    C. "Try to just get elected to departmental committees and do not worry about university committees"—NO, the faculty members should become a member of the university committee for service.

    D. **"Decrease the overload that you are teaching and concentrate that time on scholarship"—YES, this will assist the faculty to prioritize her career goals.**

36. The best method for a nurse faculty member to demonstrate Boyer's scholarship of integration is to:

   A. **Develop an interprofessional simulation experience about cultural competence—YES, this includes an interdisciplinary learning experience.**
   B. Become a consultant for schools applying for National League of Nursing's Center of Excellence Award—NO, this is application.
   C. Examine whether grouping test questions in a content area increases medical–surgical student's test scores—NO, this is discovery.
   D. Develop a value-clarification exercise that can be used with large class groups—NO, this is teaching.

37. The best method for a nurse faculty member to demonstrate Boyer's scholarship of application is:

   A. Develop an interprofessional simulation experience about cultural competence—NO, this is interdisciplinary learning experience.
   B. **Become a consultant for schools applying for National League of Nursing's Center of Excellence Award—YES, this is applying knowledge to an end user.**
   C. Examine whether grouping test questions in a content area increases medical–surgical student's test scores—NO, this is discovery.
   D. Develop a value-clarification exercise that can be used with large class groups—NO, this is teaching.

38. The best method for a nurse faculty member to demonstrate Boyer's scholarship of discovery is:

   A. Develop an interprofessional simulation experience about cultural competence—NO, this is integration.
   B. Become a consultant for schools applying for National League of Nursing's Center of Excellence Award—NO, this is application.
   C. **Examine whether grouping test questions in a content area increases medical–surgical student's test scores—YES, this is discovery, creating new knowledge.**
   D. Develop a value-clarification exercise that can be used with large class groups—NO, this is teaching.

39. The best method for a nurse faculty member to demonstrate Boyer's scholarship of teaching is:

   A. Develop an interprofessional simulation experience about cultural competence—NO, this is interdisciplinary.
   B. Become a consultant for schools applying for National League of Nursing's Center of Excellence Award—NO, this is application.
   C. Examine whether grouping test questions in a content area increases medical–surgical student's test scores—NO, this is discovery.
   D. **Develop a value-clarification exercise that can be used with large class groups—YES, this is teaching.**

40. A test item had the following statistics:

$p = 55\%$. The correct answer is B.

	A	B	C	D
Point biserial	−0.7	0.32	0.09	−0.12
Percentage	6	31	14	7

The nurse educator should:

A. Revise distractor A—NO, this is a wrong distractor and has a negative point biserial.
B. Revise distractor B—NO, this is the right distractor and has a positive point biserial.
C. **Revise distractor C—YES, this is a wrong distractor and has a positive point biserial.**
D. Revise distractor D—NO, this is a wrong distractor and has a negative point biserial.

41. Which of the following best demonstrates a nurse educator using role-modeling in a practice setting?

A. Sharing how many years she has been a nurse and how to maintain a "thick skin"—NO, this is not role-modeling, it is informing and modeling nonsupportive behavior.
B. Determining whether one student's medication calculations are correct on a whiteboard for the clinical group to see—NO, this is demonstration.
C. **Sharing in postconference a medication error the nurse educator made as a novice nurse—YES, this gives an example of her role as a novice educator and how she handled the situation.**
D. Sharing an example of a practice error a colleague had made while providing patient care—NO, this is just sharing a story or providing an example.

42. Which of the following verbs should be used when writing instructional objectives at the comprehension level of Bloom's taxonomy?

A. Compare, contrast, and critique—NO, these are not at the comprehension level; these are written at the evaluation level.
B. Design, create, and implement—NO, these are written at the synthesis level.
C. Examine, comprehend, and analyze—NO, these are written at the analysis level.
D. **Review, summarize, and explain—YES, these are written at the comprehension level.**

43. Which of the following activities is an example of active learning?

A. Attend a lecture at a local conference—NO, this is a passive learning experience.
B. Answering NCLEX-style alternative format questions on the computer—NO, this is passive.
C. Having the educator demonstrate the correct way to perform a psychomotor skill—NO, this is still a passive learning experience.
D. **Debrief a simulation experience of a small clinical group—YES, this is a more active learning experience. It involves an interactive discuss with the class.**

44. It has been brought to the nurse educator's attention that a student is performing questionable safe nursing practice in clinical. Which of the following would be a priority for the nurse educator to do?

   A. Notifying the program administrator for the student's immediate dismissal from the program—NO, this is not the solution. The educator needs to give the student time and a chance for improvement.
   B. **Document the pattern of marginal performance or unsatisfactory behavior in a formative evaluation and tell the student quite clearly what he or she needs to do to improve—YES, then have a re-evaluation date to be sure the student is compliant with the evaluation and met the goals set by both the instructor and student.**
   C. Ascertain whether the student has passed the basic clinical competency skills—NO, although knowing whether the student had passed the basic clinical competency skills may be valid in determining competency, it is assumed if the student is in clinical he or she has passed the basic competency skills.
   D. Ask the student's friends whether something is going on in clinical you should know about—NO, the educatory should ask the student, not the students friends, whether something is going on in clinical you should know about.

45. Which of the following is an example of a well-written student learning outcome?

   A. Discussing various methods of implementing and prioritizing care of a group of people—NO, this has three verbs, *discussing, implementing*, and *prioritizing*, in the objective. Each outcome should have one verb or task to do.
   B. Identifying nursing diagnosis to prevent disease transmission—NO, it is clear in that you identify a nursing diagnosis but how a diagnosis prevents the transmission of disease is not identified.
   C. Summarizing key points of a PowerPoint presentation on respiratory distress—NO, this is not a measurement of a learning outcome. It is summarizing a PowerPoint presentation.
   D. **Utilizing selected aspects of the nursing process to provide care to the geriatric population—YES, this has a verb and is specific by naming what behavior is to be done and to what population. This can be measured through a care planning or concept mapping assignment.**

46. A novice nurse educator is discussing how to measure his teaching effectiveness with his mentor. Which of the following statements indicates that the novice nurse educator understands this concept?

   A. "If the learners met the course objectives, my teaching was effective"—NO, this is not a true measure of teaching effectiveness.
   B. "Anonymous computer evaluations are biased and are an unreliable assessment of my teaching effectiveness"—NO, student evaluations, especially those that are anonymous, may be unreliable but that should not be the only evaluation method used.
   C. "All the students passed NCLEX and my course; my teaching was effective"—NO, just because students passed NCLEX is not a true measure of teaching effectiveness.
   D. **"Multiple methods will be needed to determine whether my teaching was effective"—YES, several methods are needed to determine whether teaching was effective.**

47. A new educator was texting her boyfriend in class while presenting her lecture to the students. This is an example of:

    A. **Incivility—YES, educators can be incivil to the students as well. Not giving their full attention to the class is an example of incivility.**
    B. Bullying—NO, this is not bullying students.
    C. Good use of time—NO, this is a poor use of time.
    D. Multitasking—NO, this is not giving the class your full attention.

48. Which of the following demonstrates the best way to facilitate learning for a diverse group of learners?

    A. **Utilize a variety of teaching techniques to best meet the needs of the learners—YES, this will assist different types of learners to assimilate the knowledge being presented.**
    B. Use a teaching strategy that best meets the instructors' style—NO, this only meets the needs of the instructor, not the student.
    C. Match instructors with learners from the same culture—NO, this is just helping the language barrier. It does not necessarily address learning of a diverse group of learners.
    D. Use YouTube videos—NO, this only responds to visual learners and those who are technologically up to date.

49. Which of the following is an example of role-playing in the classroom?

    A. Have the students perform a song that demonstrates blood flow through the heart—NO, this is a demonstration, not truly playing a role.
    B. Give students a question and have them act out the answer—NO, this is more like charades.
    C. **Have a student demonstrate a therapeutic communication response to another student who is exhibiting signs of depression—YES, this is an example of role-playing in which each student has a role and acts out an appropriate therapeutic response and reaction.**
    D. Have the faculty member name a disease process and have the students choose responses that are consistent with that disease process—NO, this is a matching type interaction.

50. Which of the following statements are true about utilizing a flipped classroom and its purpose in education?

    A. It enables the faculty member to have a day off—NO, that is not the point of a flipped classroom.
    B. It cuts down on the faculty member's prep work and shifts it to the student—NO, the faculty member needs to be equally prepared when the student is preparing and sharing the classroom content.
    C. **It enables the student to take charge of his or her learning by researching a clinical situation and presenting it to the class—YES, it gives the student control and enables the student to actively learn and also assists with developing good speaking and presentation skills.**
    D. It is like postconference when students find an interesting case and present it to the class for credit—NO, it is not presenting one case, it is presenting the course content assigned, which, in fact, could involve more than one case to illustrate.

51. Which of the following statements is true about using "gaming" in the classroom?

    A. **It is effective for affective and cognitive learning—YES, students need to think while gaming and it elicits emotion through competition and empathy.**

    B. It makes the classroom fun and more course content will get covered—NO, although it does make the classroom fun sometimes all the assigned content does not get covered because of the time spent on the game.

    C. The students don't like it, it makes them feel juvenile—NO, many times the students do like it, have fun, and don't feel juvenile at all.

    D. It enables the faculty member to keep better control of all students in the classroom—NO, in fact, sometimes it makes it hard for the faculty member to keep control of the classroom and it may get loud.

52. Which of the following statements is correct about problems with the use of simulation experiences? (Select all that apply.)

    A. **It is very expensive to implement—YES, initially it is expensive to purchase high-fidelity mannequins, but grants can be written to assist with cost.**

    B. **Simulation works best when a small group of learners is involved in the simulation experience—YES, simulation is best with small groups, usually less than five or six at a time, so each one gets intimate hands-on experience.**

    C. It doesn't really help prepare the students for the "real world"—NO, this is not true. Simulation does actually enable students to prepare for the real world by practicing in a safe environment with teacher support.

    D. **Learners can practice in a safe environment—YES, learners can practice in a safe environment and if mistakes are made, no patient harm is done.**

53. The chair of the education committee is known as a transformational leader. This indicates that the leader:

    A. Develops criteria within the committee to accomplish a task—NO, the leader motivates through inspiration.

    B. Provides opportunities for the committee to make choices—NO, although the leader does include the committee to be active participants, he or she role models and encourages the group to take ownership of their work. So it is much more than just making choices.

    C. Directs the flow of the committee to complete objectives and tasks—NO, this would be an authoritative leadership style. The transformational leader inspires, not controls, the flow of the committee. It is a more open system.

    D. **Energizes the committee to perform with his or her vision and guides change through inspiration—YES, the transformational leader inspires the committee by role modeling and creating a vision to guide change and facilitates the group taking ownership in what they do.**

54. Which of the following is the best way to increase the facilitation of knowledge when building learning experiences into a curriculum?

   A. **Experiential learning—YES, providing learning opportunities for students to personally experience learning the information helps long-term retention of the information.**

   B. Reviewing procedural knowledge—NO, review of procedural information is a rote-learning method and the information does not remain in the memory.

   C. Presenting information from simple to complex methods—NO, although presenting concepts from a simple to complex methodology is helpful, it does not increase the knowledge or enhance learning experiences.

   D. Provide exemplars—NO, this is not the best way of building knowledge by building learning experiences. Examples may help illustrate points, but they are not the best method of implementing learning experiences.

55. A nurse educator is teaching an online course. One of the learners has posted a response to a discussion board question that reflects a negative opinion about the profession of nursing. Other learners in the class post comments agreeing with the first opinion. What should the nurse educator do?

   A. Do nothing and let all the learners "speak their piece" and vent their feelings—NO, this could enable the discussion to become out of control and not achieve the purpose of the assignment and outcomes of the course.

   B. **Courteously question the first learner's post and open further dialogue about the topic giving illustrations of other possible conclusions—YES, when something is posted that is inappropriate or misinformed, it is the instructor's responsibility to objectively engage the negative learner, provide accurate information, and demonstrate professional solutions and discussions of how to discuss topics.**

   C. Post evidence-based research to prove the learner is grossly misinformed—NO, although evidence-based research is encouraged, providing examples and telling a student he or she is grossly misinformed is negative and may cause the learner to not participate in further discussions. Examples of "appropriate and professional" communications should be demonstrated wherever possible.

   D. Remind the learner that negative posts are inappropriate and will be deleted—NO, this will not achieve the goal of achieving positive and professional discussion. Unless it is insulting to a person or betrays confidential information, deleting the post is not the best avenue. It is the educator's responsibility to role model professional discussion behavior. If the learner continues the negativity, perhaps the educator should have a personal discussion with the learner individually.

56. A nurse educator understands that a visual leaner would prefer which of the following activities?

   A. Read a book, then write an essay—NO, this is a task for a verbal learner.

   B. Perform a skill in the simulation laboratory—NO, this is a task for a kinesthetic learner.

   C. Listen to a book on CD and write a report—NO, this is a task for an auditory learner.

   D. **Watch a movie and then discuss it with the class—YES, this is a task for a visual learner.**

57. Which of the following objectives is written at Bloom's highest taxonomy level?
    A. Define *homeostasis* in the human body—NO, defining occurs at the knowledge level, where a student just recalls what homeostasis is.
    B. Explain how the body tries to maintain homeostasis—NO, this is at the comprehension level, where a student comprehends and translates information learned based on prior learning.
    C. **Contrast homeostasis intracellularly and extracellularly—YES, this is written at the highest level. *Contrast* is written at the analysis level, where a student has to classify and relate information about a statement or question.**
    D. Demonstrate how homeostasis in the renin–angiotensin system works— NO, this is an application level, where the student must simply classify and relate information to complete a task or problem with minimal direction.

58. Which of the following behaviors exhibited by faculty might be considered uncivil by student learners in the classroom?
    A. Supporting and valuing content taught by other faculty—NO, being supportive of other faculty and not letting the student split faculty is not being uncivil.
    B. Telling the students you do not know the answer to their question but will find it out by next class—NO, this is actually an example of role modeling how to problem solve in the future and lets students realize it's OK not to know the answer to every question, but be sure to come to next class prepared with information to answer the question to keep their respect.
    C. **Coming unprepared for class and "winging" the content because you taught the course before—YES, this is an example of being uncivil. If we expect students to come to class prepared, then the faculty should be prepared as well.**
    D. Starting class late to answer student questions about an upcoming exam— NO, each faculty person should plan to start class on time, but if time is taken at the beginning of class to answer questions about an upcoming exam, this will decrease student anxiety and help with clarification of material on the exam. This is not incivil.

59. Which of the following statements is true about the role of mentoring?
    A. Mentors should be mandated to new educators upon hiring into a new faculty role—NO, mentors should be recommended.
    B. Sending new faculty to conferences in the hopes of their networking and finding a mentor is a great way to pair up novice faculty with mentors— NO, this is not the best method of finding a mentor. What if the novice faculty member is shy and not adept at networking? The novice may never find a mentor.
    C. A mentor should attend the mentee's classes regular and provide critiques of the novice educator's teaching style—NO, a mentor should attend classes only when invited by the mentee and asked for that type of feedback. Otherwise this behavior will feel authoritative and may undermine the novice faculty members' confidence.
    D. **A key component in mentoring is that the mentor should be accessible both physically and emotionally for the novice educator—YES, this availability is key to the success or failure of a mentoring relationship. The novice educator needs to know he or she has support no matter what or when—within reason, of course.**

60. A learner reports that another learner cheated by writing the arterial blood gas values on her desk before the test. The best action for the nurse educator to take first would be:

   A. Verify the story with another learner who was sitting close by—NO, do not involve other learners if possible.
   B. **Take a picture of the desk in question—YES, the first step is to gather evidence.**
   C. Ask the learner who was being accused—NO, the faculty member should gather evidence first.
   D. Tell the learner who is reporting that there is no proof—NO, this would discourage honesty.

61. The admission and progression committee in the nursing educational unit is revising the progression standards to improve program outcomes. Which of the following is not a criterion for progression in the nursing program?

   A. A minimum grade of 80% is required for nursing and science courses—NO, this is a progression criteria for learners.
   B. Learners may repeat a nursing course one time—NO, this is a progression criteria for learners.
   C. **Junior-level status must be achieved to begin the nursing program—YES, this is an admission criteria for learners.**
   D. Learners must achieve the national standard average on the standardized test—NO, this is a progression criteria for learners.

62. A novice nurse educator states that she evaluated a learner doing a procedure for the second time and the learner corrected her first mistakes but took a long time to do the procedure. The nurse educator states, "By the performance of this learner I am not sure learning has taken place." From this statement, one can deduce that the novice nurse educator subscribes to the learning theory of:

   A. **Behaviorism—YES, behaviorists believe that for learning to take place, there needs to be a change in behavior.**
   B. Cognitivism—NO, this has to do with organizing knowledge.
   C. Constructivism—NO, this is constructing new knowledge from what is already known.
   D. Realism—NO, this bases knowledge in the present and on what can be seen and heard.

63. Social forces are increasing the accountability of institutions of higher education. One of the main social forces that propels this change, which is demanding accountability in outcomes achieved, is:

   A. Increase in college-educated citizens—NO, this is not the main force.
   B. **Funding—YES, funding is the main driving force behind increased accountability.**
   C. Accessibility—NO, this is not the main force.
   D. Legal sanctions—NO, this is not the main force.

64. After administering an exam, the nurse educator is reviewing the item analysis for each of the multiple-choice questions. One question yielded the following statistics for the items:

Point Biserial = 0. 43	Correct Answer = A		Total Group = 57%	
Distractor Analysis	A	B	C	D
Point Biserial	0.43	–0.15	0.00	–0.48
Frequency	57%	23%	0%	20%

Based on this analysis, what action should be taken by the nurse educator?

A. Revise distractor A—NO, distractor A was correct and discriminated.
B. Revise distractor B—NO, distractor B was incorrect but some of the learners who did not master the content chose it as intended.
C. **Revise distractor C—YES, no one chose this distractor.**
D. Revise distractor D—NO, distractor D was incorrect but some of the learners who did not master the content chose it as intended.

65. The nurse educator intentionally involves the learners in a group activity without providing them with specific directions for accomplishing the task. The learners are left to their own ingenuity and creativity to reach the learning outcome. This type of learning is referred to as:

A. **Inquiry-based learning—YES, this is a type of discovery learning that allows learners to be self-directed.**
B. Critical thinking activity—NO, a critical-thinking activity should have directions.
C. Goal-directed learning—NO, the outcome or "goal" is known and the process is usually the assignment or purpose.
D. Problem-based learning—NO, the outcome is known and the process is usually prescribed.

66. When considering level outcomes, educators must ensure that they progress logically to eventually reflect the:

A. Philosophy of the parent institution—NO, this is usually reflected in the mission statement of the organization.
B. **Outcomes of the program—YES, the level outcomes should feed into the "larger umbrella" of the program outcomes for logical sequencing and education flow.**
C. Demographics of the community—NO, this is reflected in the mission of the school.
D. Beliefs of the faculty—NO, this is reflected in the core values.

67. Review of an item on a test reveals the following statistics:

Point Biserial = –0.13	Correct Answer = D		Total Group = 82%	
Distractor Analysis	A	B	C	D
Point Biserial	0.02	0.19	0.01	–0.13
Frequency	12%	5%	1%	82%

The likely cause for this frequency distribution is:

A. Higher scoring learners answered the question correctly—NO, because the correct answer has a negative point biserial.

B. **Higher scoring learners answered the question incorrectly—YES, because a negative point biserial indicates that learners who scored higher on the exam got the item wrong.**

C. Lower scoring learners answered the question incorrectly—NO, some of the lower scoring students chose the correct answer as indicated by a negative point biserial.

D. The distractors show clear discrimination—NO, they do not. This is shown by the correct answer having a negative point biserial.

68. One phase of service learning is reflection. Use of reflection is important for learners because it fosters the development of:

A. **Cultural competency—YES, cultural competency is developed as a part of the reflection process and integration of concepts learned.**

B. Cognitive interpretation—NO, this is not the focus of reflection although it can enhance cognitive learning.

C. Kinesthetic learning—NO, this is not the focus of reflection. Kinesthetic learning is an active "hands on" type of learning.

D. Inductive reasoning—NO, this is a logical process in which multiple premises are believed true or found true and are put together to derive a specific conclusion.

69. An example of learner misconduct that can be considered a disruptive act and should be addressed as soon as possible is:

A. Stealing a test—NO, this is criminal misconduct.

B. **Watching YouTube videos in class and laughing out loud—YES, this is disruptive and a form of incivility. It should be addressed by the educator as soon as possible.**

C. Cheating on an exam—NO, this is academic misconduct.

D. Cyberbullying—NO, this is something that happens outside of the classroom and is something that is beyond the scope of the classroom.

70. The chair of the nursing department has had complaints from learners that a novice instructor does not finish the material because she is using too many slides. The best initial response by the leader would be:

    A. Speak to the novice educator about the complaints—NO, this is not asking the learners to take responsibility for their education and understand conflict resolution and chain of command.

    B. Observe the instructor delivering a lecture—NO, this is an unnecessary step. It is also undermines the instructor's role as educator and authority. The students will then have no respect for the educator and run to the chair for any issue they have versus speaking with the nursing educator for their course.

    C. **Ask the learners to speak directly to the instructor—YES, this should be the initial first step. It role models or demonstrates to the students how to follow the chain of command. This will assist them with conflict resolution in their future careers.**

    D. Show the novice educator how to cut down the information for each class—NO, this is insulting and undermines to the educator.

71. Item analysis of an exam question revealed the following statistics:

Point Biserial = 0. 40	Correct Answer = A		Total Group = 72%	
Distractor Analysis	A	B	C	D
Point Biserial	0.40	0.03	0.04	0.12
Frequency	72%	6%	15%	7%

    How should the nurse educator interpret these results?

    A. This question needs to be revised as too many learners answered it correctly—NO, 72% of the learners chose the right answer.

    B. **High-scoring learners answered the question correctly—YES, a point biserial of 0.40 for the question and individual distractors, along with lower point biserials for incorrect answers, indicates that learners who scored higher answered the item correctly.**

    C. Lower scoring learners answered the question correctly—NO, the point biserial was positive for the correct answer.

    D. There is inadequate discrimination of the distractors—NO, the distractors did discriminate between the learners who understood the content and those who did not.

72. The novice educator is asking her mentor for an example of experiential learning. The best example to illustrate the concept of experiential learning is when learners:

    A. **Develop a community needs assessment related to chronic conditions— YES, this needs assessment involves the students in the community and encourages them to interact in a hands-on learning situation.**

    B. Practice taking blood pressures on shoppers at the mall one Saturday— NO, this is rote learning, but does provide some interactions.

    C. Develop an in-service presentation for a grammar school class about hypertension—NO, this is basically paperwork-type learning.

    D. Develop a group project about hypertension—NO, this is basically paperwork-type learning, unless it was stated that the project had a practical application piece.

73. A novice educator is asking her mentor what would be the best learning strategy to use to teach diabetes in her adult health course. The mentor should tell the mentee that the best learning strategies are those that:

A. **Keep the learners involved—YES, active learning is the most beneficial to students.**

B. Relate to the desired outcomes—NO, this is a concern for the content more than the strategy.

C. Can be easily evaluated—NO, this should not be the main concern when choosing a strategy.

D. Are comfortable for a novice educator—NO, this also is a concern but should not be the primary concern.

74. When developing or changing the curriculum, the leader's most appropriate action is to:

A. Usher the faculty through the process, handing out tasks so that resistance is decreased and time is saved—NO, delegating or handing out tasks does not promote group cohesion. Faculty should be part of the process, not handed tasks to complete.

B. Set up a meeting with each faculty member in order to decrease group resistance—NO, meeting with each faculty member takes a great deal of time and it also does not necessarily decrease group resistance. In fact it may lead to misinterpretation and inconsistent messages because all faculty members are not present.

C. **Give individuals the opportunity to express their opinions and concerns in ongoing meetings—YES, by giving individuals an opportunity to express their opinions and concerns it allows them to "own" the decisions and end product. If faculty are included in the decision-making process, this enhances the acceptance of change.**

D. Remember to remain positive in all communications about the proposed new curriculum—NO, just because the leader is positive does not mean the faculty will buy into the process and remain positive in accepting the change in curriculum.

75. The nurse educator is arranging a promotional dossier and wants to include an exemplar of the scholarship of teaching. The best evidence to include would be to use:

A. The class standardized testing scores that are above normal—NO, this does not speak to scholarship, it speaks to teaching effectiveness.

B. Individual learner projects that received an A—NO, this has more to do with individual motivation and teaching effectiveness.

C. Course evaluations in which the educator scored above normal—NO, this speaks to teaching effectiveness and not the scholarship of teaching.

D. **The syllabus of a newly developed course that integrates the faculty's research into the course—YES, developing a new course is a good example of teaching scholarship. It includes the major elements needed to promote learning.**

76. The following statistics were recorded on an item analysis of a test question:

Point Biserial = 0. 04	Correct Answer = C		Total Group = 61%	
Distractor Analysis	A	B	C	D
Point Biserial	−0.26	0.18	0.04	0.02
Frequency	18%	20%	61%	1%

These statistics indicate which of the following?

A. There was high discrimination of the distractors—NO, the correct answer has a very low point biserial.

B. Lower scoring learners answered the question correctly—NO, the correct answer has a positive point biserial.

C. The distractors are too difficult—NO, 61% of the learners chose the correct answer.

D. **There is inadequate discrimination and one of the items is flawed—YES, a point biserial of 0.04 on a test item answered correctly suggests inadequate discrimination and a flaw in the item. The item needs to be revised.**

77. A learning activity that promotes positive interdependence among learners is:

A. Clicker response questions—NO, although these questions do promote audience participation, they also promote competition.

B. Debates—NO, this promotes direct competition.

C. Peer evaluations—NO, this is an evaluation process and not a learning activity.

D. **A cooperative learning project—YES, cooperative learning enhances responsibility, critical thinking, and developing positive relationships with peers.**

78. An experienced nurse educator who has been teaching traditional undergraduate nursing students is now assigned to teach second-degree learners. Her evaluations are much lower than usual. Which of the following syllabus modifications would be appropriate to tailor her teaching toward this group of learners?

A. Increase observation clinical hours—NO, observation is not advantageous to second-degree learners. They have limited clinical time and would benefit more from hands-on clinical learning time.

B. Decrease objective testing—NO, objective testing methods are expected by second-degree learners to verify their knowledge.

C. Increase reflective journaling—NO, this type of assignment is not accepted well by second-degree learners in that they are task and knowledge oriented.

D. **Decrease number of care plan assignments—YES, second-degree learners do not appreciate multiple assignments or assignments they perceive as "busy work." They prefer limited assignments that are objectively based.**

79. Which of the following objectives is written at Bloom's highest taxonomy level?

    A. Define *homeostasis* in the human body—NO, define is at the knowledge level, where a student just recalls wht homeostasis is.

    B. Explain how the body tries to maintain homeostasis—NO, this is at the comprehension level, where a student comprehends and translates information learned based on prior learning.

    C. **Contrast homeostasis intracellularly and extracellularly—YES, this is written at the highest level of these choices. The contrast level is written at the analysis level, where a student has to classify and relate information about a statement or question.**

    D. Demonstrate how homeostasis in the renin–angiotensin system works—NO, this is an application level, where the student must simply classify and relate information to complete a task or problem with minimal direction.

80. The novice nurse educator would like to change a course in the curriculum. The best question to be asked by the members of the curriculum committee is:

    A. "Does the new course duplicate any material in other courses?"—NO, this is a concern but not the most important preliminary question.

    B. "Who will teach the new course?"—NO, this is a concern but not the most important preliminary question.

    C. "What are the student expectations for the course?"—NO, this is a concern but not the most important preliminary question.

    D. **"Was this change based on trended data?"—YES, what is the evidence that demonstrates the change is needed?**

81. Newly hired nurse educators should expect their orientations to include all of the following EXCEPT:

    A. The rights and responsibilities of faculty—NO, this should be included.

    B. The organization's role in creating an enhancing environment—NO, this should be included.

    C. **Teaching methodologies to be used in the classroom—YES, this is the choice of each individual faculty.**

    D. Overview of the curriculum—NO, this should be included.

82. An item analysis of an exam question revealed the following statistics:

Point Biserial = 0. 31	Correct Answer = C		Total Group = 35%	
Distractor Analysis	A	B	C	D
Point Biserial	0.31	−0.41	0.26	−0.02
Frequency	35%	58%	6%	1%

The nurse educator interprets these results to mean which of the following?
A. Learners who scored lower on the exam chose the correct answer—NO, the point biserial for C would be negative.
B. **Learners who scored higher on the exam chose the incorrect answer—YES, the point biserial is positive.**
C. The point biserial indicates good discrimination among the distractors—NO, item A should have had a negative point biserial because it is not the correct answer.
D. The item difficulty for the correct answer indicates the question should be revised—NO, the item difficulty is low but it discriminated well.

83. A clinical nurse educator asks her mentor what she should do about a clinical issue that is occurring in the simulation laboratory during the exam time. Learners are asking clinical questions when they are being evaluated for skill performance. The advice of the mentor that is most helpful is:
A. "Tell learners they can ask questions when they are done"—NO, this may be an option but does not provide rigor for an evaluative mechanism.
B. "Allow learners to take a break during the activity to ask questions and then resume"—NO, this interrupts the evaluation process and actually makes it a learning event.
C. **"Review the expectations with the learners and the outcomes that are being evaluated"—YES, this will clarify the reason they are doing the activities.**
D. "Tell the learners that they will fail if they continue to ask questions"—NO, this is incivil threatening.

84. Nurse educators are undertaking a curriculum revision. The nurse educators want to align the curriculum with current practice issues. The most effective method to keep up to date with practice issues is to:
A. Buy a subscription to a peer-reviewed clinical journal for each curriculum committee member—NO, often print material has a lag time and it may not be the most effective if everyone does not read the information.
B. Do a practice analysis every 3 years at the clinical facilities used for learner experiences—NO, this may be time consuming and expensive.
C. Survey alumni of the program about their transition to work and identify deficits—NO, although this is a good method, it may take a few years to get trends.
D. **Have a faculty liaison who participates in the practice counsel at each affiliate clinical facility—YES, this is a collaborative way that identifies changes as they occur in the healthcare systems.**

85. A nurse educator is developing a professional nursing role course for second-degree learners and is deciding on a learning activity to meet the outcome of professional socialization. The best learning activity for this outcome would be:

    A. **Incorporate a guest speaker who is in a specialist nursing role—YES, this provides professional practice in public and provides networking opportunities.**
    B. Develop a group project about nursing roles—NO, this is an activity that just includes the students and no outside role modeling.
    C. Increase clinical hours so the learners can observe nurses—NO, this is stressful for working second-degree students.
    D. Have the learners join the student nurse organization—NO, this is time consuming for second-degree students.

86. An item analysis for a 50-item test showed these statistics:

    Mean score = 77

    KR-20 = 0.68

    $SD = 2.9$

    These findings indicate which of the following?

    A. There were not enough items on the test—NO, the KR 20 shows that there was enough questions to evaluate the homogeneousness of the test.
    B. Items were poorly written and do not discriminate—NO, the KR 20 is good.
    C. **The test is reliable and shows clear discrimination—YES, this is known by the high KR 20 and mean test scores that were not too high or too low.**
    D. There were too many easy questions on the test—NO, the test mean would have been higher.

87. An example of a provider-directed, provider-paced educational activity is a(n):

    A. **Seminar—YES, seminars are self-paced discussions led by faculty many times.**
    B. Journal article—NO, this is a closed-ended assignment.
    C. On-demand video—NO, this is a closed-ended assignment.
    D. All of the above—NO.

88. An example of a provider-directed, learner-paced educational activity is a(n):

    A. Live webcast—NO, this is a closed-ended assignment.
    B. **On-demand video—YES, the learner can access it when needed.**
    C. Seminar—NO, this is a provider-paced assignment.
    D. All of the above—NO.

89. An academic nursing unit is interviewing for a medical–surgical instructor and is having difficulty finding applicants because of all of the following reasons EXCEPT:

    A. Salary—NO, the salaries in practice are often higher than academia.
    B. **Overqualification—YES, underqualification of candidates is usually the problem.**
    C. Lack of scholarly production—NO, many nursing faculties have scholarship.
    D. Demands of academia—NO, academia is very demanding and faculty often work in the evenings and weekends at home developing teaching material.

90. Lewin's change theory is characterized by the presence of:
    A. The motivation and capacity for change—NO, this is not explicit in the Lewin's change theory.
    B. Driving and restraining forces—**YES, this is explained in the theory.**
    C. Self-efficacy—NO, this is not explicit in the Lewin's change theory.
    D. Perceived control over opportunities—NO, this is not explicit in the Lewin's change theory.

91. The department chair of nursing is aware that the percentage of tenured nursing faculty is lower than in many other academic departments. To increase the number of tenured faculty, the most effective thing the department chair should do is:
    A. Establish faculty classes on academic progression and leadership—NO, this may be a way but it is not individualized.
    B. Assist faculty to develop long-term and short-term goals—NO, although this is part of the process, it does not capture all that is needed.
    C. Encourage faculty to shadow a tenured professor in another department—NO, this may not be effective or completely applicable to nursing.
    D. **Mentor faculty about developing an effective academic portfolio—YES, this is individualized goal setting and progress monitoring.**

92. An item analysis for a 25-item multiple-choice test administered to 60 learners showed these statistics:

    Mean score = 20.32

    KR-20 = 0.29

    $SD = 5.67$

    The findings indicate this about the test:
    A. The test is reliable and shows clear discrimination—NO, the KR 20 is low and the standard deviation is high.
    B. **More questions should be added to the test—YES, 25 items is low and usually not adequate to determine the discrimination of a test.**
    C. The questions were most likely of average difficulty—NO, this is not true as known by the mean score of the test.
    D. Scoring was subjective—NO, this is an assumption.

93. The item analysis revealed the following statistics for a multiple-choice question:

Point Biserial = 0. 22	Correct Answer = C		Total Group = 81%	
Distractor Analysis	A	B	C	D
Point Biserial	−0.45	−0.01	0.22	0.26
Frequency	12%	1%	81%	6%

On the basis of these statistics, the nurse educator should do which of the following when using this item on future exams?
    A. Nothing, as the point biserial is just a little low but within acceptable range—NO, the point biserial is fine.
    B. Revise distractor A—NO, this distractor performed well.
    C. Revise distractor B—NO, this distractor performed well.
    D. **Revise distractor D—YES, this is a wrong answer with a positive point biserial.**

94. A clinical nurse educator tells the department chair that a learner may fail for consistent low-level clinical performance and it is 1 week before the end of the semester. A priority inquiry question from the department chair to the clinical nurse educator should be:

   A. "Would you like another faculty member to assess the learner?"—NO, this undermines the instructor's expertise.
   B. **"Do you have formative evaluations completed?"—YES, this is imperative if a student was not performing to standard all along. It demonstrates a learning plan.**
   C. "What does the learner do that is below expected competency?"—NO, this undermines the instructor's expertise.
   D. "Is this the learner's second course failure?"—NO, this is important but not a deciding factor in the case at hand.

95. Which statement by a learner should alert the nurse educator to a possible learning disability?

   A. "I have never been given such low grades before and I study the same way"—NO, this is just lack of meta-cognition.
   B. "I read the book and PowerPoint slides before class as I am told to do"—NO, these are just excuses.
   C. "I do extra questions every night to practice and it helps"—NO, this is telling the instructor that he/she is adjusting.
   D. **"I understand the material in class but cannot pick the right test answer"—YES, this may designate anxiety or a processing disorder.**

96. The members of a curriculum committee discuss the manner in which learners address the faculty and respond to learning experiences. This type of value-laden discussion of behavior is part of the program's:

   A. Operational curriculum—NO, this is more public.
   B. Illegitimate curriculum—NO, this is a legitimate concern.
   C. **Hidden curriculum—YES, these issues are difficult to identify.**
   D. Null curriculum—NO, this is being taught in some manner.

97. Which of the following are not protected under copyright law?

   A. Literary works—NO, these are protected.
   B. Sound recordings—NO, these are protected.
   C. Recorded choreographic works—NO, these are protected.
   D. **Nonrecorded choreographic works—YES, these are not protected.**

98. A nurse educator has completed a funded study about the effectiveness of the use of podcasts for nursing students with an auditory learning style preference. Which of the following is the most effective way to share results of this study?

   A. **Publish in a nursing education journal—YES, this will reach the largest number of nurse educators.**
   B. Present at national meeting of nurse educators—NO, this will reach a limited number of nurse educators.
   C. Present at statewide meeting of educators in higher education—NO, this will reach a limited number of nurse educators.
   D. Send the report of the findings to the funding agency—NO, this will reach a limited number of nurse educators.

99. Review of an item on a test reveals the following statistics:

Point Biserial = –0.04	Correct Answer = B		Total Group = 82%	
Distractor Analysis	A	B	C	D
Point Biserial	0.02	–0.04	–0.01	0.04
Frequency	1%	82%	1%	16%

The report indicates item D should be reviewed. The likely rationale for this suggestion is:

A. Higher scoring learners answered the question correctly—NO, actually lower scorers answered the question correctly.

B. **The distractor was not clear—YES, higher scorers picked distractor D.**

C. Lower scoring learners answered the question incorrectly—NO, actually lower scorers answered the question correctly.

D. The distractors show clear discrimination—NO, they do not since higher test scorers chose the wrong answer.

100. The following multiple-choice question is written at which level of Bloom's taxonomy?

The nurse understands that the patient needs more teaching when the patient states:

1. "I should take two of my hypertensive pills if I forget one the day before"

2. "I should rest if I feel lightheaded"

3. "I should call my primary care practitioner if I feel too weak to walk"

4. "I should increase my fluids to 8 to 10 glasses of water each day"

A. Understanding—NO, the students need to have a better grasp of the content than just understanding.

B. Comprehension—NO, this requires higher knowledge than just comprehending the need for the medication.

C. **Application—YES, this includes nursing interventions and assessment of correct interventions.**

D. Evaluation—NO, this does not ask students to evaluate and make a decision, just to apply knowledge.

Answers to End-of-Chapter Practice Questions

CHAPTER 2 PRACTICE QUESTIONS

1. The nurse administrator observes a new faculty member in the classroom. The faculty member uses active learning strategies and provides the students with time to ask questions, but two students in the back of the class continue to look at the mobile phone devices in their laps and exchange comments to each other. Constructive advice about the classroom observation that the nurse administrator can provide would be:

   A. Address the behavior during the next class session—NO, behavior modification (Mulligan's pillar III) should be done privately.

   B. Ask all students to put their phones at the front of the classroom on the table—NO, this is not the best choice for two reasons: a) It punishes all students, even those who have not abused the cell phone policies; and (b) it takes away the safety mechanism for individuals. Cell phones are used as a first-alert devise on campuses and in public places.

   C. Provide additional active learning activities to keep all students engaged—NO, the question stem indicated that the faculty member is using active learning strategies.

   D. **Request the students sit up front with a seat in between them—YES, changing the environment to meet the learner's needs (pillar IV) is the best intervention.**

2. The nurse educator is developing a test and would like to increase the number of evaluation questions. The best format to promote evaluative thinking in students would be to add:

   A. Fill-in multiple blanks—NO, this may be challenging, but may also be knowledge based depending on the content of the question stem.

   B. Hot spot—NO, this is usually knowledge based, but can be at a higher level if there are some decisional processes involved.

   C. **Display question—YES, typically display questions have different panels of patient information, which need to be synthesized into a nursing intervention or action.**

   D. Select all that apply—NO, although these are challenging for many students, they can be written at any level of Bloom's taxonomy.

3. A nurse educator has submitted a syllabus with the following student learning outcomes. Which learning outcome is written at the lowest level of Bloom's taxonomy?

   A. Demonstrate caring to geriatric patients—NO, this is at the application level.
   B. **Discuss common health care concerns of geriatric patients—YES, this is written at an understanding level.**
   C. Evaluate geriatric patients' understanding of home safety—NO, this is at the evaluation level.
   D. Formulate a plan of care for a geriatric patient—NO, this is at the creating level.

4. During a curriculum meeting, the certified health care simulation educator states, "This semester we will do objective structured clinical examinations (OSCEs)." The philosophical foundations for this analysis would best fit:

   A. Narrative pedagogy—NO, narrative pedagogy has storytelling and reflectiveness as its foundation.
   B. **Behaviorism—YES, OSCEs evaluate skills that can be observed.**
   C. Constructivism—NO, this is cognitive knowledge that is built by the student on previously learned knowledge.
   D. Feminism—NO, this has to do with gender and social equality.

5. During a faculty interview, the nurse educator candidate states that a preferred learning activity to facilitate learner understanding is looking at the historical roots of oppression. What nursing educational philosophy or theory is indicated by this learning activity?

   A. Narrative pedagogy—NO, narrative pedagogy has storytelling and reflectiveness as its foundation.
   B. Behaviorism—NO, this evaluates skills that can be observed.
   C. Constructivism—NO, this is cognitive knowledge that is built by the student on previously learned knowledge.
   D. **Feminism—YES, this has to do with gender and social equality.**

6. A nursing faculty group is revising the core values of the undergraduate nursing program. The group wants to add the values of individualism and self-reflection. These values best reflect which of the following educational theories?

   A. **Narrative pedagogy—YES, these core values best fit with narrative pedagogy.**
   B. Behaviorism—NO, this is built on being able to observe learned knowledge.
   C. Constructivism—NO, this is cognitive knowledge that is built by the student on previously learned knowledge.
   D. Feminism—NO, this has to do with gender and social equality.

7. A faculty group is concerned about students' clinical decision-making ability and is revising its clinical learning evaluation tool using a graded scale from one (1) to four (4) with one (1) being dependent on the instructor for assistance, two (2) needing frequent cues, three (3) needing occasional cues and preforming safely, and four (4) performing safely and independently. The best policy to support the tool would be:

   A. **Have the students reach a three (3) on each criterion by the end of each semester—YES, the Institute of Medicine (IOM) and Quality and Safety in Education for Nurses (QSEN) emphasize safety at all times.**

   B. Have the students reach level one (1) in the first trimester and work up to level four (4) in the last trimester—NO, the skills should be leveled, not the scoring method.

   C. Alter the passing score depending on the specific clinical skill—NO, the skills should be leveled appropriately.

   D. Have students predetermine the level they want to achieve and then compare the outcomes at the end of the semester—NO, safety at all times is not negotiable.

8. When interviewing for a job, a nurse educator candidate verbalizes her concerns about students having a good science and math foundation. This nurse educator most likely subscribes to the philosophy of:

   A. Phenomenology—NO, this has to do with the lived experience at the time and reflecting and learning from the experience.

   B. Emancipatory education—NO, this has to do with social equality.

   C. Narrative pedagogy—NO, this has to do with storytelling and reflection.

   D. **Constructivism—YES, this is building knowledge from previously learned knowledge.**

9. A new faculty member who has come directly from a practice setting is chronically late for meetings and often does not answer e-mails in a timely manner. The faculty member does a good job with her class and contributes to committee work. The nurse administrator should address this behavior because it may be interpreted as:

   A. A knowledge deficit—NO, this is standard in any workplace.

   B. Poor role transition—NO, this is usually verbalized or observed in poor quality work.

   C. Poor work ethic—NO, this is usually demonstrated as poor quality of work.

   D. **Incivility—YES, this is peer-to-peer incivility, not respecting each other's time.**

10. The educational nurse administrator tracks the attrition rates of the nursing educational program and finds that minority students are dismissed during their junior year at twice the number of nonminority students. The faculty discusses strategies for decreasing minority student attrition and decides the best method would be:

A. Reexamine the admission criteria—NO, the admission criteria are the same for all students.

B. Start a one-to-one faulty–student tutoring program—NO, this may be costly and there may not be a diverse faculty.

C. Identify high-risk students in their sophomore year and have them go part time their junior year—NO, this may place them at financial risk.

D. **Establish a minority student nursing organization that meets monthly and provides social events—YES, this will increase their belongingness.**

CHAPTER 3 PRACTICE QUESTIONS

1. A nurse educator is interested in using a learning strategy that will allow learners to self-reflect and examine their feelings about the clinical experience. A colleague suggests that she consider incorporating:

A. **Journaling—YES, with journaling learners are able to reflect and express their feelings; faculty have better insight into the students' learning.**

B. Concept maps—NO, this encourages analytical thinking, but not reflection.

C. Group discussions—NO, peer sharing may occur, but some learners may be uncomfortable with sharing their feelings.

D. Socratic questioning—NO, this encourages discussion, but some learners may feel threatened.

2. A novice adjunct clinical instructor is observed questioning learners in the clinical setting. What would cause the course coordinator to intervene?

A. The instructor questions the learners privately, away from other staff—NO, this is appropriate, especially if an issue or problem needs addressed.

B. **Questions are asked that only require a statement of the facts—YES, questions should be asked at a higher level to promote critical thinking.**

C. Learners are questioned about medications before administering them—NO, this is appropriate for safe administration.

D. The instructor asks questions of the clinical group in postconference—NO, this encourages discussion and group problem solving.

3. A nurse educator teaching the professional course for the first time has decided to have learners begin a portfolio they will build on throughout the nursing program. What should the educator consider in adopting this learning strategy?

   A. Portfolios should not be graded—NO, grading is acceptable.

   B. Learners should include a sample of work from each course—NO, information included can show evidence of best work or growth, but samples from each course are not needed.

   C. **Guidelines for inclusion should be provided to the learners—YES, portfolios can become quite large if learners don't receive instruction on what should be included.**

   D. There is no time commitment for the faculty—NO, portfolios can be very time-consuming to grade, especially with large classes.

4. A clinical practicum-based nurse educator needs to teach all the intensive care unit (ICU) nurses about a change in the process for obtaining blood cultures. What strategy would be most effective for allowing a large number of nurses to learn the information while on duty?

   A. Return demonstration—NO, this would be very time consuming for the nurse educator and likely unnecessary for a simple change in procedure.

   B. **Self-learning packet—YES, this would allow the nurses to review the information when they are able and at their own pace.**

   C. Group discussion—NO, it is often difficult to gather all the nurses together on a unit at one time and discussion is not really necessary.

   D. YouTube video—NO, this is not the best way to convey information on the nursing unit.

5. A novice nurse educator who has returned from a faculty development conference is sharing what she has learned about active learning strategies with other faculty. What statement by the novice would require you to intervene?

   A. "Learners will have a deeper understanding of the information."—NO, this is accurate.

   B. "Active learning improves problem-solving skills."—NO, this is accurate.

   C. **"Lecture using PowerPoint slides is one type of active learning strategy."—YES, lecture is a passive learning strategy, although activities can be included to make it more active.**

   D. "Learners will be more engaged in the classroom."—NO, this is accurate.

6. A nurse educator is interested in assessing her students' understanding of course content as she is teaching. One method that is not time intensive and provides immediate feedback is:

   A. **Audience response systems—YES, these are an efficient way to gauge learner understanding.**

   B. Debate—NO, this is time consuming.

   C. Think–pair–share—NO, this is time consuming.

   D. Group discussion—NO, this is time consuming.

7. A mental health educator is planning to use theater students as standardized patients (SPs) to teach nursing students effective communication skills. It is most important to:
   A. Use only senior-level theater students—NO, this is not necessary.
   B. Allow the nursing students to choose who will be a part of the simulation—NO, all students should be participating.
   C. **Train the theater students so they are familiar with their roles and expectations—YES, particularly, if you want all students to have the same experience, it is important to train the actors for consistency.**
   D. Encourage overdramatization by the theater students—NO, this could make the scenario less than realistic.

8. After returning from a conference and learning about various teaching and learning strategies, a nurse educator is interested in flipping the classroom in one of her courses. When explaining this to her colleagues, what statement would require her mentor to intervene?
   A. "Using this method, I will be able to focus on key concepts in the classroom."—NO, this is correct; in the flipped classroom learning is more focused.
   B. "I can place the learners in groups so they benefit from peer learning."—NO, this is correct; more active learning strategies can be used in the classroom.
   C. **"Learners will love this method because there is no increase in work for them."—YES, learners are assigned prework, and they are accountable for coming to class prepared; this may be a cause for discontent.**
   D. "This is an opportunity for learners to use and develop higher level thinking skills."—NO, this is correct.

9. A nurse educator is designing a learning activity for students to examine their attitudes and beliefs about caring for transgender patients. This would be best facilitated through:
   A. Reading—NO, it is often difficult to learn through this method.
   B. Case studies—NO, this is better for problem solving.
   C. YouTube video—NO, this is a passive activity.
   D. **Role-playing—YES, this is effective for learning in the affective domain.**

10. A novice educator expresses concern to her mentor that her students are not reading their textbooks. One method that could be used for testing each student's preparation for class would be:
    A. **Warm-up exercises—YES, this would be an efficient way to test individual student preparedness for class.**
    B. Think–pair–share—NO, this will not identify individual student preparation.
    C. Self-learning module— NO, this would be a time-consuming method for testing student preparation.
    D. Questioning—NO, this would not be time efficient.

CHAPTER 4 PRACTICE QUESTIONS

1. Informatics competencies require the educator to have competency in what areas?

    A. Technical—NO, the educator must understand the functionality of the technology.

    B. Utility—NO, the educator needs to know the utilization and possibilities of technology.

    C. Leadership—NO, the educator must demonstrate vision for technology use.

    D. **Management—YES, the educator does not have to be on a managerial level.**

2. Which of the following statements regarding serious gaming is true?

    A. Needs to be done independently to be effective—NO, it can be done in groups.

    B. Provides opportunities for research—NO, it does not usually provide research options.

    C. Has minimal effect on learning but increases socialization—NO, it does have an effect on learning.

    D. **Provides a method to assess learning—YES, it usually does not provide and evaluative piece; it is constructed as a learning tool.**

3. For which of the following activities can a mobile device be utilized to support learning? (Select all that apply.)

    A. Gaming activities—NO, this does support learning.

    B. **Answer selection on a graded quiz—YES, this supports elevation.**

    C. Medication reference—NO, this supports medication comprehension.

    D. Reference books—NO, this supports learning.

4. What is the practice of posting small pieces of digital content—which could be text, pictures, links, short videos, or other media—on the Internet called?

    A. Semantic blog

    B. Virtual memos

    C. **Microblogging**

    D. Micromemos

5. What are some of the important features that e-books offer?

    A. **Embedded links—YES, this provides references.**

    B. Individualism—NO, it supports social activity.

    C. Book pages—NO, this is obtainable in hardcopy books.

    D. Index—NO, this is obtainable in hardcopy books.

6. The essential informatics competencies required by nurse educators can be categorized into all of the following EXCEPT:

    A. **Technical—YES, they need to know how to work the systems.**

    B. Procedural—NO, this is rote and lacks creativity in using technology.

    C. **Utility—YES, understanding the uses is important.**

    D. **Leadership—YES, having vision for use is also important.**

7. A wiki is:

   A. Journal entries that are presented in reverse chronological order—NO, wiki entries are in chronological order.

   B. Community sites that build relationships and connections/networks— NO, this is social media.

   C. **A collection of web pages that may be edited only by those invited— YES, this is the purpose of wikis.**

   D. A method of distributing videos and web content—NO, these are webcasts, podcasts, or voiceovers.

8. The TIGER initiative focused on the development of what?

   A. Informatics competencies for nurse educators—NO, it is for all levels of learning.

   B. **Informatics competencies for all levels of nursing education—YES, it is for students and faculty.**

   C. Informatics competencies for the clinical setting—NO, it is also for the classroom.

   D. Informatics competencies for electronic medical record managers—NO, it is for education.

9. Social bookmarking is:

   A. **Categorizing resources using user-defined keywords or tags—YES, users define the parameters.**

   B. Sharing websites with others at a conference—NO, this is too specific.

   C. A method to distribute multimedia content—NO, this is too specific.

   D. Recording short video and audio clips for education—NO, this is too specific.

10. Which of the following is an example of a microblog?

   A. Instagram.com—NO, this is communication back and forth.

   B. Pinterest.com—NO, this is an electronic billboard.

   C. Facebook.com—NO, this is social media.

   D. **Twitter.com—YES, this is a small communication blast.**

CHAPTER 5 PRACTICE QUESTIONS ANSWERS

1. Generally, online courses provide students with:

   A. Less control over the content—NO, they have more control over the content at times.

   B. Less control over the time and place learning occurs—NO, online courses provide students with self-management of their learning.

   C. **An individualized, learner-centered learning experience—YES, online courses are more individualized and often self-paced.**

   D. More opportunities to interact with classmates—NO, this is usually not the case.

2. An online instructor provides a written transcript for a video that he is including in his course. The instructor is incorporating which of the following quality design standards identified by QualityMatters™ (2016)?

   A. Course technology—NO, this is not related to the quality design.
   B. **Accessibility—YES, online educators must respond to students in a timely manner.**
   C. Learner interaction and engagement—NO, this is not a standard.
   D. Learner support—NO, this is not a standard.

3. In an online course, which of the following will provide one-on-one interaction with the faculty:

   A. Asynchronous office hours—NO, they will not be online together.
   B. **Synchronous office hours—YES, this will provide time online at the same time.**
   C. Discussion board—NO, this is usually available to the entire class.
   D. Practice meet—NO, this is usually involving more than two people.

4. Within an online course, the term *alignment* refers to:

   A. The structure of the course content and navigation—NO, this is self-explanatory.
   B. Adherence to accessibility requirements—NO, this is capacity.
   C. How course content links with established practice standards—NO, this is currency.
   D. **How learning outcomes are linked with course materials and assessments—YES, this is important to make sure the learning outcomes are met.**

5. In an online course, which of the following will provided one-on-one interaction with the faculty?

   A. Asynchronous office hours—NO, the student and faculty are on at different times.
   B. **Synchronous office hours—YES, they are on at the same time.**
   C. Discussion board—NO, the student and faculty are on at different times.
   D. Practice meet—NO, the student and faculty are on at different times.

6. Designing an online course to be usable by all people to the greatest extent possible is called:

   A. Usable design—NO, this is not the term.
   B. Accessible design—NO, this is not the term.
   C. **Universal design—YES, this is the term.**
   D. Versatile design—NO, this is not the term.

7. Ensuring learners can perform requirements with a minimal amount of effort and achieve the course goals is called:

   A. Learnability and efficiency—NO, learnability has to do with the individual student, not the course.
   B. Consistency and effectiveness—NO, consistency does not guarantee efficiency.
   C. **Efficiency and effectiveness—YES, both are needed to achieve the goals of the course in the best possible manner.**
   D. Usability and efficiency—NO, usability does not equate to efficiency.

8. Ensuring that learning objectives are aligned with course materials and learning activities that directly support the assessments for the course is called:

A. Curriculum—NO, this is the entire learning package.
B. Synchronous—NO, this is online classes that meet all at once.
C. **Alignment—YES, this is the term used for developing outcomes.**
D. Coordination—NO, this is not the term.

9. Providing alternative means of access to course materials in formats that meet the needs of diverse learners is called:

A. Support—NO, this is needed for all learners.
B. **Accessibility—YES, this is especially important for diverse learners.**
C. Interaction—NO, this is needed for all learners.
D. Engagement—NO, this is needed for all learners.

10. Courses that deliver less than 30% of content online are considered:

A. Blended—NO, this is more than 50% online.
B. Hybrid—NO, this is 50/50 usually.
C. **Web-facilitated—YES, online just assists making course material available.**
D. Dual—NO, this is presenting a course two ways.

CHAPTER 6 PRACTICE QUESTIONS

1. A nurse educator who is assigned to an open skills lab observes a learner practicing Foley catheter insertion with a step out of the proper sequence. When the nurse educator corrects the learner, the learner responds, "This is how I was taught the skill during clinical skills lab." How should the nurse educator address this issue with the faculty?

A. Tell the learner that he or she may have heard the information incorrectly and demonstrate the correct sequence—NO, this is how you would address it with the learner.
B. Look up the skills checklist used in the clinical skills lab for Foley catheter insertion—NO, this should be correct.
C. **Speak to the faculty member directly to ascertain what is being taught in the skills lab—YES, open the discussion to find out the other faculty member's understanding of the procedure.**
D. Report this information to dean/director of the nursing program—NO, this is not following chain of command and skips over the person who is involved.

2. What is the best way to teach a senior-level learner the proper technique to administer a medication delivered by intravenous (IV) push in the nursing skills lab?

A. **Ensure a working IV arm is available with the proper simulated medication vial and the correct needle and syringe—YES, this best simulates the real clinical environment.**
B. Use a midfidelity manikin with a working IV attached—NO, this does not simulate all aspects of the real clinical environment.
C. Have the learner verbalize the proper sequence of IV push medication administration—NO, this does not practice psychomotor skill.
D. Have an injection pad available and a simulated vial of the prescribed medication—NO, this does not simulate all aspects of the real clinical environment.

3. Which of the following methods develops critical thinking skills in the clinical skills laboratory environment?

   A. Learners are able to choose the correct supplies from a variety of needles and syringes when practicing intramuscular (IM) injections—NO, this is at the comprehension level.

   B. Learners gather all necessary supplies and equipment prior to performing tracheotomy care and suctioning—NO, this is linear procedural learning.

   C. **Learners are given a medical record and history from a simulated patient and need to administer medication—YES, this requires decision making.**

   D. Learners are required to teach a nursing skill to their peers in the clinical skills laboratory—NO, this is linear procedural learning.

4. The nurse educator asks a learner to describe a health assessment. The learner describes his understanding of how an assessment is performed when he makes which of the following statements?

   A. **Components used in an assessment are based on the independent judgment of the nurse—YES, this is correct understanding.**

   B. Routinely, the nurse will always do an in-depth full-body assessment—NO, many do a focused assessment.

   C. In-depth assessments are always referred to as head-to-toe assessments—NO, this is not always true, they are not always interpreted as the same thing.

   D. Prior to a nurses' assessment, an advanced practice nurse should do a full screening of all body systems—NO, this is not necessary or true.

5. A learner is assigned to perform a task during a clinical experience. Which of the following would be a responsibility of the learner?

   A. Perform the task with the staff nurse present—NO, this is not always necessary if the learner has done it before or has been deemed competent in the skills lab.

   B. **Perform only those tasks that the learner has been deemed competent to perform—YES, if a learner has not been taught a task and it has not been verified that they can do it, it should not be done.**

   C. Have the instructor present during the task to be sure the learner doesn't make any mistakes—NO, this is not always necessary if the learner has done it before or has been deemed competent in the skills lab.

   D. Only perform the task after observing the staff several times—NO, this is not necessary or practical.

6. The first line of defense against infection is intact skin. Which statement made by the learner indicates a need for further teaching?

   A. "Hand washing is to prevent infection through contact transmission"—NO, this is correct.

   B. "It's okay to use antibacterial gel instead of soap and water in some instances"—NO, this is correct.

   C. **"It isn't necessary to wash your hands prior to patient care as long as you wash them before you leave the room"—YES, this is incorrect.**

   D. "You should always wash your hands prior to and after using gloves"—NO, this is correct.

7. The nursing learner has been assigned a patient in isolation and realizes this patient is in respiratory isolation. Which of the following indicates that the learner correctly understands the need for self-protection with personal protective equipment (PPE)?

    A. Regular PPE is hanging on the door and can be used by anyone entering the room—NO, this is not true.

    B. **Respiratory isolation requires a specialized protective mask before entering the room—YES.**

    C. Anyone can use any available mask for protection—NO, they are individualized.

    D. Patients are not contagious unless they are actively coughing while you are in the room—NO, droplets can be in the air.

8. A learner comes to the laboratory without a laboratory coat and is unprepared to practice the skill for the day. The nurse educator should first:

    A. Send the learner home—NO, this should be done after the discussion.

    B. Have the learner make up the day later that week—NO, this should be done after the discussion.

    C. **Discuss the behavior with the learner—YES, this is the first step, and then follow the program's disciplinary action policy.**

    D. Write the learner a disciplinary warning—NO, this should be done after the discussion.

9. Which of the following is an example of peer-to-peer review in the skills lab?

    A. Senior students practicing urinary catheterization repeatedly until proficient—NO, there is no peer-review in this process.

    B. Freshman students comparing websites on EBP on their mobile devices—NO, there is no peer-review in this process.

    C. **Junior students learning how to speak empathetically by example from the senior students—YES, senior students demonstrating skills to junior-level students is an example of peer-to-peer review.**

    D. Observing faculty experts demonstrating complex skills in a simulated clinical environment—NO, there is no peer-review in this process.

10. When a learner is faced with caring for a transgender patient, what would be the best way for the learner to address this patient?

    A. Tell the patient you will care for him or her regardless of what the patient's preferences are—NO, this should not even be stated.

    B. Ask someone else to care for the patient—NO, it is the nurses duty to care for the patient.

    C. **Ask the patient politely how he or she would prefer to be addressed—YES, this demonstrates respect.**

    D. Offer the patient psychiatric counseling for gender confusion—NO, this is not necessary and is judgmental.

CHAPTER 7 PRACTICE QUESTIONS

1. When choosing a clinical unit, the faculty member would consider all of the following environmental conditions EXCEPT:

   A. How actively the students are able to participate in the care of patients—NO, students must be able to do many of the treatments and procedures.

   B. **Whether or not new ideas may be implemented—YES, students need to be able to try current practice ideas within policy guidelines.**

   C. The ratio of staff nurses to patients—NO, although important, this is not necessary.

   D. Students are able to express their own ideas and opinions—NO, students need to feel free to express themselves.

2. When the student says _____, the clinical environment is considered to be a negative one.

   A. The nurses on this unit consider my feelings and listen to me—NO, this illustrates the components of a positive learning environment.

   B. **The nurse manager has decided that I should take a different patient—YES, this infers that the unit is not student centered.**

   C. My clinical faculty thinks of innovative activities for the students—NO, this illustrates the components of a positive learning environment.

   D. The nurses on this unit go out of the way to help the students—NO, this illustrates the components of a positive learning environment.

3. When conducting a postconference, the faculty feels that the student is reflecting on practice when the student states:

   A. **I gave my patient time to consider her options for the day, but I should have been more directive—YES, this infers that the student has reflected on her patient as an individual.**

   B. Our textbook says that the correct dose for that drug is always the same no matter what—NO, this follows procedures without thought.

   C. The nurse manager says we should treat all the patients the same way because it indicates that we do not have favorites—NO, this follows procedures without thought.

   D. The patient was uncomfortable but the staff did not think I should move her—NO, this follows procedures without thought.

4. Critical reflection via debriefing enables the faculty member to help the students in all ways EXCEPT:

   A. Examining information to see all of reality—NO, this is not encouraging inner reflection.

   B. Promoting knowing what to knowing how—NO, this is not included in reflection.

   C. Reframing the context of a situation—NO, this is externalizing the situation.

   D. **Ignoring past learning—YES, reflective practice includes past learning.**

5. The clinical nurse educator realizes that dedicated educational units (DEUs) include which of the following qualities: (Select all that apply.)

   A. **Promote quality care and patient safety—YES, DEUs promote quality and safety of care.**

   B. Are confusing to students—NO, research does not indicate any confusion with students.

   C. **Allow students the chance for enhanced mentorship—YES, there is one-on-one mentorship.**

   D. **Permit students to practice with communication and teamwork—YES, students on DEUs are able to practice with communication and teamwork.**

6. A clinical nurse educator is on a renal unit with senior-level students. There is a low patient census today. All of the following are alternatives that may be considered for students EXCEPT:

   A. Observational assignment that meets the course outcomes—NO, observational experiences are an option if they meet the course outcomes.

   B. Dual assignments—NO, this may be appropriate, especially for complex patients.

   C. Case studies—NO, case studies may be used if they include conditions that are consistent with course outcomes.

   D. **Cancellation of the clinical day—YES, cancellation should not occur.**

7. The clinical nurse educator receives a phone call from a family member that a student has posted information about a patient on social media. What is the most appropriate response?

   A. **This is a HIPAA violation and must be reported—YES, it is a HIPAA violation.**

   B. HIPAA does not include social media—NO, HIPAA includes social media.

   C. Maybe no one else will find out about this, so I will just keep it to myself—NO, this must be reported.

   D. Have the student apologize to the patient—NO, this incident must be reported and an apology by itself is not adequate.

8. The students in the clinical group feel that postclinical conference is a "waste of time" and want to do something else. How should the clinical nurse educator respond? (Select all that apply.)

   A. We will start doing a shorter postclinical conference because it is not beneficial to you—NO, this is not appropriate.

   B. **Postclinical conference gives you a chance to reflect on your day—YES, postclinical conference allows for debriefing and reflection.**

   C. Postclinical conference allows you to learn from the instructor—NO, postclinical conference allows for learning from peers.

   D. Student-led postclinical conferences are not an option—NO, it is possible for students to assist with leading postclinical conferences with educator support.

9. During the first 2 weeks of the semester, the clinical nurse educator has noticed that one student has had difficulty with assessing patients in the clinical learning environment. What is the best response by the nurse educator?

    A. I will wait until the student's summative evaluation to discuss this because the student may be nervous—NO, it is better not to wait until the end to provide feedback.
    B. **I will provide feedback to the student after each clinical day and assess whether improvement occurs—YES, this is appropriate to provide frequent feedback and assess whether the student is improving.**
    C. I will keep careful notes on this and communicate with the course coordinator at the end of the course—NO, it is important to keep notes and communicate with the course coordinator in an ongoing fashion.
    D. I will wait until the midterm clinical evaluation to discuss this—NO, it is better to provide the student with feedback each week.

10. The nurse educator in a women's health course has scheduled a clinical day in a women's homeless shelter. Another educator is concerned because it is not a traditional clinical setting and the shelter does not have a nurse. All of the following are appropriate responses EXCEPT:

    A. The women at the homeless shelter have unmet health care needs, and I want the students to learn more about their experiences—NO, this will allow the students to learn about vulnerable populations.
    B. I feel that the clinical setting meets the course learning outcomes objective related to health disparities—NO, this will allow the students to learn about health disparities.
    C. The hospital is having an accreditation visit and this is an alternative clinical site that fits well with my course—NO, this is an appropriate alternative clinical activity.
    D. **I will schedule a traditional clinical day because there are no nurses at the shelter—YES, students do not have to complete all of their hours in acute-care settings with nurses.**

CHAPTER 8 PRACTICE QUESTIONS

1. When discussing HPS simulation, what does *HPS* stand for?

    A. Health care procedure simulation—NO
    B. **Human patient simulator—YES.**
    C. Health care process simulator—NO.
    D. Human procedure simulation—NO.

2. What is a standardized patient (SP)?

    A. **An actor trained to portray a patient—YES.**
    B. A type of HPS manikin—NO, it may involve a manikin but is an actor.
    C. A computer program for health care diseases—NO, this is a different type of simulation.
    D. A virtual reality serious game—NO, this is a different type of simulation.

3. What attribute is not associated with fidelity?
   A. Realism—NO, this is included in fidelity of simulation.
   B. Capabilities—NO, this is included in fidelity of simulation.
   C. Complexity—NO, this is included in fidelity of simulation.
   D. **Risk-taking—YES, this is not part of fidelity.**

4. What is the process by which the standardized patients (SPs) learn the simulation scenario?
   A. Simulation feedback—NO, this is the process in which they discuss how the student felt and what the student did correctly and incorrectly.
   B. Role-play—NO, this is the actual enactment of the scenario.
   C. Scenario review—NO, this can happen but it is not the initial learning process.
   D. **SP training—YES, training includes the SP understanding the healthcare issue and the expectations.**

5. Possible resources for standardized patients include the following:
   A. **Volunteers—YES, as long as they are consented.**
   B. Faculty—NO, the student should not know the person.
   C. Students—NO, the student should not know the person.
   D. Immunosuppressed patients—NO, this may compromise their health.

6. Which of the following is an example of a basic part-task trainer (PTT)?
   A. **Pelvis that can be used for Foley catheter insertion—YES, this will teach anatomical positions and procedures.**
   B. Pelvis that can birth a baby with complications such as bleeding—NO, this is an HPS.
   C. An intravenous (IV) arm connected to a virtual patient—NO, this is a hybrid simulation.
   D. Nasogastric insertion setup connected to a virtual patient—NO, this is a hybrid simulation.

7. Following a standardized patient (SP) simulation experience the learner has the opportunity to meet with the SP one on one. What is this process called?
   A. Debriefing—NO, this is done by faculty with a group of students.
   B. Evaluation—NO, this is an evaluation process usually between one faculty member and one student.
   C. **Feedback—YES, feedback is the one-to-one interaction between the SP and the student.**
   D. Review—NO, this is not the terminology.

8. Which of the following is an example of complex a part-task trainer (PTT)?
   A. Patient torso with multiple lung sounds—NO, this is considered just a PTT.
   B. **Laparoscopic trainer connected to virtual patient—YES, this is a trainer that does one thing but is more complex because it is an internal procedure.**
   C. IV cushion with multiple injection sites—NO, this is considered just a part-task trainer.
   D. Pelvis with male and female genitalia—NO, this is considered just a part-task trainer.

9. Which of the following are essential for a debriefing facilitator?

   A. Has observed someone else debrief—NO, actually education in debriefing is needed.

   B. Received a report of how the scenario went—NO, the debriefer needs to observe the scenario.

   C. **Select and use a specific model for debriefing—YES, this provides consistency.**

   D. Be ready to explain better interventions than what was done—NO, the learners should reflect.

10. Where can a faculty obtain simulation scenarios for a human patient simulator (HPS) manikin?

    A. Free from a vendor—NO, these are usually for sale

    B. **Design their own—YES, this makes it specific to the learners.**

    C. Run the scenario on the fly—NO, this may not meet the learning outcomes.

    D. Take it from medicine—NO, these have different objectives.

CHAPTER 9 PRACTICE QUESTIONS

1. The nurse educator needs additional understanding when she states that the following is incivil behavior:

   A. The student falls asleep in class—NO, this is incivil.

   B. The student is texting on her cell phone while in class—NO, this is incivil.

   C. The student rolls his eyes at the professor—NO, this is incivil.

   D. **The student is taking notes on the computer—YES, this is appropriate.**

2. Which of the following methods is a positive way to socialize a newly licensed nurse into the nursing profession?

   A. Invite the new nurse to go out drinking with "the gang"—NO, although that might be including the new nurse, it is done in a negative, noncoping manner.

   B. Say to the new nurse "I got your back"—NO, although that sounds nice it gives mixed messages for the new nurse may not know what exactly "I got your back" means.

   C. **Invite the new nurse to attend a professional nursing conference with you—YES, this is the most positive way of including the new nurse and promoting education and growth by attending a professional conference.**

   D. Be nice to the nurse, but when you are with senior nurses say what you really think of her abilities—NO, this is being unprofessional and will not lead to an honest work relationship.

3. The nurse educator is working in an institution and notices a new nurse and her preceptor interacting on a weekend shift. The nurse educator notices that the preceptor is in fact bullying the new nurse who quietly stands by and does not react when her preceptor embarrasses her in front of their patient. What would be the best strategy to employ to correct this behavior?

   A. Ask the patient whether he or she likes the care he or she is receiving—NO, do not involve the patient into the mix of the interaction.

B. Tell your nurse manager on Monday that you don't think the preceptor should have new orientees anymore—NO, although telling the nurse manager you have concerns is not wrong, you should intervene if someone is being bullied and embarrassed in front of a patient. By telling the manager on Monday it will allow this behavior to continue all weekend.

C. Do nothing as this is not your preceptee—NO, ignoring the situation will not help the preceptee.

D. **Ask to speak with the preceptor in private and share with her your perceptions and offer a suggestion as to how she might better interact with the student—YES, ask to speak with the preceptor in private and professionally point out that you noticed she was correcting and making her orientee feel embarrassed by correcting her directly in front of the patient. Gently suggest that in the future she correct the orientee in private, just as you are discussing the situation with the preceptor now.**

4. Which of the following is an acceptable teaching strategy when teaching low-literacy patients?

A. Create a professional authoritative relationship with them because you are the educator—NO, a trusting open relationship is best and will facilitate learning.

B. **Use repetition to reinforce information—YES, using repetition of information will reinforce content for better learning.**

C. Use the direct question-and-answer method—NO, this may make them uneasy and may inhibit the learning session.

D. Give them large amounts of information at a time as availability of a translator is limited—NO, in fact small bits of information should be presented at a time. Remember, people with poor reading and comprehension skills are easily overwhelmed.

5. Which of the following statements is true about learning styles?

A. When a teacher uses a variety of teaching methods, it confuses the learner and the student learns less—NO, using a variety of teaching methods makes the learner feel less stressed and enables concept understanding in that you do not know which method will work for each student.

B. Learners feel less stressed when using just one style of learning—NO, sometimes when using only one style the learner is more stressed. This is particularly so if the teaching method being used is not congruent with the learner's individual style.

C. **Using learning methods that are consistent with the learner is considered the best way to effect the best learning achievement—YES, using the teaching method that is consistent with the learning style is the best way to effect learning achievement.**

D. The educator applying learning styles theory to each learner allows the educator to recognize whether learners will process information correctly—NO, this is not a true statement. Processing information and learning styles are two different things. It is important to realize that everyone processes information in different ways.

6. The nurse educator has a learner in the class who has an accommodation for increased time for testing. The educator needs to:

    A. Understand the nature of the disability—NO, the educator just needs to make the documented accommodations and this would not maintain confidentiality.

    B. Meet privately with the learner—NO, the educator just needs to make the documented accommodations.

    C. **Accommodate the learner—YES, the educator needs to accommodate the learner as indicated.**

    D. Keep a copy of the letter from the physician—NO, the educator just needs to make the documented accommodations from the learning center, the learning center keeps the physician diagnosis.

7. The nurse educator is teaching a large class that is very diverse. Which population of learners is at an increased risk for failure? Learners who:

    A. Decided to pursue a second career—NO, second-degree learners usually self-direct their leaning and do well.

    B. Just graduated from high school—NO, although some younger learners may be at risk because of their new-found freedom at college, this does not apply to all of them.

    C. **Speak English as a second language—YES, learners who speak English as a second language are at increased risk of being unsuccessful in the program as well as on the NCLEX-RN®.**

    D. Transferred from another nursing program—NO, although many transfer learners could be at risk this is also not universal because not all learners transfer because of poor grades; many transfer because of relocation.

8. The nurse educator is discussing graduation with learners. One of the learners says that being responsible for patients without the instructor is very frightening. Which statement by the nurse educator would be most appropriate?

    A. "The nurse manager will be available to guide you in decision making that is related to patient care"—NO, this is not necessarily true; nurse managers are often consumed with administrative responsibilities.

    B. "Most hospitals have an orientation program that will make sure you are prepared"—NO, although orientation programs assist greatly they are not helpful once the learner is on his or her own in the patient care unit.

    C. "The procedure manual is always available to assist you in making patient care decisions"—NO, although the procedure manual is helpful, it may not cover every individual decision-making process.

    D. **"Your mentor will provide a structured process to guide your decisions and behaviors"—YES, the mentor working alongside the learner provides guidance during everyday patient care, decision making, and teaching.**

9. The nurse educator assesses the written work of a millennial learner and is surprised that among the references the learner uses is a(n):

    A. Textbook—NO, learners often use textbooks in paper or electronic format to find information and verify answers.

    B. Internet source—NO, this is common.

C. **Encyclopedia—YES, millennial learners usually use the web for referencing and electronic sources.**

D. Article—NO, journals are available electronically and are used for up-to-date information and evidence.

10. Learners are encouraged to become members of the National Student Nurses Association (NSNA). The framework of this organization indicates that the learner will gain experience:

A. **Making decisions and being accountable for those decisions—YES, the framework for this organization is shared governance; therefore, learners will have the opportunity to discuss their opinions and make decisions. The group members are responsible for the outcome of decisions.**

B. Following regulations determined by elected officers—NO, this is not the main purpose of the organization.

C. Learning how to engage in social activities while in school—NO, this is not the main purpose of the organization.

D. Discussing health information and presenting projects—NO, this is not the main purpose of the organization.

CHAPTER 10 PRACTICE QUESTIONS

1. According to Bringle and Clayton (2012), the optimal service learning (SL) design includes:

A. A formal buddy assignment—NO, this is not always productive.

B. Separation from a formal academic course—NO, it can be part of a course.

C. **Benefits to the community—YES, it should benefit the student and the community.**

D. Mandatory core competencies—NO, this is a forced situation and not conducive to learning.

2. A student is going to travel to Cuba for a service learning (SL) experience. To build intercultural competence predeparture, which of the following will help the most?

A. Dining weekly in restaurants in a Hispanic neighborhood—NO, this may not be an authentic experience.

B. Binge watching HBO's *Havana* series—NO, this is fiction.

C. **Attend the predeparture training session offered by the study abroad office—YES, this will teach actual cultural practices.**

D. Take a conversational Spanish course—NO, this would help but not teach the culture specifically.

3. An example of implementing a global classroom would be to:

A. **Collaborate with students and faculty using video-teleconferencing—YES, this video linking with other students and/or faculty takes the classroom out of your institution and links it with another classroom anywhere in the world.**

B. Assign research articles to students to review nursing around the globe—NO, this just has the student review research articles on an assigned topic.

C. Have students find a research article about nursing in another country—NO, this just has the student find a research article on an assigned topic.

D. Have a class utilizing Internet videos about other countries—NO, this is utilizing videos in one classroom and does not integrate classrooms across the globe.

4. Which of the following exemplifies study-abroad opportunities?

A. A student going to take blood pressures in a well clinic in another country—NO, this would be a service learning (SL) opportunity.

B. **A student taking a course in research at the University of Sydney, Australia—YES, this would be an example of a student taking a course and studying abroad for which the student may or may not get credit.**

C. Participating in an online virtual class from his or her apartment—NO, that is online learning.

D. Going to South America to help rebuild homes after a hurricane—NO, that is SL or a service mission.

5. Which of the following programs enables students to spend a year in a different country learning at an institution of higher learning?

A. **Studying abroad—YES, studying abroad involves spending more than a few weeks and involves taking classes at an institution of higher learning.**

B. Faculty enhancement program—NO, a faculty enhancement program, enables faculty to meet other faculty in other countries.

C. Service learning—NO, service learning is usually more limited in time and the students provide a service or skills for an underprivileged population.

D. Global classroom—NO, although the global classroom allows students to take a course at an institution of higher learning, there is no need to leave the country in which you reside. This type of learning can be done from home using web-based resources.

6. Which of the following is an important element for students to utilize when returning from an international learning experience to enable them to share and verbalize feelings and experiences?

A. Write a paper summarizing the experience—NO, this is just a summary assignment in which the students write about their experience. It is a one-way communication tool.

B. **Conduct a debriefing experience—YES, a debriefing session is an important two-way communication process and allows students to verbalize their feelings and experiences in a safe and supportive environment with people who have experienced the same thing.**

C. Do a role-play to reenact the experience—NO, role-play is acting out a given situation. It does not necessarily allow others to comment until after the role-play is completed.

D. Write a case study of an individual they met and present it—NO, this is the most removed and does not allow for one-on-one interaction and support.

7. Which of the following statements best reflects what *cultural competence* means?

   A. Understanding people react differently depending on their religion—NO, that is understanding reactions according to religion, not culture.

   B. Being aware that language plays a key role in one's ability to access health care—NO, this does not have anything to do with being culturally competent. This refers to language barriers.

   C. **Allowing the nurse to recognize the impact of globalization of individual health and nursing practice—YES, this allows a nurse to fully understand the relationship of culture in relation to nursing care and the individual's health options.**

   D. Having a cognitive understanding of what each member of the health care team's role is in different areas of the world—NO, this is role definition.

8. A university has an exchange program with a university in Europe. The best description of a well-managed exchange program is:

   A. The foreign university will accommodate English-speaking students—NO, many universities have classes in English.

   B. The foreign university is gaining tuition funds by participating—NO, usually the tuition is a wash-out; the student pays the price he or she would normally pay.

   C. **The foreign university will grant course credit—YES, usually the courses are transferable.**

   D. The foreign university cannot grant transferable courses—NO, courses can be transferred.

9. A nurse educator is taking a group of interprofessional students on a service learning (SL) trip. A safety feature that is encouraged is to:

   A. Take cash for exchange purposes—NO, cash is easy to lose or get stolen.

   B. Carry school texts for reference—NO, this weighs down students.

   C. Be generous with people who beg for cash or goods—NO, this is not acceptable to many foreigners.

   D. **Develop a social media site—YES, this will help keep people back home up to date with the students' whereabouts.**

10. During a debriefing from a service learning (SL) experience, which student comment best indicates cultural awareness:

    A. "This experience allowed me to see how others live"—NO, this is just observational.

    B. **"I think we should go back, the people need more resources from us"— YES, this student demonstrates a sense of civic duty and responsibility.**

    C. "I think we made a difference today"—NO, this is focused on the student.

    D. "This experience was different than what I expected"—NO, this is observational.

11. The culture of service learning (SL) is currently developed in learners by:
    A. Nurse educators, in order to emphasize the caring aspects of nursing—NO, it is developed in primary and secondary schools.
    B. Parents, to better prepare their children for the world—NO, it is usually introduced in schools.
    C. **Primary and secondary schools, to develop global citizens—YES, primary and secondary schools are advocates of service learning.**
    D. Organizations, to increase fund-raising—NO, it is usually introduced in schools.

12. The best format to publicize service learning (SL) done by learners and faculty would be to:
    A. Produce flyers about the trip—NO, this is not the most effective or professional method.
    B. **Hold an SL conference with poster presentations—YES, the learners can tell about their experiences in a professional format.**
    C. Post an advertisement in the local newspaper—NO, this is not the most effective or professional method.
    D. Comment on the experiences on Facebook—NO, this is not the most effective or professional method.

CHAPTER 11 PRACTICE QUESTIONS

1. The program evaluation committee is reviewing the nursing program evaluation data. The nursing program has established an 86% pass rate as the benchmark for graduates taking the National Council Licensure Examination (NCLEX) for the first time. This goal has not been met for the past 3 years. Which of the following recommendations would be a *priority* for the committee to make?
   A. Increase the passing-grade benchmark for each nursing course to 93%—NO, this will just shift the perceptions of what a passing grade was to a higher grade and not necessarily increase rigor.
   B. **Require a minimum GPA of 3.0 in the natural science and nursing courses—YES, the evidence supports this.**
   C. Lower the NCLEX pass-rate benchmark for first-time takers to 78%—NO, this is not an acceptable passing rate.
   D. Institute a pre-RN assessment test with a minimum benchmark for admission into the nursing program—NO, there is no evidence to support this change.

2. The clinical educator is preparing to write the summative evaluation for the learners in her clinical group. The educator believes in the constructivist philosophy of evaluation. Therefore when completing the evaluation, she will do which of the following?
   A. Determine whether the objectives of the course have been met—NO, this is not building knowledge from real situations.
   B. Compare the learner to others to determine level of development—NO, this is not building knowledge from real situations.
   C. **Seek input from clinical staff regarding the learner's clinical performance—YES, this is investigating learning built in the real situation.**
   D. Assign a grade of pass/fail for the clinical performance—NO, this is not building knowledge from real situations.

3. The nursing curriculum committee is revising the curriculum to be more congruent with changes in health care delivery. The *most important* consideration of the committee should be which of the following?

 A. **Be sure the new curriculum is aligned with the mission and philosophy of the governing institution—YES, this is always the foundational information needed for curriculum evaluation.**

 B. Develop curriculum objectives and program outcomes—NO, this is done after the curriculum and the organization's mission is aligned.

 C. Establish benchmarks for first-time pass rates on the National Council Licensure Examination (NCLEX)—NO, this is not part of curriculum development but part of establishing policies and standards.

 D. Require a standardized exit exam with a benchmark pass rate of 85%—NO, this is not part of curriculum development but rather part of establishing policies and standards.

4. The nurse educator is reviewing the item analysis on a course test for a multiple-choice question. The following statistics were calculated for one item:

Point Biserial = −0.27	Correct Answer = B		Total Group = 88.24%	
Distractor Analysis	A	B	C	D
Point Biserial	0.27	−0.27	0.00	0.00
Frequency	12%	88%	0%	0%

The educator realizes the cause for this frequency distribution is that:

 A. The distractors were not clear—NO, two distractors were chosen by learners.

 B. The distractors were too hard for learners to choose—NO, 88% of the learners chose the correct answer.

 C. **Learners who scored lower on the exam got the item correct—YES, the point biserial for the correct distractor is negative.**

 D. Learners who knew the content answered the item correctly—NO, the point biserial would have been positive.

5. The following statistics were calculated on a multiple-choice question on an examination:

Point Biserial = 0.61	Correct Answer = C		Total Group = 76.47%	
Distractor Analysis	A	B	C	D
Point Biserial	0.59	0.00	0.61	−0.24
Frequency	6%	0%	88%	6%

The reason for this frequency distribution is that:

 A. Learners who scored lower on the exam got the item correct—NO, the point biserial was positive.

 B. The distractors were not clear—NO, three distracters were used and the correct distractor had a positive point biserial.

 C. This item has been used on previous exams—NO, there is no evidence of this.

 D. **Learners who scored higher on the exam got the item correct—YES, the correct distractor had a positive point biserial.**

6. The item analysis revealed the following data for a multiple-choice question:

Point Biserial = 0.19	Correct Answer = D		Total Group = 5.88%	
Distractor Analysis	A	B	C	D
Point Biserial	−0.25	0.39	−0.35	0.19
Frequency	41%	41%	12%	6%

Based on these statistics, the professor should do which of the following when using this item on future exams?

A. Nothing, as the upper third of the class answered the item correctly—NO, only 6% of the class chose the correct option.

B. Revise distractor A—NO, distractor A had a negative point biserial.

C. **Revise distractor B—YES, this distractor was wrong and had a positive point biserial so many of the better learners for this test chose it.**

D. Revise distractor C—NO, this is a wrong distractor with a negative point biserial.

7. An item-analysis report for a multiple-choice exam revealed that the KR-20 was 0.56. Based on this statistic, which of the following interpretations can be made regarding this exam?

A. **The exam is reliable in measuring learner knowledge of the material—YES, this is an appropriate KR-20 for an instructor-made classroom test.**

B. There are too few items on the exam—NO, the KR-20 is appropriate.

C. The items are poorly written and do not discriminate—NO, the KR-20 is appropriate so this is not reflected in the statistics.

D. There is an excess of very easy questions—NO, the KR-20 is appropriate, so this is not reflected in the statistics.

8. A professor administered a multiple-choice exam and performed an item analysis, which revealed the following data:

Point Biserial = 0.56	Correct Answer = A		Total Group = 52%	
Distractor Analysis	A	B	C	D
Point Biserial	0.56	−0.31	−0.44	0.02
Frequency	52%	18%	18%	12%

The likely cause for this frequency distribution is:

A. The distractors are too hard—NO, this item discriminated.

B. **Learners who scored highest on the exam got the item correct—YES.**

C. The distractors are too easy—NO, only 52% chose the correct distractor.

D. Learners guessed the answer to this question—NO, there is no evidence that there was a four-way split of grades.

9. The following statistics were obtained in an item analysis for a multiple-choice exam:

Point Biserial = 0.00	Correct Answer = C		Total Group = 100%	
Distractor Analysis	A	B	C	D
Point Biserial	0.00	0.00	0.00	0.00
Frequency	0%	0%	100%	0%

What action should be taken based on this data?

A. No action is needed as all learners answered the question correctly—NO, this test item did not discriminate.
B. Revise distractor C—NO, there are other issues with the item.
C. Add another distractor to the choices—NO, there are other issues with the item.
D. **Rewrite all of the distractors—YES, they all need to be looked at again.**

10. Which of the following activities would be the *best* strategy to engage the visual learner at the cognitive and affective levels?

A. Audiotaping a lecture—NO, this would work best for the auditory learner.
B. Writing a case study—NO, this is tactile (writing) and cognitive.
C. **Developing a concept map—YES.**
D. Writing an essay—NO, this is tactile (writing) and cognitive.

CHAPTER 12 PRACTICE QUESTIONS

1. When developing an interprofessional curriculum, the planning committee should:

A. **Communicate with and include community members to decide on areas that need improvement—YES.**
B. Try to align the entire curriculum with the various programs—NO, One or two courses is enough.
C. Allow each discipline to plan its own clinical activities—NO, the students should participate together.
D. Invite students at the same level in their own programs to participate—NO, students should be at varying levels.

2. A teaching strategy appropriate for an interprofessional education course would include all EXCEPT a(n):

A. Interdisciplinary case study—NO, this could be completed by members of one profession.
B. Low-risk simulation experience—NO, this does not necessarily have more than one professions involved.
C. Panel presentation by an interprofessional team of experts—NO, this is not interactive learning for students.
D. **Concept map from each discipline—YES, the disciplines should work together to create an active learning environment.**

3. Which technique may have the potential for "transforming" nursing education?

   A. Simulation—NO, simulation alone and without debriefing is not enough.
   B. Journaling—NO, journaling by itself would not meet the criteria.
   C. **Debriefing—YES, the National League for Nursing and the International Nursing Association for Clinical Simulation and Learning have suggested that this technique, done properly could transform nursing education.**
   D. Questioning—NO, this is a good method for higher level thinking, but would not transform the curriculum.

4. Which is an example of first-order change?

   A. **The faculty moves the pediatric content to a different semester—YES, this change does not effect the entire system.**
   B. The new curriculum stresses concepts, not diseases—NO, this is second order.
   C. The library becomes completely electronic—NO, this is second order.
   D. Testing is done completely via simulation—NO, this is second order.

5. The Preparation for the Professions Program (PPP) has identified three dimensions of apprenticeships for professional education. They include the following: (Select all that apply.)

   A. **Acquired skill-based learning that includes clinical judgment—YES, this is one of the recommendations.**
   B. Dependence on authority—NO, this is not one of the recommendations.
   C. **Intellectual training—YES, this is one of the recommendations**.
   D. **Ethical standards— YES, this is one of the recommendations**.

6. Which course would be appropriate for a conceptual curriculum?

   A. Respiratory care in the intensive care unit—NO, this is specific to one set of problems.
   B. **Respiratory care over the life cycle—YES, the concept of respiration is described in all developmental stages.**
   C. Pediatric respiratory problems—NO, this is specific to children.
   D. Issues in respiratory care—NO, this may not include all areas of respiratory care.

7. An objective that is appropriate for the first nursing course in a baccalaureate nursing program is:

   A. **List the nutritional needs of clients of all ages—YES, that is the objective written at the lowest level (remembering).**
   B. Choose foods appropriate for a low-sodium diet—NO, this is a higher level objective (applying).
   C. Analyze the nutrients in a diabetic diet—NO, this is analyzing.
   D. Develop a nutritional plan for a client with kidney disease—NO, this is creating.

8. Graduates of any program should be able to:

A. Develop research questions related to patient safety—NO, they practice according to evidence, but do not design the studies to support the evidence.

B. **Practice according to ethical standards—YES, all nurses practice using standards.**

C. Feel confident that they have mastered the practice of nursing—NO, we are continually learning.

D. Provide care that is appropriate to individuals—NO, they include at least families in their care.

9. Competencies for graduates of baccalaureate programs include all EXCEPT:

A. Human flourishing—NO, this should be part of the curriculum.

B. Professional identify—NO, this should be part of the curriculum.

C. **Research expertise—YES, they identify questions in need of study.**

D. Nursing judgment—NO, they make judgments substantiated with evidence.

10. Which is the most appropriate topic for a simulation used in an interprofessional education (IPE) course with several disciplines?

A. **Disaster training—YES, this is appropriate for public health, medical, nursing, and emergency medical technician students.**

B. Difficult childbirth—NO, this is most appropriate for obstetricians, nurse midwives, and neonatal nurses.

C. Cardiac failure—NO, this is most appropriate for physicians and nurse practitioners.

D. Infectious disease training—NO, this is most appropriate for public health, nursing, and medical students.

CHAPTER 13 PRACTICE QUESTIONS

1. A majority of faculty have identified a need for mentorship to accomplish which of the following:

A. Improvement in classroom teaching—NO, this is assisted with mentoring but many nurse educators arrive with experience.

B. **Work–life balance—YES, this is needed to prevent burnout.**

C. Preparing for retirement—NO, this is a human resource responsibility.

D. Identifying venues for professional presentations—NO, this is done as part of the faculty role but mentors can assist.

2. Mentoring a late-career faculty member may include:

A. Encouraging and supporting the faculty to identify and test innovative pedagogies—NO, this is more appropriate for a mid career faculty member.

B. Providing guidance in transitioning into academic leadership positions—NO, this is more appropriate for a mid career faculty member.

C. **Encouraging the faculty to identify new faculty members who show potential as leaders in nursing and nursing education—YES, this is appropriate for a late-career faculty member to do. After identifying a faculty member who shows potential, the late-career faculty can enter in a mentorship relationship to support this individual's professional development.**

D. Encouraging faculty to propose new solutions to problems and to evolve as educators and scholars in local, regional, and national arenas—NO, this is more appropriate for a mid career faculty member.

3. Early-career faculty need mentorship in the following areas:
    A. Help in identifying and testing innovative pedagogies—NO, this is more appropriate for a midcareer faculty member.
    B. Help in identifying academic leadership positions—NO, this is more appropriate for a midcareer faculty member.
    C. **Help navigating political and administrative environment—YES, this is appropriate for the novice faculty member.**
    D. Help identifying national venues for scholarly presentations— NO, this is more appropriate for a midcareer faculty member.

4. The novice nurse educator needs additional mentoring about student boundaries established when he tells his mentor that he:
    A. Shares personal stories that emphasize a content point—NO, this is okay as long as the storytelling is appropriate and relevant.
    B. Demonstrates a positive attitude with students—NO, this is appropriate.
    C. Shows enthusiasm for students learning new techniques—NO, this is appropriate.
    D. **Discusses the personnel responsibilities that limit his time—YES, this is not for student discussion.**

5. Nurse educators understand that one of the main consequences of lack of mentorship is a decrease in:
    A. Understanding of the curriculum—NO, this is not the main consequence of lack of mentorship.
    B. **Socialization into the role—YES, new educators must be socialized into the role.**
    C. Dissatisfaction of faculty—NO, lack of mentorship increases dissatisfaction.
    D. Attrition of faculty—NO, lack of mentorship increases attrition.

6. A new faculty member is constantly comparing the current teaching methods of the faculty to methods used by faculty at her previous educational unit. The mentor's best response would be to:
    A. Encourage the new faculty member to return to the previous position— NO, encouraging them to leave does not help build a team.
    B. Ask the faculty member to stop comparing—NO, this may be viewed as nonsupportive.
    C. Have the faculty member present ideas in a lunch conference—NO, it is a good idea but too early in the faculty's career.
    D. **Explain to the new faculty member that there are many methods that work well—YES.**

7. The director of the educational unit asks a seasoned faculty mentor to mentor a new hire and the seasoned faculty member objects. The best way to handle this situation would be to:
    A. **Document the situation and find someone who is willing—YES, this should be discussed at evaluation time because it is an expected professional obligation.**
    B. Insist that the faculty mentor do it—NO, this will not encourage a supportive mentor–protégé relationship.

    C. Terminate the faculty mentor who refuses—NO, this is not a good idea with a faculty shortage.

    D. Tell the faculty mentor that it is a professional reasonability—NO, this will not encourage a supportive mentor–protégé relationship.

8. A faculty member tells another faculty member, in the hallway, that his skills are out of date because he no longer practices clinically. The director of the educational unit would best respond to this comment by telling:

    A. The faculty member who made the comment that it is incivil—NO, this will set up further conflict.

    B. The faculty member who does not work clinically that it would be a good idea to seek out a per diem clinical position—NO, this is not necessary.

    C. Both faculty members to take their conflict behind closed doors—NO, this may not resolve the issue.

    D. **Both faculty members that competency is not based solely on clinical practice—YES, this is what they need to understand.**

9. The novice nurse educator understands that faculty role expectations include:

    A. Completing a terminal degree—NO, this depends on the type of educational unit they are employed in.

    B. Concentrating on teaching and not service—NO, all areas need to be addressed.

    C. Attending conferences in the future—NO, although conferences are very helpful to novice nurse educators.

    D. **Incorporating ethical and legal principles into teaching practice—YES, this is an expectation.**

10. An important orientation activity for nurse educators is:

    A. Developing a curriculum matrix to follow—NO, this is done by the curriculum committee members.

    B. **Attending departmental meetings—YES, this is a very important learning tool.**

    C. Doing a university-wide scavenger hunt—NO, meeting faculty from other departments is more helpful.

    D. Socializing with other faculty—NO, this is important but not the initial priority.

CHAPTER 14 PRACTICE QUESTIONS

1. Davis's technology acceptance model involves consideration of which of the following:

    A. **External factors—YES, external factors need to be considered.**

    B. Early majority—NO, this not associated with Davis's theory.

    C. Thought leaders—NO, this not associated with Davis's theory.

    D. Community members—NO, this may be part of the external factors but is not inclusive.

2. Strom (2001) identifies which of the following strategies for successful change implementation:

   A. Use only one intervention to support change—NO, Strom calls for multiple interventions.
   B. Keep site visits at minimum—NO, Strom calls for multiple interventions.
   C. **Send frequent reminders—YES, this keeps the change in everyone's mind and vision.**
   D. Communicate a shared vision—NO, this is not an element.

3. Donabedian (2005) conceptualizes evaluation into three dimensions that include:

   A. People—NO, the model involves structure, processes, and outcomes.
   B. Places—NO, the model involves structure, processes, and outcomes.
   C. **Processes—YES, this is one of the three dimensions.**
   D. Constructs—NO, the model involves structure, processes, and outcomes.

4. Which of the following practices is likely to be utilized by the transactional leader?

   A. Enlisting others in a common vision by appealing to shared aspirations—NO, this would be transformational.
   B. **Using a rewards/punishment system—YES, they use a patriarchal award and punishment system that is dehumanizing.**
   C. Experimenting and taking risks—NO, this would be transformational.
   D. Sharing power—NO, this would be transformational.

5. Under the realm of motivation, Grenny and colleagues' (2008) sources of influence include:

   A. Creating social support—NO, this is not the primary influence.
   B. **Linking to mission and values—YES, this is essential.**
   C. Overinvesting in skill building—NO, this is not the primary influence.
   D. Changing the environment—NO, this is not the primary influence.

6. There are things that a manager can do to "manage" organizational culture. These include which of the following?

   A. **Purposeful recruitment, selection, and replacement—YES, each individual contributes to the organizational culture.**
   B. Conduct a performance needs assessment—NO, this is not interventional.
   C. Establish partnerships outside one's usual circles—NO, this is not focused on internal culture.
   D. Plan and implement policies and procedures—NO, these are just managerial tasks and do not usually affect culture.

7. The theory that describes change as a dynamic balance of forces working in opposing directions is:

   A. Lippitt's Phases of Change Theory—NO, this theory discusses specific stages.
   B. Prochaska and DiClemente's Change Theory—NO, this theory discusses innovation.

    C. Theory of planned behavior—NO, this is a systematic theory.

    D. **Lewin's Three-Step Change Theory—YES, this theory talks about opposing forces.**

8. The theory that is describes change from the perspective of the person moving through stages of change is:

    A. Social cognitive theory—NO, this discusses influences of change.

    B. **Prochaska and DiClemente's Change Theory—YES, this discusses innovation and stages.**

    C. Theory of reasoned action—NO, this theory discusses intentions to change.

    D. Theory of planned behavior—NO, this theory links beliefs to behavior.

9. Contextual factors of the change process include all of the following except:

    A. Situational/environmental factors—NO, these change.

    B. Leadership—NO, this also changes and is not individualized.

    C. Communication or incentives—NO, this can also vary.

    D. **Personal traits—YES, it is the personality of the leader that affects the change process.**

10. The National Center for Cultural Competence states that the integration of high-level cultural competence skills/strategies is a priority for health organizational policies because nurses must do which of the following?

    A. Be sensitive to others' beliefs and values—NO, this is part of it but does not encompass all that is needed.

    B. **Eliminate health disparities among people from diverse racial, ethnic, and cultural backgrounds—YES, cultural diversity in workforce should reflect the population.**

    C. Consider individual/group needs, preferences, or experiences—NO, this is part of it but does not encompass all that is needed globally.

    D. Be able to develop communications/materials at the appropriate level, language, and literacy—NO, this is part of it but does not encompass all that is needed.

CHAPTER 15 PRACTICE QUESTIONS

1. A nurse educator's area of expertise is mentoring. Which of the following indicates the educator is meeting expectations for scholarship of discovery?

    A. Serves as a mentor in a mentoring program of a national organization—NO, this would be the scholarship of application.

    B. **Conducts research about the characteristics of a mentor—YES, according to Boyer, the scholarship of discovery involves systematic inquiry.**

    C. Offers workshops about being a mentor—NO, this would be the scholarship of teaching.

    D. Serves on a national committee to develop mentoring guidelines—NO, this is the scholarship of application.

2. The promotion and tenure committee at a school of nursing is reviewing a nurse educator's dossier for promotion to associate professor. Which of the following indicates the nurse educator is demonstrating the scholarship of teaching? The dossier indicates the nurse educator:

   A. Has received consistently excellent student reviews of teaching over six semesters—NO, this is the scholarship of application.

   B. Has created and implemented a scenario to be used in a simulation—NO, this is also application.

   C. Has improved her teaching following a peer review—NO, this is application.

   D. **Has published three articles about innovative teaching in peer-reviewed journals—YES, scholarship of teaching involves disseminating work in appropriate journals.**

3. Which of the following indicates a nurse educator is developing in the role of scholar?

   A. **Identifies the need for evidence about best practices for clinical placement of students—YES, the role of the scholar is to identify issues and problems requiring evidence for practice.**

   B. Participates in a "journal club" at the school of nursing—NO, this is promoting dissemination of information and can occur in all realms of scholarship.

   C. Is asked to be a mentor for new faculty—NO, this is part of the role of nurse educator.

   D. Teaches a research course in a graduate program—NO, this is part of the role of nurse educator.

4. Which is a characteristic of scholarship?

   A. Funding from a federal organization—NO, funding is not related to scholarship, but can be helpful in funding a research project.

   B. **Peer review—YES, scholarly activities, including teaching, must be documented, visible, and capable of being reviewed by peers.**

   C. Implementing a new teaching strategy—NO, merely implementing a strategy does not constitute scholarship. The use of the strategy must be reported; documented, for example, in a manuscript or presentation; or peer reviewed.

   D. Reporting the use of a teaching strategy on a curriculum vitae (CV)—NO, reporting scholarship is not sufficient, it must be peer reviewed.

5. Boyer's model of scholarship is most appropriately used to guide which of the following decisions?

   A. Determining an area of research to pursue—NO, Boyer's model of scholarship is used to make decisions about appointment, performance review, promotion and tenure, and organizing a dossier.

   B. **Awarding promotion and tenure—YES, Boyer's model of scholarship is used to make decisions about appointment, performance review, promotion and tenure, and organizing a dossier.**

   C. Selecting a nursing organization to join—NO, this is not the correct use of the model.

   D. Choosing a mentor—NO, this should be done on experience and expertise.

6. Which indicates a nurse educator is demonstrating integrity as a scholar?

   A. Publishes results of an attitude survey administered to students—NO, the nurse educator must obtain intuitional review board approval prior to publishing the results of any survey administered to students.

   B. Includes only recent publications in the reference list of a manuscript—NO, all references to any source material or ideas not original to the author must be included in the reference list.

   C. **Ensures that all persons who contributed to the writing and reviewing of the manuscript are listed as authors—YES, all persons involved in writing the manuscript must be listed as such.**

   D. Tells a student that he or she cannot be considered as an author on a manuscript because the work was done in his or her role as student—NO, anyone who contributes to the development and writing of a manuscript must be considered as an author. Student status is not a reason to deny the student authorship credit.

7. A nurse educator is seeking funding to conduct a pilot study of the effects of peer testing in the educator's classroom. The nurse educator should first seek funding from:

   A. **The university's research fund for teaching and learning—YES, this is a small classroom study that involves advancing the science of teaching and learning. The small grants fund at the university is the most appropriate for this study.**

   B. Health Resources and Services Administration (HRSA)—NO, this is for a large external grant.

   C. National Institutes of Health (NIH)—NO, this is for a large external grant.

   D. Robert Wood Johnson Foundation—NO, this is for a large external grant.

8. A nurse educator administers a standardized learning-style inventory to incoming students and is planning to correlate the findings with the students' grade point average (GPA). The nurse educator should first:

A. Administer the learning-style inventory and request the GPA for each student from the student services office—NO, this needs IRB approval.

B. Administer the learning-style inventory and ask each student to self-report his GPA—NO, this is inappropriate if the participants do not consent and are not knowledgeable about why they are divulging the information.

C. **Seek review and approval from the Institutional Review Board (IRB) to conduct this study—YES, this study requires protection of human subjects and permission from the students to have access to their grade point average; approval from the IRB is required. Having a colleague with research skills is helpful, but is not required to conduct this study.**

D. Find a colleague with research skills to be a coinvestigator for this project—NO, this project needs to be approved first.

9. A faculty member who is a full professor is collaborating with a faculty member who is an assistant professor, a nursing doctoral student, and a doctorally prepared statistician who is not a nurse to conduct research that will result in a paper to be submitted for publication. The group agrees that each member will write a significant component of the paper according to his or her expertise. Who should be listed as author on the paper?

A. The full professor—NO, this does not recognize the expertise of the other contributors.

B. The two faculty members—NO, this does not recognize the expertise of the other contributors.

C. Only the nurses—NO, this does not recognize the expertise of the other contributors.

D. **All members of the team—YES, all members of the team who contribute to the writing of the paper must be included as authors on the paper.**

10. A nurse educator who has a DNP degree and is a psychiatric nurse practitioner with an appointment as clinical assistant professor is receiving an annual review from the department chair following the first year of teaching. Which of the following provides the best evidence that the nurse educator has met the requirement for continued employment in the area of scholarship of teaching? The nurse educator:

A. Received student reviews of teaching of 4.8 on a 5-point scale—NO, although this is helpful, it is not the best evidence.

B. Attended two conferences related to using simulations—NO, although this is helpful it is not the best evidence.

C. **Presented the findings from a study of student response to stress during clinical assignments—YES, presenting and publishing work is the best example of meeting requirements for the scholarship of teaching; scholarship of teaching is an expected role of a nurse educator and appointment on a clinical track.**

D. Has received the outstanding teacher award presented by the student nurses association at the school—NO, although this is helpful, it is not the best evidence.

CHAPTER 16 PRACTICE QUESTIONS

1. Learners of nursing understand the mandate of today's health care society best when they are taught:

    A. **Interprofessional collaboration—YES, interprofessional collaboration and communication will decrease health care mistakes and cost.**

    B. Fundamental skills—NO, fundamental skills alone will not teach them what is need in the clinical arena.

    C. Information technology—NO, this is only one aspect.

    D. Triage management—NO, again this is only one aspect.

2. Developing a curriculum based on current demographics would best include which of following?

    A. Complementary therapies—NO, although this is important, it is one type of therapy.

    B. Childbearing choices for women with previous cesarean births—NO, although this is important, birth rates are decreasing.

    C. Health issues of HIV-positive patients—NO, although this is important.

    D. **Geriatric concepts of aging—YES, this is the fastest increasing population.**

3. The nurse educator is putting together an academic portfolio for review and includes a curriculum vitae (CV). In what order should the information appear?

    A. **Education, work history, courses taught, references—YES.**

    B. Education, work history, honors, licensure—NO, licensure should come before honors because it is necessary for employment.

    C. Licensure, education, work history, references—NO, education is first.

    D. Work history, education, licensure, honors—NO, education is first.

4. When designing a curriculum, which answer would meet the criteria needed for today's health care system? It would be a curriculum that:

    A. Develops a concept-based curriculum— NO, this is not necessary to meet the culture of safety.

    B. Includes combined classes with junior and senior nursing students for role modeling—NO, this does not meet the culture of safety.

    C. **Builds on standardized skills that are practiced and then demonstrated back, in order to pass—YES, competency-based skills meet the culture of safety.**

    D. Delivers a community-based curriculum concept throughout the program—NO, this does not meet the culture of safety.

5. The 2010 Carnegie Foundation study calls for nurse educators to increase:

    A. Rehabilitation content—NO, this was not in the report.

    B. Psychomotor domain learning—NO, task development is not an issue.

    C. **Research on nursing education—YES, more research about nursing education is needed.**

    D. Scholarship related to active learning strategies—NO, this was not the report's focus.

6. Sigma Theta Tau International Nurse Faculty Leadership Academy (NFLA) was founded as a result of data that nurse educators stay in academia because of:

   A. A research degree versus a practice degree—NO, many academic organizations use both as terminal degrees.
   B. **Mentoring—YES, lack of mentoring increases attrition.**
   C. Faculty practice—NO, many faculty like faculty practice days to keep up their skills.
   D. Salary—NO, although salaries are lower than practice this was not identified as a detriment.

7. Programs of nursing use an accreditation agency in order to:

   A. **Tell the public that standards are met—YES, this ensures the public that the program meets standards.**
   B. Ensure faculty governance—NO, it looks at this but does not ensure it.
   C. Establish NCLEX-RN® scores above the national average—NO, it looks at this but does not ensure it.
   D. Increase student satisfaction—NO, students rarely know specifics about accreditation.

8. Tenure criteria differ from institution to institution and are mostly dependent on:

   A. The professional department of the faculty applicant—NO, many tenure processes are centralized.
   B. The current governance system—NO, the tenure process is usually historically long standing.
   C. The faculty applicant's years of service—NO, tenure is usually time limited to the 7th year.
   D. **The Carnegie Classification of the institution—YES, different levels of institutions expect different standards for tenure.**

9. The Community of Inquiry Framework identifies three core elements associated with role adjustment to online learning, which include all of the following except:

   A. **Discourse presence—YES, this is not a core element.**
   B. Teaching presence—NO, this is included.
   C. Social presence—NO, this is included.
   D. Cognitive presence—NO, this is included.

10. Teaching portfolios should include all of the following items except:

    A. CV—NO, this is included.
    B. **Current student support letters—YES, this may involve a conflict of interest, alumni are a better choice to write support letters.**
    C. Examples of syllabi—NO, this is included.
    D. Teaching philosophy—NO, this is included.

Index

AACN. *See* American Association of Colleges of Nursing

AAUP. *See* American Association of University Professors

abuse, types of, 191–192

academic community, institutional environment and, 331

academic excellence, reaching for, 3–4

academic institutions, roles, rules, and responsibilities for, 113, 114

Academic Nurse Educator Certification Program (ANECP), 15

academic responsibilities
- research/scholarship, 340
- service, 340–341
- teaching, 339

academic setting
- characteristics of, 247
- collaboration/partnerships/innovation in, 338–339
- college/university, 335
- faculty governance in, 336
- mission relating to, 336
- organizational climate in, 336–337
- school of nursing, 336

accessible technologies, 105

accommodative learners, 180–181

accreditation, 334–335
- model for evidence-based evaluation, 220
- and regulations, for curriculum design accreditation, 246

achievement testing, 222

achievement tests and assessments, guidelines for, 222–224
- classroom tests, developing, 224–225
- criterion-referenced tests, 225
- identifying and defining learning outcomes of, 226–228
- item analysis relating to, 231–232
- item discrimination, 232–234
- item revision, 234–235
- nondiscriminating questions, 234
- norm-referenced tests, 225
- outcomes, 226–228

planning of, 225–235
- test questions, determination of, 228–231
- validity and reliability of, 11, 230–231

action orientation, 292

active learners, 178

active learning
- activity, 47, 48
- advantages and disadvantages, 56
- strategies, 47, 48, 59–71

additive curriculum, 253

administrative intervention CQI, 311

administrative roles, competent instructor, 105

admission criteria/policies, 216

adult learners, 181–182

advanced beginner, levels of nursing expertise, 25

affective domain
- in clinical practice, 149
  - altruism, 149
  - autonomy, 149
  - human dignity, 149
  - integrity, 149
  - social justice, 149
- of learning, 38

affective, learner's behavior, 153

affiliative leadership style, 294

"ah ha" moments, clinical domain, 144

alternative assignments, 146

altruism, 149

American Association of Colleges of Nursing (AACN), 149, 182, 260–262, 265–269, 334
- baccalaureate outcomes of, 265–269

American Association of University Professors (AAUP), 250, 342

American Nurses Association (ANA), 283

Americans with Disabilities Act, 89, 187

ANA. *See* American Nurses Association

analytical learners, 180

ANA *Scope and Standards for Nursing Professional Development,* 284

andragogy, 30
- and pedagogy, 30

anecdotal notes, 152

Printed in the United States
By Bookmasters